VETERINARY PHYSIOLOGY

NIPA GENX ELECTRONIC RESOURCES & SOLUTIONS P. LTD.
New Delhi-110 034

About the Author

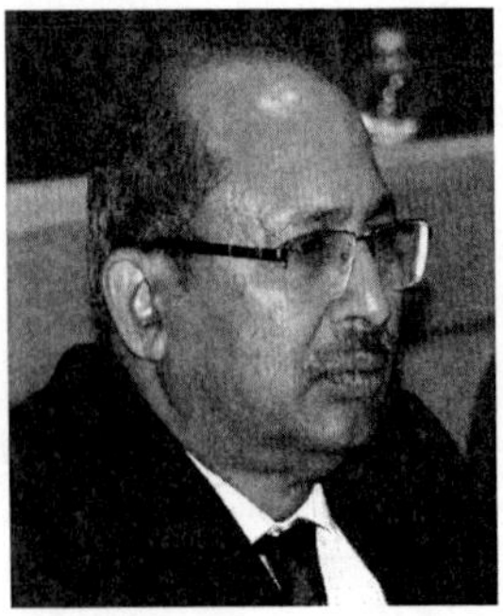

Dr. S.K. Jindal was Professor of Veterinary Physiology and Biochemistry, Post Graduate Institute of Veterinary Education, Research, Jaipur, Rajasthan, India. He has earlier served as Principal Scientist and Head and Acting Director, ICAR-Central Institute for Research on Goats, Makhdoom, Farah,Mathura and Senior Scientist and Head, ICAR- Central Institute for Research on Buffaloes, Hisar, Haryana and as Scientist S-1 at ICAR-Indian Veterinary Research Institute, Izatnagar, Bareilly, U.P. He obtained his Masters and Doctorate degree from ICAR-National Dairy Research Institute, Karnal-Haryana, India. He also obtained his post-doctoral training in reproductive biotechnology at California, USA and University of Louisiana, USA.He has been conferred with fellowship award of Indian Society of Goat and Sheep Production and Utilization.He has served as a member of Editorial Board of International Journal of animal Science and referee for a number of International and National journals like Animal Reproduction Science, Indian Journal of Animal Science etc. He has more than 42 years of research experience in physiology with specialization in lactation endocrinology, semen cryobiology and reproductive biotechnology.

He has also published more than 100 research articles in the peer-reviewed national and international journal, and authored or co-authored 9 books. He is a member of many national and international scientific societies.

VETERINARY PHYSIOLOGY

Dr. S.K. Jindal

NIPA GENX ELECTRONIC RESOURCES & SOLUTIONS P. LTD.
New Delhi-110 034

NIPA GENX ELECTRONIC RESOURCES & SOLUTIONS P. LTD.

101,103, Vikas Surya Plaza, CU Block
L.S.C.Market, Pitam Pura, New Delhi-110 034
Ph : +91 11 27341616, 27341717, 27341718
E-mail:newindiapublishingagency@gmail.com
www: www.nipabooks.com

For customer assistance, please contact
Phone: + 91-11-27 34 17 17 Fax: + 91-11- 27 34 16 16
E-Mail: feedbacks@nipabooks.com

ISBN: 978-93-90591-40-4

Composed and Designed by NIPA.

Preface

This Veterinary Physiology is intended to be useful for elementary physiology course in colleges of agriculture, zoology, veterinary and animal sciences. In particular I have tried to cover the VCI syllabus. Hope the efforts will be of some use to students. In all chapters, the aim has been to present a clear and concise account of the functioning of various systems of domestic animals. Where appropriate, examples from human and nondomestic animals such as rat and rabbit have been cited. Physiology has now grown into a vast discipline. Lot of new information is added to the physiology literature almost everyday and it is almost impossible to keep track of all the new information. So specialized books and journals need to be consulted from time to time. I have listed selected text books on physiology as an appendix An appendix on physiological literature has been added as appendix IV for those who intend to persue physiology in higher studies. List of Nobel Prize winners has been given to encourage you to ask questions as to why and how something happens in the body. If you know how and why than you are better equipped to handle an emergency or to manipulate the process to your advantage. For example if you know basics of reproduction, you can manipulate reproduction to the advantage of mankind. Physiology of lactation can help you better to augment milk production by better breeding, feeding and management and better control of factors limiting milk production say mastitis. For example we have seen remarkable advances in animal productivity in the past century.

I am of the opinion that whatever is written in a book is not the final word. There are many if and but. The student while remembering the basic principles, definitions etc must question why and how to most phenomenon occuring in the body. It you know why, it will be easy for you to remember and use your knowledge in a clinical setting or day to day life. For example by adding paneer to your diet, you are adding protein to your nutrition. Similarly, feeding of urea to ruminant animals augments or supplements the nitrogen in their diet. Providing a good housing to animals, decreases their heat load in a hot weather and increases productivity. Providing sufficiently clean water to lactating animals is very important in their thermoregulation and milk production as milk contains a very large percentage of water. I request the indulgence of learned readers to send in their valuable suggestions for improvement. I am indebted to my teachers, colleagues and friends.

I am especially thankful to my colleagues at PGIVER namely Dr. Pawan Mittal, Dr. Barkha Gupta, Dr. G.S. Gottam, Dr. Desh Raj Bilochi, Dr. Amit Pandey for many helpful discussions. My senior colleagues at PGIVER namely Dr. V.K. Gupta, Dr. G.S. Manohar, Dr. Rajpurohit, and Dr. R.S. Dabar were constant source of inspiration, guidance, and support in various ways.

I am also thankful to Dr. G.N. Purohit, Dr. Chetna Gangwar who kindly went through an earlier draft of the manuscript and gave suggestions.

Book writing is something which uses many sources of information and it becomes impossible to thank each one of them individually. I wish to thank all of them from the core of my heart. I also thank all the scientists and sources whose contributions have been used but I failed to convey acknowledgement and gratitude. I have used google scholar and other references and am grateful for contribution of numerous scientists whom I am deeply indebted.

Last but not the least I am especially grateful to my wife Mrs. Sadhana Jindal and my family for their constant encouragement.

S.K. Jindal

Contents

1

Nature and Scope of Physiology

The word physiology initially meant for that branch of biology which deals with the function of living organisms.Physiology can be defined as the study of mechanisms of body functions. Physiology is concerned with the way the various systems of the body function and the way each contributes to the functions of the body as a whole.Thus, physiology not only seeks to define the functions of living organisms like feeding, digestion, respiration, transport of gases in the blood, circulation and functions of the heart, excretion and kidney functions, muscle and movement, reproduction etc but also seeks to answer to 'why' and 'how' all these functions are regulated. Physiology is also to know about how the living organisms adjust to the adversities of the environment, obtain enough water to live or avoid too much water, escape freezing to death or dying from excessive heat, move about to find suitable surroundings, food and mates and how they obtain information about the environment through their senses. Physiology also involves how body defences are mobilized during disease and stress to ensure survival. Physiology investigates the processes and mechanisms that allow a living thing to survive, grow, and develop. Thus, physiology tries to explain the phenomenon of life in terms of physical and chemical laws. In this book we have taken the mechanistic view that most of the phenomenon in the animal body can be explained in terms of various physical and chemical laws.

Physiology provides important insights and practical applications in medicine, veterinary medicine, agriculture, nutrition, and industry.

Veterinary and agriculture students are more interested about the body functions of domestic animals which are useful to mankind in one way or other so that judicious manipulation of these functions can yield more meat, milk and fibre and also to fight disease and stress situations more effectively. They are interested to know about the mechanism of milk formation and secretion, physiology of muscle growth, hair and fibre growth as well as skin. Most of the domestic animals falls within the general category of ruminants which distinguish them from other classes of animals in having a compound stomach and in their ability to utilize the complex carbohydrate cellulose with the help of microbes inhabiting the rumen, a property quite unique in the animal kingdom. In this way, they provide an important part of man's day to day life by converting the useless cellulose to easily consumable and highly nutritious feed stuffs like meat and milk.

Physiology cannot be explained separately than the mechanism of **cell physiology** since individual cells are the basic units of both the structure and the function of living things. However, we do not wish to say that there are no differences in cell function in a liver cell and nerve cell. On the other hand these differences in cell function generally represent specialization of one of more of the fundamental common properties. Thus the excitability of nerve and muscle cells represents a specialization of electrical phenomenon common to the membranes of virtually all cells. The secretion of protein hormones by certain gland cells of the body is a specialized form of the genetically controlled protein synthesis found in all cells. These specializations have all occurred as a part of evolution and have resulted in the adaptation of certain cells for specific roles.

Physiology is as ancient as human existence on this earth. It is a ancient as well as original science. Physiology is the study of mechanisms of body functions. Basic body functions include provision of oxygen and nutrients to the cells and organs, removal of metabolites and waste products, maintenance of body temperature , locomotor functions, reproduction, lactation and special sensory functions. Knowledge of physiology is essential to understand pathology and repair of body functions. In fact this knowledge is key to progress of all mankind .

Physiology is truly an interdisciplinary science. The animals which man has domesticated over the years to meet his own needs for food, clothing, power or companionship include cattle, buffalo, sheep, goats, horses, pigs, cats, dogs and poultry. Domestic animals like most other animal forms existing on earth including human beings, are the result of a long evolution and therefore related to each other and indeed to all living beings. Much has been learned or better understood about the physiology of these animals through comparative study on the other animal forms, though many a time these animals have served as experimental models for studies designed to gain knowledge about human physiology. Dog and goat for a long time yielded to such experimentation. The domestic animals have been used for obtaining information on their physiology per se only recently and most experiments have been designed to understand better the mechanisms related to production potential of these animals in terms of meat, milk and wool. Knowledge is also gained by the study of sick and abnormal individuals or through surgery.

The study of physiology is not independent of other related disciplines like animal biochemistry, animal biotechnology, animal nutrition, animal genetics and breeding, livestock production and management, animal anatomy, chemistry and physics but is indeed complementary and supplementary.In fact physiology is the mother science on which several disciplines of veterinary, human and related disciplines derive strength. The application of chemistry to physiology initially named as physiological chemistry evolved further to become biochemistry and subsequently biotechnology as independent disciplines. The application of physiological knowledge related to digestion and some parts of chemistry ie essential and non essential nutrients became specialized as nutrition. Now we know of essential and non essential vitamins, minerals, amino acids, fatty acids and their supplementation in food and feeds become a part of nutrition. Nutrient bioavailability is largely a domain of physiology where a lot has been done and achieved.

Animal ethology (study of behavior) is a comparatively recent discipline whi ch has contributed abundantly to our understanding of the behavior of animals in relation to their productivity.

The place of domestic animals in nature is objectively described by placing them along with other living organisms in the accepted scheme of classification as formulated by the biologists. The domestic animals belong to the Animal Kingdom, which like the plant kingdom, is divided into a number of major categories, the Phyla. The animal Phyla range from the relatively simple protozoa mostly single celled forms, to the chordata which encompasses backboned animals, including domestic animals and human beings. This scheme of classification is based on the concept of evolution of life and the animals are classified on the basis of closeness or the distance of their relationship. The life cycle of the animal (Ontogeny) is said to repeat the evolutionary development of the animal (Phylogeny).

The domestic animals belong to the phylum Chordata, subphylum Vertebrata, characterised by the presence of a backbone or vertebral column. They are further classified to belong to class Mammalia and subclass Eutheria. The cow, buffaloes, goat, sheep etc. belong to order Ungulata in sub class Eutheria. The horse and asses belong to order Perissodactyla. The cats and dogs belong to order Carnivora. The poultry belong to the order Galliformes in Class Aves.

Systems of Body and Their Physiological Functions

The body of domestic animals is like the body of human beings and other animal forms, in that it consists of many organs, each organ having its own particular function to perform. Each organ is made up predominantly of a particular type of tissue. The tissues are a group of specialized cells bunched together. Anatomy is the study of the structure of the body. Physiology (study of function) is closely related to anatomy (study of structure), biochemistry (chemical processes of living things), comparative anatomy (similarities and differences between species), and embryology (development of embryos). Microscopic anatomy is subdivided into cytology (the study of cells) and histology (the study of tissues).

There are four basic tissues in the body namely epithelial tissue, connective tissue, muscle tissue and nervous tissue. Connective tissue may get further differentiated in soft adipose tissue or hard tissue such as cartilage and bone. The muscle tissue can be either skeletal muscle, smooth muscle or cardiac muscle.

The cell is the unit of the tissue. The cells are adapted to perform the special functions of the organ. Organs are made up of group of tissues that work together for common purposes. The organs are organised into several systems according to the functions they perform. Some of them are outlined below.

Blood and lymph are fluid tissues: Blood is the main transport system. It carries oxygen (O_2) and nutritive substances and antibodies to the tissues and removes carbon dioxide (CO_2) and waste products from the tissues. The physical properties of water in the blood helps to maintain body temperature.

Circulatory System / Cardiovascular system : Cardiovascular system is primarily blood, blood vessels and heart. Primary function of the cardiovascular system is to transport of essential nutrients that are essential for life and health including the oxygen and nutrients required for cells of the body. Heart is the chief organ of circulation of the blood. The blood is pumped by the heart along the arteries to the capillaries and is returned by venules and veins.If heart stops contracting and circulation ceases, the animal becomes unconscious within 30 seconds and within a few minutes irreversible damage to the brain occurs. The condition of inadequate blood flow to a tissue is called ischemia.

Respiratory System : The respiratory system consists of the lungs and the passages through which air reaches them. The passages are nasal cavities, the pharynx, the trachea, the bronchi and their intrapulmonary continuations. Oxygen (O_2) from the air is taken into the lungs and from there it diffuses into the blood which carries it to the tissues. The CO_2 which is produced by tissue tissues is carried by the blood from the body tissues to the lungs and breathed out in the expired air.

Digestive System : It consists of alimentary canal and the glands associated with it. It deals with the digestion and absorption of food. The digestive system of ruminants differ from that of non-ruminants. The food supplies energy to the body and supplies nutrients for its growth and maintenance.

Excretory System / Urinary System : Excretion is the removal of waste products of metabolism from the body. Consists of kidneys, ureters, urinary bladder and urethra. The kidney helps to keep the composition of the blood constant by excretion of waste products. Kidney also helps in maintenance of blood pressure.

Physiology and its Branches

Skin : Skin is the outermost covering of the body. Skin protects the body and it is concerned with general sensation and it plays an important role in the regulation of body temperature. It acts as a physical barrier against entry of microorganisms and other substances. The appendages of skin include hairs, nails, sebaceous glands and sweat glands. A sebaceous gland is a microscopic exocrine gland in the skin that opens into a hair follicle to secrete an oily or waxy matter, called sebum, which lubricates the hair and skin of mammals. Sweat glands, also known as sudoriferous glands are small tubular structures of the skin that produce sweat. Sweat glands are a type of exocrine gland, which are glands that produce and secrete substances onto an epithelial surface by way of a duct.

Endocrine Glands or Ductless Glands : These glands produce special chemical substances known as hormones which pass directly into the blood stream. These hormones control the various body functions.

Reproductive System : This system is concerned with the preservation of species. The function of male reproductive organ is to produce sperms and male sex hormones. The function of female reproductive system is to produce ova and female sex hormones.

Special Sense Organs : include tongue (taste), nose (smell), eye (sight) and ear (hearing). Through these organs, the animal remains aware of the external environment.

Nervous System : It consists of the brain, spinal cord and the nerves arising from them. They are concerned with the quick control of bodily functions and coordination.

Locomotor System : This includes the parts concerned with the movement of the body. This comprises bones, joints called ligaments and muscles. The basic framework of the body is provided by a large number of bones that collectively form the skeleton. At joints, the bones are united to each other by fibrous bands called ligaments. Overlying and usually attached to the bones are various muscles. Three distinct types of muscles can be identified which are skeletal muscles, smooth muscles and cardiac muscles.

The functions of various systems are not exactly independent but are delicately interrelated.

The study of various body systems is very important for animal health and production. The various parts of the body must work together in near-perfect harmony to maintain the life and well-being of an animal.Knowledge of normal physiology of various systems of body is critical to our ability to keep our animals in best of health and productivity and to be able to manage the health and survival in case of disease or stress.

Homeostasis

All mammals including domestic animals are able to regulate the condition of their internal environment within narrow limits. Claude Bernard, the French scientist first described it as the 'Constancy of the internal milieu'. Homeostasis is the maintenance of the overall stability of physiological processes of the body. It is monitored by the brain and nervous system and regulated by the physiology and activity of individual organs. Homeostasis is a universal phenomenon in animals, allowing them to survive in stressful and varying environments. Thus the chemical milieu of the tissues, cells, body temperature, blood and intracellular ionic composition are contained within narrow limits in spite of wide fluctuations in the external environment.

Thus all the cells of the body except those on the surface are provided with a fluid environment of relatively constant temperature, hydrogen ion concentration and osmotic pressure. Because of this, many body activities like the working of enzymes or the functioning of nerve cells etc are carried out under optimum conditions. Activities of several systems of the body are called for in the maintenance of this intricate process of homeostasis through a set of checks and balances like positive and negative feedback mechanisms. Thus kidney, endocrine, nervous, circulatory tissue are intimately concerned with the process of homeostasis. The concept of homeostasis is key to the understanding of most body functions and mechanisms.The whole body systems are responsible for homeostasis. Homeostasis requires normal functioning of the body's cells, tissues, organs and systems and thus make possible the functioning of the body as a living being.

Cell, Tissue and Organ

Since the 1830's when Schwann introduced the concept of cellular theory, it has been accepted that all animals are composed of cells. Thus cells are the basic units of biological systems just as atoms are of chemical systems. Cells could not be seen until microscopes were invented in the 17th century. A microscope is an instrument that makes an enlarged image of a small object, thus revealing details too small to be seen by the unaided eye. The magnifying power of a microscope is an expression of the number of times the object being examined appears to be enlarged . Common microscopes are optical, or light microscopes in which glass lenses are used to form the image. Optical microscopes can be simple, consisting of a single lens, or compound, consisting of several optical components in line. The other microscopes are electron microscope, which uses a beam of electrons in its image formation. The transmission electron microscope (TEM) has magnifying powers of more than 1,000,000×. TEMs form images of thin specimens. The scanning tunneling microscope (STM), which can create images of atoms, and the environmental scanning electron microscope (ESEM), which generates images using electrons of specimens in a gaseous environment, use other physical effects that further extend the types of objects that can be examined.

Cells are the structural and functional units of all living organisms. Domestic animals and human beings are multicellular organisms containing many different types of cells, which vary in size, shape, and specialized function.

A typical cell has two major parts (1) Nucleus (2) Cytoplasm. The cytoplasm is surrounded by cytoplasmic membrane and nucleus is surrounded by nuclear membrane. The fluid portion inside the cell is called cytosol or protoplasm. In the evolution of multicellular organisms, cells become specialized and organized into different systems, e.g. cardiovascular, muscle, kidney and so on.

Structure of a Mammalian Cell

Living organisms can survive only if the cells of which they are made up of, can absorb the required nutrients, can excrete waste products, can synthesize and secrete the substances necessary for sustaining life processes, like digestive enzymes, hormones, neuro transmitters etc. Absorption, excretion and secretion, all involve the movements of substances through cellular and intracellular membranes. Thus membrane function is key to all the body functions including electron transport, protein synthesis, muscle contraction, sensory reception, acid base balance, impulse conduction and endocrinological regulation. The plasma membrane defines the periphery of the cell, separating its contents from the surroundings. The membranes of animal cells make up some 40 to 90% of the total mass in various cell types.

The structure of all the membranes is having certain features in common. The biological membrane is a central lipid layer sandwiched between two protein layers.

The concept of unit membrane as proposed by Robertson in 1959 had an important impact in elucidating the complexity of cell function in terms of membrane biochemistry. It was formulated to account for electron microscopic and X ray diffraction data, while at the same time incorporating much of the information accumulated over many years about the physiological nature of membranes particularly plasma membranes. This theory says that there is one basic structure common to all membrane. The membrane which bounds the cell and other intracellular membranes contain approximately 400 g lipid (mainly phospholipid) and 66 g protein per kg. These components are thought to be arranged as per the fluid mosaic model of membrane structure as postulated by S.J. Singer and G.L. Nicholson in 1972.Essentially the phospholipids are thought to form a bilayer with hydrophilic hydrocarbon center : this accounts for the high electrical resistance and low permeability to highly polar molecules. The proteins are thought to be embedded in the lipid bilayer (hence the term mosaic) with some completely spanning the bilayer and others not. This accounts for the asymmetry of membranes both in terms of chemical characteristics and the directional nature of the transport systems. The lipid bilayer is not rigid and both lipid and protein molecules are thought to diffuse laterally in the membrane, hence its fluidity and flexibility. These latter properties are influenced by the fatty acid composition of the lipid bilayer, the greater the degree of unsaturation of fatty acids, the more fluid and flexible the membrane is.The lipid bilayer greatly restricts the diffusion of polar substances across membranes. Therefore, the concentration of substances within the cell (most of which are ionized) can differ markedly from those of extracellular fluid. Lipid layer of the cell membrane is a semipermeable membrane and allows only the fat-soluble substances to pass through it. Protein layers of the cell membrane are electron-dense layers. These layers cover the two surfaces of the central lipid layer. Protein layers give protection to the central lipid layer. The protein substances present in these layers are mostly glycoproteins. Transport proteins in the plasma membrane allow the passage of certain ions and molecules; receptor proteins transmit signals into the cell; and membrane enzymes participate in some reaction pathways. Fatty acids can be transported into and out of the cell membrane by diffusion.

Membrane Transport

The lipid bilayer of biological membranes is intrinsically impermeable to ions and polar molecules. Permeability is conferred by two classes of membrane proteins, **pumps** and **channels**. The transport is either **active transport** ie they require energy and are is exemplified by pumps and passive transport as through diffusion exemplified through channels. The passive transport is through concentration gradients and do not require ATP or energy.

Within the cell membrane are two major compartments: The cytoplasm and The nucleus. The cytoplasm contains structures that consume and transform energy and perform the cell's functions. The internal volume enclosed by the plasma membrane, the cytoplasm, is composed of an aqueous solution, the cytosol, and a variety of suspended particles with specific functions. Cytoplasm of the cell is the jellylike material formed by 80% of water. It contains a clear liquid portion called cytosol.

The nucleus contains the cell's genetic material and the structures that control cell division and reproduction. The hereditary information that is encoded in DNA is called genome. Genome is complete set of genes.

DNA, RNA, and proteins are informational macromolecules; the precise sequence of their monomeric subunits contains information. Most chemical reactions in the cell are aided by enzymes—biocatalysts that, like all other catalysts, greatly enhance the rate of specific chemical reactions without being consumed in the process. Enzymes are globular proteins that work as catalyst for chemical reactions. Enzymes are specific to their substrates.

Mitochondria are tiny structures inside every cell that provide the cell with energy in the form of ATP. Mitochondria are called 'powerhouse' of the cell. In the presence of oxygen organisms are capable of using the Kreb's Cycle. The reason oxygen is required is because the NADH and [FADH2] produced in the Kreb's Cycle are able to be oxidized in the electron transport chain (ETC) thus replenishing the supply of NAD+ and [FAD]. Organisms derive the majority of their energy from the Kreb's Cycle, also known as the TCA cycle. The Kreb's Cycle is an aerobic process consisting of eight definite steps. In order to enter the Kreb's Cycle pyruvate must first be converted into Acetyl-CoA by pyruvate dehydrogenase complex found in the mitochondria.

Cytoplasmic organelles are the cellular structures embedded in the cytoplasm. These organelles include rough endoplasmic reticulum, smooth endoplasmic reticulum, golgi apparatus, lysosomes, peroxisomes, mitochondria, ribosomes, nucleus. Each of these organelles have specific functions. For example nucleus functions include control of cellular activities and storage of hereditary material ie DNA and RNA.

Basic principle common to all biomolecules in the body is the intimate relation between structure and function. DNA is a double-stranded nucleic acid. The remarkable properties of DNA allow it to function as a very efficient and robust vehicle for storing information. DNA structure is a double helix composed of two intertwined strands arranged such that the sugar-phosphate backbone lies on the outside and the bases on the inside. DNA forms the component of chromosomes, which carries the hereditary information. The hereditary information that is encoded in DNA is called genome. Each DNA molecule is divided into units called genes. Gene is a portion of DNA molecule that contains the message or code for the synthesis of a specific protein from different amino acids. Three bases along a DNA chain encode a single amino acid. The specific correspondence between a set of three bases and 1 of the 20 amino acids is called the genetic code.

An important nucleic acid in addition to DNA in the cell is **ribonucleic acid** (RNA). RNA is a linear polymer made up of a limited number of repeating monomers, each composed of a sugar, a phosphate, and a base. RNA has three basic roles in the cell. First, it serves as the intermediate in the flow of information from DNA to protein, the primary functional molecules of the cell. The DNA is copied, or transcribed, into messenger RNA (mRNA), and the mRNA is translated into protein. Second, RNA molecules serve as adaptors that translate the information in the nucleic acid sequence of mRNA into information designating the sequence of constituents that make up a protein. Finally, RNA molecules are important functional components of the molecular machinery, called ribosomes, that carries out the translation process.The most active site of protein synthesis is the ribosome. Genetic information of nuclear DNA is transmitted to the site of protein synthesis by tRNA.

The Golgi complex forms glycoproteins.

The digestive enzymes of cellular components are confined to lysosomes. Lysosomes are also called 'suicide bags'.

Metabolic processes inside the cell need to be viewed in the context of the whole organism. An essential characteristic of multicellular organisms is cell differentiation and division of labor. The specialized functions of the tissues and organs of complex organisms impose characteristic fuel requirements and patterns of metabolism.

Tissues are related cells that are joined together. Tissue is defined as the group of cells having similar functions for example muscle tissue, nerve tissue, epithelial tissue and connective tissue. The cells in a tissue are not identical, but they work together to accomplish specific functions.There are four basic tissues of the body namely epithelial tissue,muscle tissue, connective tissue, and nervous tissue.

Epithelial tissues line the outer surfaces of organs and blood vessels throughout the body, as well as the inner surfaces of cavities in many internal organs. An example is the epidermis, the outermost layer of the skin. There are three principal shapes of epithelial cells: squamous, columnar, and cuboidal. Connective tissue provides support, binds together, and protects tissues and organs of the body. Examples of connective tissue include adipose, cartilage, bone, tendons, and cartilage, and adipose (fat) tissue. Muscle tissue is characterized by properties that allow movement. Muscle cells are excitable; they respond to a stimulus. Muscle tissue is composed of cells that have the special ability to shorten or contract in order to produce movement of the body parts. The three types of muscle tissue are skeletal, smooth, and cardiac. Nervous tissue is found in the brain, spinal cord, and nerves. It is responsible for coordinating and controlling many body activities. Nervous tissue consists of two cells: nerve cells and glial cells.

Organs are the body's recognizable structures (for example, the heart, lungs, liver, eyes, and stomach) that perform specific functions. An organ is made of several types of tissue and therefore several types of cells. The eye contains muscle cells that open and close the pupil, clear cells that make up the lens and cornea, cells that produce the fluid within the eye, cells that sense light, and nerve cells that conduct impulses to the brain. The heart contains muscle tissue that contracts to pump blood, fibrous tissue that makes up the heart valves, and special cells that maintain the rate and rhythm of heartbeats.

Hormonal and neuronal signals integrate and coordinate the metabolic activities of different tissues and optimize the allocation of fuels and precursors to each organ.

Receptors are protein molecules inside the target cell or on its surface that receive a chemical signal. A receptor is a protein which binds to a specific molecule. The molecule it binds is known as the ligand. Receptors bind to specific ligands, which activate numerous cellular processes. Receptors are protein molecules in the target cell or on its surface that bind ligands. There are two types of receptors: internal receptors and cell-surface receptors. Internal receptors, also known as intracellular or cytoplasmic receptors, are found in the cytoplasm of the cell and respond to hydrophobic ligand molecules that are able to travel across the plasma membrane. Once inside the cell, many of these molecules bind to proteins that act as regulators of mRNA synthesis to mediate gene expression. Gene expression is the cellular process of transforming the information in a cell's DNA into a sequence of amino acids that ultimately forms a protein. When the ligand binds to the internal receptor, a conformational change exposes a DNA-binding site on the protein. The ligand-receptor complex moves into the nucleus, binds to specific regulatory regions of the chromosomal DNA, and promotes the initiation of transcription. Internal receptors can directly influence gene expression without having to pass the signal on to other receptors or messengers.

Cell-surface receptors are cell surface, membrane-anchored proteins that bind to external ligand molecules. This type of receptor spans the plasma membrane and performs signal transduction, converting an extracellular signal into an intracellular signal. There are three general categories of cell-surface receptors: ion channel-linked receptors, G-protein-linked receptors, and enzyme-linked receptors.

Ion channel-linked receptors bind a ligand and open a channel through the membrane that allows specific ions to pass through. G-protein-linked receptors bind a ligand and activate a membrane protein called a G-protein. The activated G-protein then interacts with either an ion channel or an enzyme in the membrane. Enzyme-linked receptors are cell-surface receptors with intracellular domains that are associated with an enzyme.

Different types of body cells normally divide and grow at different rates. The cells lining the intestines divide about once every 24hr. whereas adult nerves and muscles cells are unable to divide at all. Even the same type of cell may be able to multiply rapidly under certain conditions but slowly under others. Liver cells normally divide infrequently and at a rate just sufficient to replace those which have been damaged and die, but if a part of the liver is surgically removed, the remaining cells divide rapidly and multiply until the amount of tissue that was removed has been replaced. Many types of cells which do not divide or divide infrequently in the body multiply rapidly when removed and cultured in an **artificial medium outside the body**. For example cells removed from embryonic chicken heart tissue have continued to grow and divide in a test tube for over 30 years, whereas if they had remained in the chicken, they would have stopped dividing when the heart was fully formed. Cell differentiation is often accompanied by loss of the ability to divide, as shown most clearly in the case of adult nerve and muscle cells. Cancer is an uncontrolled multiplication of cells in the body.

History of Physiology

Studying the history of physiology allows you to have a glimpse into just how we discovered everything we know about physiology today. Many scientists bypass history and its importance. But learning the scientific methods and the history of science is the embodiment of scientific knowledge. Hippocrates (ca. 460–370 BCE) described the human brain as being in two halves divided by a thin vertical membrane, as it was in other animals. A school of anatomy was founded in Alexandria in the early third century and became the first of its kind carrying out human dissection. Herophilus identified the brain as the organ at the centre of the nervous system. Herophilus was born in 335 BCE, studied in Alexandria. He remained there during the reigns of the first two Ptolemaios Pharaohs and is said to be the first anatomist to perform a systematic dissection of the human body. Erasistratus concentrated on physiology and mechanisms rather than pure anatomy. Aristotle (384–322 BC) from Greek became known as the father of comparative anatomy through his dissections performed on a variety of animals, including mammals, reptiles and insects. Aristotle was the first person to study biology systematically.

William Harvey born in 1578 in England was the first to correctly describe the circulatory system, identifying the blood flow returning to the heart and the heart acting as a muscular pump. Harvey also proposed the idea of capillary anastomoses joining the arterial and venous systems, although their existence was not proven until after his death by Marcello Malpighi in 1661.

Hooke also designed a microscope and wrote the now famous 'Micrographia' and Antonie van Leeuwenhoek-the Father of the Microscope developed this work.

1895 saw X-rays observed for the first time by German physicist Wilhelm Roentgen.

In later years, Godfrey Hounsfield expanded the use of X-rays by developing computer software that could integrate multiple radiographic images to give a three-dimensional view inside the body. This was the discovery of computed tomography (CT). The invention of CT had vital practical applications, and as a result, Hounsfield was awarded the Nobel Prize for Physiology or Medicine in 1979.

Ian Donald pioneered the use of ultrasound in obstetrics and gynaecology in a paper published in 1958. The inventors of MRI shared the Nobel Prize in Medicine or Physiology in 2003.

Land-marks in the History of Physiology

- The study of human physiology as a medical field originates in classical Greece, at the time of Hippocrates (late 5th century BC).
- Claudius Galenus (c. 130–200 AD), known as Galen of Pergamum, was the first to use experiments to probe the functions of the body.
- Jean Fernel (1497–1558), a French physician, introduced the term "physiology".
- Santorio Santorio in 1610s was the first to use a device to measure the pulse rate (the pulsilogium), and a thermoscope to measure temperature.
- In 1791 Luigi Galvani described the role of electricity in nerves of dissected frogs.
- In 1858, Joseph Lister studied the cause of blood coagulation and inflammation that resulted after previous injuries and surgical wounds. He later discovered and implemented antiseptics in the operating room.
- Claude Bernard's (1813–1878) further discoveries ultimately led to his concept of milieu interieur (internal environment).

- In 1954, Andrew Huxley and Hugh Huxley, alongside their research team, discovered the sliding filaments in skeletal muscle, known today as the sliding filament theory.

History of Physiology

Cardiovascular Physiology	
Harvey (1628)	First Discovered about circulation of blood. William Harvey, an English physician published his observations on the anatomy and physiology of the heart.
Halez Stephen (1932)	First to measure the blood pressure.
Laennec (1819)	Invented Stethoscope
Fick (1870)	Measured cardiac output by dye dilution
Frossman (1929)	Catherterization of the heart
Mosso (1875)	Plethysmograph
Ludwig (1847)	Kymograph
Einthoven (1900-1903)	Electrocardiogram (ECG)
Koch (1925)	Role of the carotid sinus.
Respiration	
Knowltron & Starling (1912)	Heart lung preparation
Hering & Brever (1868)	Role of the vagus in the expansion of and contraction of the lung.
Lumsden (1923)	Pneumotaxic centre
Haldane, J.S. (1905)	Regulation of respiration
August Krogh (1920)	How blood flow is regulated in capillaries.
Autar Paintal (1969)	J-receptors in the alveopar walls
Digestive Physiology	
DeGraff (1664)	Cannulated the pancreatic duct.
Spleanzani (1777)	Fed tubes filled with sponges and showed that the liquid squeezed out of them would digest meat.
Prout (1823)	Found HCl in gastric juice.
Beaumont (1825-33)	First gastric fistula in man-observeds ecretiono fg astic juice, stomach movements.
Bassow (1842)	First experimental gastric fistula in animals.
Ludwig (1851)	Nerve supply to the salivary gland.
Ivan Pavlov (1891)	Performed research on "conditional responses" that involved dogs' saliva production in response to a bell and visual stimuli.
Cannon (1898-1902)	Stomach and intestinal movement.
Anand and Brobeck (1951)	Neural control of food intake.
Cannon (1911)	Studied swallowing and esophageal transport by X-ray
Chatfield (1941)	Location of salivary center in the medulla.
Endocrinology	

Paracelsus (1493–1541)	Paracelsus (1493–1541) was the first person to propose a relationship between goitre and minerals (particularly lead) in drinking water. Iodine was later discovered by Bernard Courtois in 1811 from seaweed ash.
Astley Cooper (1840)	First removed thyroid
Kendal (1914)	Isolated thyroxine
Smith (1926)	Hypophysectomy
Starling (early years of 20th century)	Coined the word hormone
Banting and Best (1922)	Discovered Insulin
Evans and Long (1921)	Discovered Growth hormone
H. Ramussen and L.C. Craig(1959)	Parathyroid hormone was first isolated
William Rutte (1985)	Insulin receptor cloned
A.V.Schally (1971)	Isolation and identification of a gonadotropin-releasing hormone (GnRH or LHRH) of hypothalamic origin
Reproductive Physiology	
Antonie van Leeuwenhoek 1677	Sperms were first observed in 1677 by Antonie van Leeuwenhoek using a microscope.
Speemen 1930	Cloning hypothesis
Philips and Lardy (1940)	Egg yolk as a semen diluter to protect the sperm cells against damage during cooling.
Polge et al 1949	Cryo-protective properties of glycerol for human spermatozoa
Almquist et al (1949)	Introduced the addition of the antibiotics penicillin and streptomycin to semen to control pathogenic microorganisms.
Willet et al 1953	Calves born after surgical transplantation of fertilized bovine eggs.
Chang 1954	First IVF (of rabbit oocyte)
Donaldson and Hansel 1965	LH is luteotropin for the bovine CL
Wilmut & Rowson 1973	First successful cryopreservation of embryo i.e. birth of calf from frozen embryo
Steptoe & Edwards 1978	First test tube (IVF) baby
Brackett et al.1982	First test tube (IVF) calf
Pierson and Ginther 1984	Ultrasonography of ovary to monitor follicle and CL development
Willadsen 1986	Birth of cloned lamb derived from 8 -16 cell sheep embryo
Kommadath et al 2013	Identified genes that affect estrous behaviour
Nervous Physiology	
Hippocrates 460 -379 B.C.	Hippocrates discussed the epilepsy as disturbance of brain and also indicated that the brain is involved with sensation and is the seat of intelligence.

1764	Domenico F.A. Cotugno, describes the spinal, subarachnoid and cerebrospinal fluid and reported that ventricular and spinal fluids are connected.
1903	Ivan Pavlov coins the word, conditioned reflex.
1906	Golgi and Cajal won Nobel Prize for describing the structure of nervous system.
1911	George Barger and Henry Dale discover nor-epinephrine

The modern veterinary physiology teaching and research in India got its impetus from the start of veterinary schools where departments of veterinary physiology, pharmacology and biochemistry departments were established. The first civil veterinary school was established in Babugarh (Hapur) in Uttar Pradesh, in the year 1877. Subsequently, the first veterinary college was started in Lahore (1885), now in Pakistan. The Bombay veterinary college was established in 1886. Subsequently veterinary colleges were established in Calcutta in 1893 and Madras in 1903 In 1989, the first veterinary university in India, Tamil Nadu Veterinary and Animal Sciences University (TANUVAS), was formed. The Institutions which had strong physiology departments in the beginning were Indian Veterinary Research Institute, Haryana Agricultural University, Punjab Agricultural University, Madras Veterinary college etc. Some of the earlier stalwarts got their training at CDRI, AIIMS, Bose Institute also. Before a full fledged M.V.Sc. in veterinary physiology was started, an Associate IVRI course trained a few pioneers. The intial pioneers trained many more and the process continued and now we have strong physiology departments in all the Institutes and veterinary colleges and a National Institute of Animal Nutrition and Physiology was established by ICAR at Bengaluru in 1995.

The first animal physiology society i.e. Society of Animal Physiologists of India was established in 1985. Initial researches in physiology were conducted on blood, environment, heat tolerance, climatology and lactation physiology. Later reproductive endocrinology, reproductive biotechnology, stem cell and cloning technology were perfected at various ICAR institutes and University Departments.

Physiological Terms

Some of the physiological terms and their meanings are listed below which will help in understanding the subject in the subsequent chapters.

Abdominal cavity	In vertebrates that part of the body cavity containing the digestive organs, and in mammals separated from the thoracic cavity by the diaphragm.
Ablation	Removal
Acclimatization, acclimation	The process of adaptation to a new environment, for example with altered ambient temperature, pressure or (with aquatic animals) salinity.
Acoustic	Related to sound or sound waves.
Adrenergic	Related to adrenaline.
Aerobic	In oxygen – usually refers to organic chemical reactions or to microorganisms that operate in the presence of oxygen.

Alimentary	Relating to food or the gastro-intestinal tract
Alveolus	The terminal air sacs in the lungs, where gas exchange takes place with the blood.
Anabolism (anabolic)	The constructive chemical processes in living organisms involve formation of complex molecules from simpler ones, and the taking up and storage of energy.
Anaerobic	Without oxygen; usually refers to organic chemical reactions or microorganisms that operate in the absence of oxygen- eg rumen microorganisms.
Anoxia	A condition without oxygen.
Annulus	Ring shaped
Apoptosis	The process of regulated cell death
Aqueous	Associated with water
Articulation	An area where adjacent bones are in contact (via cartilage or fibrous tissue) at a joint.
Aqueous	Associated with water.
Artery	Elastic, thick walled vessels carrying blood at relatively high pressure away from the heart.
Average	Mean
Bilirubin	A chemical breakdown product of hemoglobin.
Buccal	Toward the cheeks
Chronic	Continuous, or existing for a long time.
Conjunctivitis	Inflammation of the conjunctiva
Cortex	The skin, or outer part of an organ (e.g. The cerebral cortex or adrenal cortex)
Cryptocrine	It involves the secretion of a hormone into a closed environment. This system requires a very special intimacy between cells. E.g. Between sertoli cells and spermatids.
Endocrine	Pertaining to cellular secretions that enter the bloodstream and have their effects on distant tissues.
Enzyme	A biomolecule, mostly protein, that catalyzes a specific chemical reaction. It enhances the rate of the reaction by providing a reaction path with a lower activation energy.
Enzyme-linked immunosorbent assay (ELISA)	A sensitive immunoassay that uses an enzyme linked to an antibody or antigen to detect a specific protein.
Epithelial cell	Any cell that forms part of the outer covering of an organism or organ.
Erythrocyte	A cell containing large amounts of hemoglobin and specialized for oxygen transport; a red blood cell.
Fatigue	A reduction in a response as a result of repeated or prolonged stimulation or activity. In the context of muscle function, it usually means a reduction in the amount of force that the muscle can produce
Fibrin	A protein factor that forms the cross-linked fibers in blood clots.
Foramen	An opening through a bone, usually a passage for blood vessels and nerves.

Gametes	Reproductive cells with a haploid gene content; sperm or egg cells.
Glycogenolysis	The enzymatic breakdown of stored (not dietary) glycogen.
Glycoprotein	A protein containing a carbohydrate group.
Gustatory	Relating to taste
Half-life	The time required for the disappearance or decay of one-half of a given component in a system.
Hemocrine	Secretions transported through blood *autocrine :* secretions act on the same cell
Hemoglobin	A heme or iron containing protein in erythrocytes; functions in oxygen transport.
Hepato-	Related to the liver
Hormone receptor	A protein in, or on the surface of, target cells that binds a specific hormone and initiates the cellular response.
Humoral	Relating to body fluids
Hypo-	Below, less than normal. E.g. Hypotonic = less concentrated than isotonic. Hypoxic= less oxygenated than normal. Hypodermic= below the skin.
Hypoxia	The metabolic condition in which the supply of oxygen is severely limited.
Immune response	The capacity of a vertebrate to generate antibodies to an antigen, a macromolecule foreign to the organism.
In vitro	"in glass"; that is, in the test tube.
In vivo	"in life"; that is, in the living cell or organism.
Interstitial	Relating to the interstices, or spaces in between things (usually cells). The interstitial space is the extracellular compartment
Intracrine	Hormone synthesis and receptors binding occurs intracellularly.
Juxtacrine	In this case hormone is synthesized as a membrane bound precursor. Although this precursor is usually cleaved to yield a soluble peptide, it may also remain attached to the plasma membrane, where it retains its biological activity.
Labial	Towards the lips. The labial surfaces of incisors are observed when a person smiles.
Lingual	Towards the tongue.
Luminal	Where hormone is released into the lumen of the gut.
Lyse	To break, dissolve or destroy. Often refers to cells bursting, for example, due to a hypotonic extracellular solution
Malignant	A condition that gets worse if not treated. Particularly refers to a tumour that invades and destroys other tissues
Mechanism	The sequence of events, steps and interactions involved in a process
Metabolism	The chemical reactions that occur in the body.
Micturition	Urination
Motility	Movement, particularly of cells or parts of cells.
Myocardium	The muscle tissue of the heart.
Necrosis	A form of cell death that results from acute cellular injury.

Nephro	Renal -relating to kidney. E.g. Nephritis= inflammation of kidney.
Neurocrine	Where neurons contact its target cells by axonal extensions & then release the hormone in synaptic cleft between cells.
Neuroendocrine	Where hormones are released by the nerve is blood born.
Non-invasive	A technique that doesn't require entry into the tissue being studied, or damage to it e.g. Ultrasonography
Olfactory	Relating to smell.
Osteoporosis	A condition that is characterized by a decrease in bone mass and density, causing bones to become fragile.
Ovum	The female gamete
Paracrine	Secretions act on the adjacent cell *solinocrine :* secretions come in the cavity
Peptide	Two or more amino acids linked together by a bond called a peptide bond.
Physiological	Characteristic of the normal workings of the tissue. If an experimental condition or a type of stimulation is said to be 'physiological', this means that it is within the range of conditions normally experienced by the tissue within the animal.
Prandial	Relating to a meal.
Proteinuria	Presence of protein in urine, sometimes indicative of kidney or heart disorders.
Puberty	The condition of becoming first capable of reproducing sexually.
Pulmonary	To do with the lungs
Pylorus	The narrow end of the stomach (pylorus) leading to the duodenum.
Reflex	A response to a stimulus in which the signals are relayed by neurons, and are not normally subject to voluntary control.
Renal	Relating to the kidney.
Ringer solution	Named after Sidney ringer, who discovered that calcium ions are an essential component of the physiological environment of cardiac cells. A simple saline solution that is sufficiently similar to the normal environment of a tissue that the tissue continues to behave fairly normally when immersed in it.
Saline	A solution of salts, usually one suitable for bathing or injecting into tissues. The simplest saline for clinical and mammalian use is 0.9% NaCl (approx. 150mm), which is roughly isosmotic with cells. More elaborate solutions for maintaining tissues in good physiological conditions are often named after scientists who worked out their formulae, e.g. Ringer, krebs.
Sebaceous	Containing or secreting fatty matter.
Serum	The fluid that separates from blood when it clots. Approximately equivalent to the plasma without much of its dissolved proteins.
Shaft	The long, straight section between the ends of a long bone.
Solinocrine secretions	Several hormones secreted directly into the lumen of git, respiratory and reproductive tracts e.g. Gastrin, somatostatin, vip, calcitonin, secretin, serotonin etc.
Stasis	Cessation of movement. E.g. Homeostasis, haemostasis.
Subcutaneous	Just below the skin.
Thoracic	That part of the body cavity carrying the heart and lungs
Tinnitus	Sensation of dizziness

Tonicity	Osmolarity, a hypotonic solution (e.g. A more dilute solution, with lower osmolarity) makes cells swell; a hypertonic solution makes them shrink.
Toxin	A poisonous or harmful substance
Trauma	A painful, harmful, or destructive event, or the wound caused by such an event.
Trophic	Relating to nutrition or growth
Vertigo	Sensation of dizziness
Virulent	Ability to cause disease.
Zygo-	Denoting a joining or pairing. Eg Zygote

2

Blood

Blood is the fluid pumped by the heart that circulates throughout the body via the arteries, veins, and capillaries . Blood is a body fluid in animals and human beings that delivers necessary substances such as nutrients and oxygen to the cells and transports metabolic waste products away from those same cells. Hematology is the science or study of blood, blood-forming organs and blood diseases.

Blood is very important for the body as is evident from the fact that the loss of blood from the body makes it weak and may even cause death. Physiologically the blood is a red tissue composed of cells suspended in a pale yellow fluid, plasma. Blood is made up of several parts, including red blood cells, white blood cells, platelets and plasma.

Blood and lymph are important connecting fluids among the diverse anatomical structures of the mammalian organisms. Thus blood is the liquid vehicle by which the major organic nutrients are transported from the intestine where they are absorbed, to the liver where they are processed and thence to other organs. Similarly blood is the liquid vehicle for the transport of waste materials from various organs to the kidney and gastrointestinal tract from where they are eliminated. Thus, the blood is the major transport carrier of nutrients, metabolites, oxygen, hormones, waste products etc. inside the body. Blood is a fluid connective tissue which transports substances from one part to another part of the body.

Clinical blood analysis is usually the first to be carried out in case of disease as its analysis can detect anemia, clotting problems, blood cancers, immune system disorders, infections and many other disorders.

Properties of Blood as a Body Fluid

As a transport medium, blood serves the following major functions of the animal body.

1. **Nutritive function**: Blood carries nutritive substances from the gut to the tissue where they are utilized.
2. **Respiratory functions**: It transports O_2 from lung to the tissue and CO_2 from tissue to lung.
3. **Excretory function**: It transports various metabolic waste products to the excretory organs (kidney, skin, intestine and lungs).
4. **Transport function**: Various hormones, enzymes, antibodies are transported by blood.

5. **Protective functions**: It plays an important role in the defence mechanism of the body. The body defends against infection by increasing the number of certain types of white blood cells (neutrophils and monocytes), which engulf and destroy invading microorganisms. This army is in the form of cells, called white blood corpuscles or leucocytes (Neutrophils and monocytes).
6. Maintenance of body temperature.
7. **Storage functions**: It can store various nutrients such as glucose, protein, electrolytes and water for use in emergency conditions.
8. Blood helps in maintenance of fluid balance and pH equilibrium in the body. Blood is an important medium to maintain homeostasis of various electrolytes in the body.

The blood is composed of two parts, the cells and the fluid part or plasma. The cellular constituents of blood include erythrocytes or red blood corpuscles, leukocytes or white blood corpuscles and thrombocytes or platelets.

- Red blood cells (Erythrocytes), which carry oxygen to the tissues
- White blood cells (Leucocytes), which fight infections
- Platelets (Thrombocytes) smaller cells that help blood to clot

The cellular constituents of blood vary with the species as well as with the age and physiological stage of the animal. About half of blood volume is composed of blood cells:

Blood is conducted through blood vessels (arteries and veins). Blood is prevented from clotting in the blood vessels by their smoothness, and the finely tuned balance of clotting factors.

The extracellular constituents or plasma are composed of water, electrolytes, proteins, lipids, glucose, enzymes and hormones etc. The blood undergoes coagulation on exposure to air leaving clear watery fluid, called serum. Blood serum is equivalent to blood plasma minus fibrinogen and other clotting factors.

The serum is nothing but plasma minus fibrinogen and other clotting factors. The serum is a clear yellowish fluid. The yellow color is due to the presence of small quantities of bilirubin, a bile pigment and of carotenoids.

The blood serum of cattle is yellow due to the presence of more carotenoids whereas that of buffalo is white due to the absence of carotenoids. The blood clot consists of a network of fibrous strands of fibrin in which are enmeshed in the cellular elements of the blood. Blood clotting is a protective mechanism against excessive loss of blood from the body. The lymph also clots, although, somewhat more slowly than blood.

The solutions having the same effective osmolality as body fluids are called isotonic solutions. The suspension of erythrocytes in isotonic solutions does not result in any volume change in the cells. This is because of the osmotic equilibrium between inside and outside of the cell across the cell membrane. The osmotic pressure of blood is equivalent to that of 0.9% sodium chloride solution or that of 5% dextrose solution. Such a solution is called isotonic solution and is approximately 300 milliosmoles/liter.

The erythrocytes respond by swelling (endosmosis) in hypotonic solutions resulting in breakage of cells. In hypertonic solutions there occurs shrinkage of erythrocytes (exosmosis).

The other reasons for hemolysis are freezing and thawing, stirring and agitation, high temperatures, substances that lower surface tension like saponin, soaps and bile salts, alcohol, ether, chloroform and acetone by damaging cell membrane.

Abnormally high or low counts may indicate the presence of many forms of disease, and hence blood counts are among the most commonly performed blood tests in medicine, as they can provide an overview of a patient's general health status. Complete Blood counts have been used for clinical purposes. Automated equipment to carry out complete blood counts was developed in the 1950s and 1960s. Most blood counts today include a CBC count (i.e.: complete blood count) and differential leukocyte count (DLC) that gives the percentage of each WBC type, such as neutrophils, eosinophils, basophils, monocytes, and lymphocytes. Blood tests such as blood count tests help doctors check for certain diseases and conditions. They also help check the function of body organs and show how well treatments are working. Problems with blood may include **bleeding disorders**, **excessive clotting** and **platelet disorders**. If you lose too much blood, you may need a transfusion.

Metabolism and Fate of Erythrocytes (R.B.C)

The erythrocytes or red blood corpuscles are non-motile, non-nucleated (except in birds which are nucleated) and biconcave (dog) or discoid (cattle, sheep and goat) or slightly biconcave (cat and horse) cells in circulating blood. During the maturation of erythrocyte the nucleus is large in size initially and contains chromatin. But, as RBCs mature, the size of the nucleus decreases, until it finally disappears with the condensation of the chromatin material.

RBCs of Cold Blood Animals and Birds are Elliptical and Nucleated

RBCs of Mammals these are non-Nucleated and non-motile

(Every cell in the body has a nucleus except mature erythrocytes)

The principal functions of erythrocyte metabolism in the mature erythrocyte include maintenance of adequate supplies of adenosine triphosphate (ATP), production of reducing substances to act as antioxidants, and control of oxygen affinity of hemoglobin by production of adequate amounts of 2,3-diphosphoglycerate (2,3-DPG)

Composition: In adult animals RBC contains 62-72 percent water and approximately 35% solids, of which 95% is hemoglobin and the rest 5% constitutes proteins in the stroma and cell membrane, phospholipids (Lecithin, Cephalin and Sphingomyelin), cholesterol, neutral fats, glucose, enzymes (cholinesterase, phosphatase, carbonic anhydrase, peptidases and enzymes concerned with glycolysis) vitamins as a part of coenzymes and minerals - phosphorus, Sulphur, chlorine (intracellular anion) magnesium, potassium (intracellular cation) and sodium (cation of extracellular fluid).

Size: The mean diameter of erythrocytes in dry smear varies from 4 μ (goat) to 7 μ (dog). Average thickness will be around 2 μ. The total erythrocyte surface area is relatively constant to the body weight which varies in most of the domestic animals from 56-68 Sqcm/kg body weight and for chicken the value is 44 whereas the body surface area of a man will be 2 Sqm and that of 500 kg cow will be around 5 Sqm.

Number: The number of erythrocytes varies among and within species and even within individuals. Variations also exist between venous and arterial blood. Other factors that influence the numbers are breed, age, sex, nutrition, various physiological stages like estrous cycle, pregnancy, lactation and egg production, adrenaline production due to freight etc. , changes in haemoconcentration , ambient temperature, altitude and other climatic factors. The erythrocyte counts are higher in Bos indicus as compared to Bos taurus. Crossbred cattle have values more in tune with Bos taurus (European cattle). Among the Indian cattle and buffaloes, the buffalo's blood shows the highest number of erythrocytes.

Erythropoiesis is the process which produces red blood cells (erythrocytes), which is the development from erythropoietic stem cell to mature red blood cell. Erythropoiesis is a complex physiological process to maintain oxygen level in the body through production of red blood cells . The number of erythrocytes is regulated so that they can provide sufficient tissue oxygenation. The rate of erythropoiesis is controlled by tissue need for oxygen. It is stimulated by decreased O_2 in circulation, which is detected by the kidneys, which then secrete the hormone erythropoietin. Erythropoietin is a hormone, which regulate the process of erythropoiesis. It is produced by the justaglomerular apparatus of the kidney. The justaglomerular apparatus is a specialized structure formed by the distal convoluted tubule and the glomerular afferent arteriole. It is located near the vascular pole of the glomerulus and its main function is to regulate blood pressure and the filtration rate of the glomerulus. A host of growth factors and the element iron are necessary ingredients that are used by erythroid precursor cells for effective erythropoiesis. Essential for the maturation of red blood cells are Vitamin B_{12} (cobalamin) and Vitamin B_9 (Folic acid). Lack of either causes maturation failure in the process of erythropoiesis. Vitamin B_{12} (Cyanocobalamin) also known as extrinsic factor– function in maturation of RBCs. Folic acid (essential for synthesis of DNA and RNA of RBCs) and Fe, Cu, CO are the minerals that are essential for erythropoiesis. The erythropoiesis control is affected mainly by hematopoietic growth factors ie **cytokines**.

During mammalian development, erythropoiesis consist of two major events. Primitive erythropoiesis is initiated in the yolk sac with the generation of large erythroblasts and definitive erythropoiesis, which takes place in fetal liver with the development of enucleated erythrocytes.

Erythropoiesis begins with the commitment of a small pool of hematopoietic pluripotent stem cells to primitive and multipotent nonlymphoid lineages referred to as CFU-GEMM (colony forming Units-GEMM). In the adult bone marrow, the erythropoiesis initiates with the appearance of proerythroblast or rubriblast as the first stage of differentiation. The rubriblast differentiates into early, intermediate and late normoblasts stages, at which time the nucleus is expelled and the cell becomes a reticulocyte. The reticulocyte gets expelled from the bone marrow to enter into circulation and become fully mature RBCs.

During folate deficiency, iron deficiency or vitamin B_6 deficiency, the developing erythroid cells gets destroyed in the bone marrow and this process is called as ineffective erythropoiesis. Erythropoiesis-stimulating agents (ESAs) (e.g. erythropoietin or epoetin), are genetically engineered erythropoietin recombinants that were introduced in the late 1980s for anemia management in patients undergoing hemodialysis.

Erythropoietin is the principal hormone that regulates erythropoiesis and its transcription is mediated by hypoxia inducible factor-1 (HIF-1). In addition to erythropoietin, the erythropoietic machinery requires a constant supply of iron, vitamin B_{12}, and folic acid. Inadequate supplies of any of these constituents result in anemia, which is a deficiency in oxygen-carrying erythrocytes. Megaloblastic anemia is caused by inadequate folic acid or vitamin B_{12} absorption, which is required for purine and pyrimidine formation in the synthesis of DNA.

During prenatal life erythropoiesis, the formation of erythrocytes, takes place in yolk sac which later in prenatal life is taken up by liver, spleen and lymph nodes. During postnatal life erythrocytes are continuously formed in bone marrow as nucleated cells (to certain extent in spleen in birds) at a rate to balance destruction in blood circulation.

Rubriblast by passing through various developmental stages such as prorubriblast, rubricyte metarubricyte and reticulocyte develop into erythrocyte in the bone marrow. They enter bone marrow capillary to join blood stream by diapedesis, a process of penetration without rupturing the capillary wall, mostly after extruding the nucleus (1-3% enter as nucleated reticulocytes).The erythrocytes thus develop in the bone marrow of the adult, by mitosis and differentiation, from a common line of progenitor cells, the pluripotent stem cells.

For the formation of blood and blood cells (hematopoiesis) and for their maturation adequate availability of various vitamins (B_{12}, folic acid, thiamine, riboflavin, pyridoxine, nicotinic acid, pantothenic acid, biotin and ascorbic acid) minerals (iron, copper and cobalt), amino acids, water and energy are essential. Due to hypoxia or oxygen debt in tissues due to various diseases, hemorrhage or hemolysis, a humoral factor (hormone) erythropoietin is produced in the kidney and in tissues with low oxygen supply, which stimulates hematopoiesis. Polycythemia is the presence of an unusually large number of erythrocytes in circulation. Plasma from animals rendered anemic by various means induces polycythemia when injected into normal animals. This effect is due to the secretion of erythropoietin. Erythropoietin is a mucoprotein with a molecular weight of 46000 Dalton.

Life span of erythrocytes from the time they enter blood stream till they are destroyed vary from species to species. A great number of erythrocytes are destroyed daily. In an animal weighing 450 kg with a blood volume of 8 percent of body weight having 300 trillion erythrocytes with a life span of 100 days, around 3 trillion in a day or 35 million in a second are destroyed.

The reticuloendothelial system or macrophage system is a part of the immune system that consists of the phagocytic cells located in reticular connective tissue. The Kupffer cells of the liver and tissue histiocytes are also part of the macrophage system. The cells are primarily monocytes and macrophages, and they accumulate in lymph nodes and the spleen. Reticuloendothelial cells are stellate or Kupffer cells found in the walls of blood sinuses of the liver, spleen, bone marrow and lymph nodes. They have phagocytosis capacity and release all kinds of cytokines, chemokines, and soluble biological mediators. Kupffer cells play an important role in liver diseases. Kupffer cells, play a role in eliminating macromolecules, immune complexes, toxins, and degenerated cells from circulation. Kupffer cells also could remove the senescent or damaged erythrocytes. Kupffer cells have various functions in liver injury and repair.

These cells are instrumental in the destruction of old exhausted erythrocytes. As the erythrocytes are destroyed, the iron moiety (0.334% of Hb or 0.04-0.05% of blood) of haemoglobin is conserved for the new haemoglobin production and iron that is not utilized immediately is stored in liver and spleen. The pigment part of the haemoglobin is converted into bile pigments, bilirubin and biliverdin which are excreted in bile by liver. The protein portion is either utilized in new haemoglobin formation or in the formation of other body proteins.

The production of biliverdin from heme is the first major step in the catabolic pathway, after which the enzyme biliverdin reductase performs the second step, producing bilirubin from biliverdin. In the liver, bilirubin is conjugated with glucuronic acid by the enzyme glucuronyltransferase, making it soluble in water: the conjugated version is the main form of bilirubin present in the "direct" bilirubin fraction.

Bilirubin is excreted in bile and urine, and elevated levels may indicate certain diseases. It is responsible for the yellow color of bruises and the **yellow discoloration in jaundice**. Its subsequent breakdown products, such as stercobilin, cause the brown color of faeces. A different breakdown product, urobilin, is the main component of the straw-yellow color in urine.

Serum bilirubin is usually less than 1 mg/dL and primarily unconjugated. Elevated levels of bilirubin may indicate liver damage or disease. Degree of elevation correlates with prognosis in primary biliary cirrhosis, alcoholic hepatitis, and liver failure. Disorders of bilirubin metabolism and excretion resulting in **jaundice** are some of the most common disorder of the liver and hepatobiliary system.

Hemoglobin-Chemical Structure, Synthesis, Physiological Functions

Hemoglobin is an oxygen-binding protein found in erythrocytes which transports oxygen from the lungs to tissues. It is a respiratory protein of all vert-ebrates, which is localized exclusively in erythrocytes. It transports oxygen from the lungs to all parts of the body, by virtue of its property to combine reversibly with molecular oxygen.

Haemoglobin is a conjugated iron containing protein with a molecular weight of about 65,000 daltons. It is composed of four heme groups attached to a protein called globin. It comprises four peptide strings, two α-subunits and two β-subunits, containing

574 amino acids total. It has a common cyclic tetrapeptide called a porphyrin. To form heme groups, one iron is firmly chelated by the electron pairs of the nitrogen atoms of the four pyrrole residues. A molecule of hemoglobin, consists of nearly 600 amino acid subunits in four long chains, folded into globular shapes and associated in a structure 5.5 nm in diameter.

Amino acid glycine and acetate form a four carbon compound with additional glycine. This compound unites with glycine to form pyrrole. Four pyrrole molecules form into protoporphyrin which in turn unites with iron to form heme. Four heme molecules unite with protein globin to form haemoglobin.

Oxygenated hemoglobin is bright red. The color of hemoglobin depends on the number of oxygen molecules bound to the hemoglobin molecule. When hemoglobin is saturated with oxygen , it is bright red, while it is dark bluish-red when no oxygen is bound.

Arterial blood, which is normally almost completely saturated with oxygen, is bright red. Venous blood is darker because it has less oxygen molecules bound to hemoglobin. Blood never actually turns blue, but skin can take on a bluish cast as a result of certain diseases and disorders. This blue color is called cyanosis.

Biosynthesis of haemoglobin, the pigment of erythrocytes starts in the erythrocytes (Rubriblasts) and continues in the subsequent stages of cell development till the nuclear material is present. Haem & globin produced at two different sites in the cells. Hb is synthesized in the cytoplasm of intermediate normoblasts. Haem is synthesized in the mitochondria. Globin is the protein part of Hb and it is synthesized in ribosomes.

There are multiple steps involved in heme synthesis. Eight enzymes accomplish this process, four of which work in the mitochondria and four in the cytosol. The process starts in the mitochondria, where ALA (aminolevulinic acid) synthase links glycine and succinyl coenzyme A to form ALA. Steps 2-5 occur in the cytosol. Next, ALA dehydratase takes two molecules of ALA and produces porphobilinogen (PBG). In the third step, porphobilinogen deaminase takes four molecules of PBG and produces hydroxymethylbilane. Next, uroporphyrinogen III cosynthase takes hydroxymethylbilane and produces uroporphyrinogen III. In the fifth step, uroporphyrinogen decarboxylase takes uroporphyrinogen III and produces coproporphyrinogen III. The final three steps of heme synthesis occur in the mitochondria. Coproporphyrinogen III is then transformed to protoporphyrinogen IX by coproporphyrinogen oxidase. The seventh step occurs when protoporphyrinogen oxidase converts protoporphyrinogen IX to protoporphyrin IX. The eighth and final step of heme synthesis is the addition of Fe to protoporphyrin IX by ferrochelatase, producing a heme molecule.

Derivatives of Hemoglobin (Methemoglobin; Carboxyhemoglobin; Sulfhemoglobin)

Hemoglobin derivatives are altered forms of hemoglobin. Hemoglobin derivatives are formed by the combination of different ligands with the heme part, or change in the oxidation state of iron.

Oxyhemoglobin (HbO_2): The main function of hemoglobin is to transport oxygen from the lung to the tissues. In lungs the partial pressure of oxygen is 100 mm of Hg, at this pressure hemoglobin is 95-96% saturated with oxygen. On binding with O_2 in the lungs hemoglobin is converted to oxy-hemoglobin (HbO_2). O_2 is bound to heme iron.

$Hb + O_2 \rightarrow HbO_2$

Haemoglobin combines with oxygen while blood passes through pulmonary capillaries to form a bright red oxyhaemoglobin owing to the oxygen combining capacity of the iron content of haemoglobin which in turn loses oxygen to tissues while blood passes through systemic capillaries to form purplish red haemoglobin. One gram of haemoglobin carries 1.36 ml of oxygen or 15 gm of haemoglobin in 100 ml blood may carry 20 ml of oxygen.

Myoglobin or myohaemoglobin or muscle haemoglobin contains one heme group and one iron molecule with approximate molecular weight of 16,700 daltons has a greater affinity for oxygen than blood haemoglobin and serves as a brief oxygen store and rapidly releases oxygen when muscle fibres contracts which are replenished while resting.

Carboxyhaemoglobin or Hemoglobin also binds to CO_2 in the tissues. CO_2 is bound to the α-amino group at the N-terminal end of each of the four polypeptide chains of hemoglobin to form carbaminohemoglobin. As one CO_2 binds O_2 is released.

Carbonmonoxyhemoglobin is bright cherry red, results when haemoglobin combines with carbon monoxide present in inspired air. Carbon monoxide has 200 times more affinity with haemoglobin due to which it prevents the carriage and supply of oxygen to tissues.

Methaemoglobin is formed by oxidation of ferrous iron of haemoglobin to ferric state and occurs in blood in minute quantities. Though non toxic it cannot function as respiratory pigment. Reducing compounds like ascorbic acid, glutathione etc in erythrocytes prevent accumulation of methaemoglobin. Larger amounts are formed after the administration of certain drugs like nitrites, aminophenols, sulphonamides etc. In RBC the iron of hemoglobin is normally in ferrous (Fe_2+) form, but it is readily oxidized to the ferric (Fe_3+) form by hydrogen peroxide formed by RBC cell metabolism, to yield met-hemoglobin. Ferric iron is incapable of binding O_2 therefore the functions of hemoglobin are disturbed. Normally 1.7 to 2.4 % of total hemoglobin will be in the form of met-hemoglobin. Increase in the percent of met-hemoglobin is prevented by the peroxidase action of a naturally occurring peptide known as glutathione present in the RBC. Met-hemoglobin is dark brown in colour.

The percent of met-hemoglobin can increase if the person consumes drugs like ferricyanide, nitrite, quinines, hydroxylamine's, acetanilide and sulfonamide. Higher levels of met-hemoglobin is observed clinically in factory workers who inhale (or contact through skin) aromatic nitro and amino compounds and in patients taking large amounts of acetanilide and sulfonamides. The symptoms are cyanosis (blue skin) and dyspnoea (labored breathing).

Met-hemoglobin can be used to overcome cyanide poisoning. By injecting met-hemoglobin it combines with cyanide to form cyanmethemoglobin preventing cyanide poisoning.

Once the oxygen diffuses across the alveoli, it enters the bloodstream and is transported to the tissues where it is unloaded, and carbon dioxide diffuses out of the blood and into the alveoli to be expelled from the body. Although gas exchange is a continuous process, the oxygen and carbon dioxide are transported by different mechanisms.

An enzyme present in red blood cells, carbonic anhydrase, aids in the conversion of carbon dioxide to carbonic acid and bicarbonate ions. When red blood cells reach the lungs, the same enzyme helps to convert the bicarbonate ions back to carbon dioxide, which we breathe out.

Reduced Hemoglobin (HHb)

Oxy-hemoglobin moves to the tissue where the partial pressure of O_2 is 26 mm of Hg due to which oxygen is released into the tissues and in turn H+ binds to Hb and forms reduced hemoglobin.

$HbO_2 + H^+ \rightarrow HHb + O_2$

Carbaminohemoglobin: Carbaminohemoglobin is a compound of hemoglobin and carbon dioxide, and is one of the forms in which carbon dioxide exists in the blood.

Methemoglobin: Methemoglobin is a hemoglobin in the form of metalloprotein, in which the iron in the heme group is in the Fe3+ (ferric) state, not the Fe2+ (ferrous) of normal hemoglobin. Methemoglobin cannot bind oxygen, which means it cannot carry oxygen to tissues.

Carboxyhemoglobin: Oxy-hemoglobin can bind to carbon monoxide (CO). The affinity of CO to Hb is 200 times more than that of oxygen. It is then unsuitable for oxygen transport. Even normal, non- oxygenated hemoglobin can bind with CO to form carboxyhemoglobin. [Hb + CO $\rightarrow$ HbCO]. CO has got an affinity of 200 times more than that of O_2 towards Hb. Hemoglobin can bind more readily to CO than to O_2. Even if there is a little amount of CO in air, it can displace oxyHb to form carboxyHb. Due to this there will be tissue hypoxia because the oxygen binding capacity is reduced and there is also reduced O_2 releasing capacity i.e. it cannot release O_2 though it may be bound to O_2.

Breathing the automobile exhaust in closed space is the commonest cause for CO poisoning. City dwellers have at least 1% of carboxyhemoglobin which can increase to 8% depending upon the pollution. Over-traffic can increase carboxyHb to 40% which leads to death. Clinically such patients show cherry red colour of skin. CO poisoning can be treated if a high amount of O_2 is provided continuously at high pressure, then at such high concentrations and pressure HbCO is dissociated forming HbO_2 + CO. When treatment continues for 2 hours CO is expelled out.

CO is a colorless, odorless, tasteless gas generated by incomplete combustion. CO poisoning is a major occupational hazard for workers in mines. One of the primary symptoms of carbon monoxide exposure in both pets and humans is nausea. In the brain, CO binds to cytochrome c oxidase, which results in impairment of ATP synthesis and increased production of reactive oxygen species. Erythropoietin is a cytokine that originally was identified for its role in erythropoiesis and more recently was shown to be produced in the central nervous system. Erythropoietin offers neuronal protection when administered systemically to animals with cerebral ischemia.

Ferrihaemoglobin : the reduced form of haemoglobin, combines reversibly with oxygen to form oxyferrohemoglobin according to the reaction.

$Hb_4 + 4\ O_2 = Hb_4\ (O_2)_4$

Anemia

Anemia means a deficiency of red blood cells, which can be caused by either too rapid loss of blood or by too slow production of red blood cells or deficiency of haemoglobin in the red cells. Anemia results in an absolute decrease in the red cell mass as measured by RBC count, hemoglobin concentration, and PCV. Anaemias cause decreased efficiency of the transport of oxygen to the tissues because of decreased haemoglobin. Anaemic animals fatigue rapidly and their endurance is weakened. Supplementation of iron can relieve anemia in domestic animals.

Anemia is classified as regenerative or nonregenerative. In a regenerative anemia, the bone marrow responds appropriately to the decreased red cell mass by increasing RBC production and releasing reticulocytes. In a nonregenerative anemia, the bone marrow responds inadequately to the increased need for RBC. Anemias due to hemorrhage or hemolysis are usually regenerative. Anemias that are caused by decreased erythropoietin or an abnormality in the bone marrow are nonregenerative.

Clinical signs in anemic animals depend on the degree of anemia, the duration (acute or chronic), and the underlying cause. Acute anemia can result in shock and even death if more than a third of the blood volume is lost rapidly and not replaced. In acute blood loss, the animal usually presents with tachycardia, pale mucous membranes, bounding or weak pulses, and hypotension. The cause of the blood loss may be obvious, eg. trauma. If no evidence of external bleeding is found, a source of internal or occult blood loss must be sought, eg. a ruptured splenic tumor, coagulopathy, GI ulceration or parasites, or other neoplasia. If hemolysis is present, the patient may be icteric.

Patients with chronic anemia have had time to adjust, and their clinical presentation is usually more indolent with vague signs of lethargy, weakness, and anorexia. These patients will have similar physical examination findings, pale mucous membranes, tachycardia, and possibly splenomegaly or a new heart murmur, or both.

The reticulocyte count is usually reported as a percent of the RBC mass. This value should be corrected for the degree of anemia in order to evaluate the degree of regeneration. An absolute reticulocyte count (measured by RBC/µL × reticulocyte percentage) of >50,000/µL or >60,000/µL in cats or dogs, respectively, is considered regenerative. In order to correct the percent reticulocytes, this formula can be applied: A corrected reticulocyte percent >1% indicates regeneration in the dog and cat. After acute blood loss or hemolytic crisis, reticulocytosis usually takes 3-4 days to become evident.

Causes of Anaemia

1. Blood loss
2. Bone marrow aplasia (aplasia means lack of development of an organ or tissue or of the cellular products from an organ or tissue).
3. Deficiency of vitamin B^{12} or folic acid.
4. Haemolysis of red cells.
5. Deficiency of iron in the diet.

Anemia in domestic animals can be caused by trypanosomiasis and paratuberculosis. Gastrointestinal nematodes of ruminants (cattle, sheep and goats) are ubiquitous and can cause severe anemia. Attempts have been made to categorise the anemic status of small ruminants based on the conjunctiva mucosa color on a scale from 1 (optimal eye color, red) to 5 (pale eye color, white).

Anemias may be classified according to number and size of cells and the haemoglobin content.

1. **Normocytic and normochromic anaemia :** In such anaemia, there is a decrease in number of cells but the cells retain their normal size and haemoglobin content. Such anaemia is a result of acute haemorrhage because plasma volume is replenished long before the RBCs are restored.
2. **Microcytic and hypochromic anaemia** : In such anaemia the decrease in number of cells is accompanied by a decrease in cell size and haemoglobin content. This anaemia is caused by a deficiency of iron in the diet.
3. **Macrocytic and hyperchromic :** In such anaemia the decrease in number of cells is accompanied by an increase in cell size and haemoglobin content. Such a condition is characteristic of pernicious anaemia caused by lack of extrinsic factors (Vitamin B_{12}) or intrinsic factor produced in gastric mucosa.
4. **Aplastic anaemia** : It is caused by malfunctioning of bone marrow; may result from excessive X radiation or from unknown cause.
5. **Sickle cell anaemia :** Cells are abnormal in shape (sickle shaped) and normal oxygen transport function is disrupted. This condition is hereditary in nature.
6. **Megaloblastic anaemia :** Megaloblastic anemia is a condition in which the bone marrow produces unusually large, structurally abnormal, immature red blood cells (megaloblasts). Megaloblastic anemia results from inhibition of DNA synthesis during red blood cell production. When DNA synthesis is impaired, the cell cycle cannot progress from the G2 growth stage to the mitosis stage. This leads to continuing cell growth without division, which presents as macrocytosis. Megaloblastic anemia has a rather slow onset, especially when compared to that of other anemias. The defect in red cell DNA synthesis is most often due to hypovitaminosis, specifically vitamin B_{12} or cobalamin.

Polycythemia is a disorder characterised by increased erythrocytes and it may be caused by dehydration by an overactive bone marrow. Hypoxia or high altitude, markedly increase the RBC number: however after some time animals adapts to high altitude, the number decreases and may approach those observed at sea levels. Polycythemia is common in patients with hemoglobin desaturation secondary to hypoxia. In response to hypoxemia, increased erythropoietin production in Polycythemia causes increased oxygen transport which is supposed to be beneficial.

Blood Transfusions

Blood transfusion has been practiced for centuries for saving the lives of human beings and animals. Richard Lower in 1665 transfused the blood in a dog for the first time in history. With the help of latest techniques and equipment developed after 1950, blood transfusion became more popular in veterinary medicine. Advancement in techniques of separating the components of blood has given the clinician an opportunity to use the component as per the demand of the patient. Transfusion medicine may be a life saving modality in case of emergency or critically ill animals.

Blood transfusions has been practiced since long back to improve oxygen carrying capacity and rectify the clinical signs of anemia. Frequently, the need for blood transfusions is acute, as in acute hemolysis or hemorrhage; transfusions are also appropriate in treatment of acute or chronic anemias. Animals with hemostatic disorders often require repeated transfusions of either whole blood, red cells, plasma, or platelets. In Human beings normally blood transfusions are commonly reported in the following conditions.

- **Haemorrhage**
- **Trauma**
- **Burns**
- **Anaemia**

Sometimes infusion of Sodium chloride solution (0.9%) and glucose (5%) is used as a substitute for blood transfusion. Human blood plasma has been used in exceptional cases for transfusion if blood is not available.

Major and minor cross matching tests are done for agglutinating and/or hemolytic reactions between donor and recipient. For dog and cat agglutinating tests are sufficient whereas in equines agglutinating and hemolytic tests are required because of presence of agglutinating as well as hemolytic antibodies in equines. Several precautions must be taken while transfusing blood including sterile conditions, proper temperature and proper rate of transfusion. Two anticoagulants namely Citrate-phosphate-dextrose-adenine (CPDA-1) and Acid-citrate-dextrose (ACD) are commonly used for storage of blood.

Blood transfusions must be given with care because they have the potential for further compromising the recipient. The diversity of blood groups in animals and the lack of commercially available blood-typing reagents make complete typing and matching difficult but should not preclude the clinical use of transfusions. In horses and dogs, the blood group antigens most commonly implicated in transfusion incompatibilities are known; by selecting donor animals that lack these groups, or that match the recipient, the risk of sensitization of the recipient to the most important antigens can be minimized. Previously sensitized recipients can be detected by crossmatching, which will preclude administration of incompatible blood. In the USA, >99% of cats are of blood group A, so the risk of incompatible transfusion is low. Any incompatible transfusion in cats results in rapid destruction of transfused cells, so typing or crossmatching should be done before any transfusion.

Whole blood frequently is not the ideal product to be administered. If the need is to replace the oxygen-carrying capability of the blood, then packed RBC are more appropriate; if replacement of circulatory volume is needed, crystalloid or colloid solutions may be used to replace volume, with packed RBC added as needed. Platelet numbers rise rapidly after hemorrhage, so replacement is rarely needed. Plasma proteins equilibrate from the interstitial space, so plasma is not needed except in massive hemorrhage. Animals that require coagulation factors benefit most from administration of fresh-frozen plasma or cryoprecipitate if the need is specifically for factor VIII, von Willebrand factor, or fibrinogen. Platelet-rich plasma or platelet concentrates may be of value in thrombocytopenia, although immune-mediated thrombocytopenia usually does not respond to administration of platelets because they are removed rapidly by the spleen.

Risks of Transfusion

The most serious risk of transfusion is acute hemolysis. Fortunately, this is rare in domestic animals. Dogs rarely have clinically significant preformed antibodies, so only those that have received repeated transfusions are at risk. The most common hemolytic reaction in dogs that have received multiple transfusion is delayed hemolysis, seen clinically as shortened survival of transfused RBC and a positive Coombs' test. Even crossmatch-compatible RBC given to horses or cattle survive only 2-4 days. Repeated transfusions can cause acute hemolysis. Non immune causes of hemolysis include improper collection or separation of blood, freezing or overwarming of RBC, and infusing under pressure through a small needle. Other complications include sepsis from contaminated blood, hypocalcemia from too much citrate, and hypervolemia (especially in animals with pre existing heart disease or in very small animals). Urticaria, fever, or vomiting are seen occasionally. Transfusions can also spread disease from donor to recipient, such as RBC parasites (eg, *Haemobartonella*, *Anaplasma*, or *Babesia*) and viruses (eg, retroviruses such as feline or bovine leukemia, equine infectious anemia, or other viruses). Other diseases, such as those caused by rickettsia or other bacteria, can also be spread if the donor is bacteremic.

Extracellular Constituents

The non cellular portion of the blood is the blood plasma of which about 10 per cent consists of various organic and inorganic solutes. The plasma proteins make up three fourth of the solutes.

Plasma

Plasma constitute 55-70 percent of blood which consists of **water**, gases (oxygen, carbon dioxide and nitrogen), proteins (albumins, globulins and fibrinogens), glucose, lactate and pyruvate, lipids (fat, lecithin and cholesterol), non protein nitrogen compounds (amino acids, urea, uric acid, creatine, creatinine, and ammonium salts) inorganic substances (sodium, potassium, calcium, magnesium, chloride, sulphate, phosphate and traces of iron, manganese, cobalt, copper, zinc and iodine) and enzymes, hormones, vitamins and pigments.

Blood hematological parameters are an important index for metabolic processes in the body under varying physiological conditions. Physiological variations in the blood parameters are of great significance for clinical hematology and animal production as blood constituents are indicative of stress during various physiological stages. Pregnancy and lactation are physiological periods that result in increased metabolic demands. Although homeostatic mechanisms keep substances in the blood at relatively constant levels, some changes in the concentrations of hematological parameters occur indicative of the metabolic stress during pregnancy and early lactation.

Plasma Proteins

Proteins, macromolecules built from one or more unbranched chains of amino acids linked by peptide bonds, are the major components of the blood serum or plasma and have many different functions. Proteins are involved in almost all of the reactions occurring in the organism. Proteins are involved in the regulation of cellular activity and the immune system.

Plasma proteins perform the following major **functions** in the animal body.

1. Maintain colloid osmotic pressure of blood
2. Maintain normal blood pressures
3. Influence the suspension stability of erythrocytes
4. Regulate the acid base balance of blood.
5. Provide the antibodies.
6. Affect the solubility of carbohydrates, lipids and other substances
7. Transport of electrolytes and other substances such as lipids & fatty acids as well as some trace metals, vitamins and hormones . Blood proteins act as carriers of lipids, hormones, vitamins and minerals in the circulatory system.
8. Blood proteins are involved in the regulation of cellular activity and the immune system
9. Provide amino acids for protein synthesis in tissues when amino acid concentration of the later falls below that of plasma.
10. Certain blood proteins are essential for haemostasis and have important functions in platelet adhesion and aggregation, as well as coagulation
11. Blood proteins play important roles as enzymes, complement components or protease inhibitors.

All the major proteins in the blood serum are formed by **hepatocytes** in the **liver**. The major exceptions are the immunoglobulins that are produced by the immune system consisting of the reticuloendothelial tissues, lymph nodes and bone marrow. The measurement of serum proteins may be an important diagnostic tool for the detection, diagnosis, and monitoring of various diseases and pathological processes.

More than 10,000 proteins may be present in blood but the major proteins are albumin, globulins and their concentrations can be measured in g/ml. The blood plasma contains 6-8 g per 100 ml protein of which 3.0-3.5 g per 100 ml is albumin, 3.5-4.0 g per 100 ml is globulin and 0.5 gm per100 ml is fibrinogen. The normal concentration of globulins in human blood is about 2.6-4.6 g/dL. Protein concentrations in serum are controlled to balance their physiological role in immune function, coagulation, molecular transport and inflammation etc.

Albumin predominates globulins in man, sheep, goat, rabbit and dog, whereas both are almost equal in horse, pig and cow. Albumin constitutes 35 to 50% of total serum protein. Albumin plays an important role in maintaining homeostasis, in transport of substances, and acts as a free-radical scavenger. Albumin is responsible for about 75% of the osmotic pressure of plasma and is a major source of amino acids that can be utilised by the animal's body when necessary. Muscle, liver, and kidney are the main sites of albumin catabolism.

Plasma proteins are large molecules with the following molecular weight. The fibrinogen has got the highest molecular weight. The protein molecules are soluble in water because of the presence of polar residues like NH_2 and COOH.

- Albumin 69,000 daltons
- Globulins 90,000 -1,56,000 daltons
- Fibrinogen 5,00,000 daltons

In very young animals/infants the total protein content is low due to low gamma globulins.

A/G ratio is usually calculated as it is indicative of the health status of animals. The albumin/globulin ratio is the amount of albumin in the serum divided by the globulins. The ratio is used to identify causes of change in total serum protein. A/G ratio in canines usually varies from 0.8 to 2.0. Decreased A/G may be due to increased globulins during infection and inflammation. Decreased A/G due to decrease in albumin may point towards severe liver disease or disorder because albumin and fibrinogen is synthesized mostly by reticuloendothelial cells of the liver.

The antibodies gamma globulins are lacking in the newborn as the fetus cannot synthesize them and the placenta is impermeable to these protein molecules and thus has to obtain them through colostrum.

The globulins are of three types mainly alpha, beta and gamma.

The gamma globulins or immunoglobulins are important in resistance of the body against foreign substances and disease producing organisms. These proteins are formed in the spleen and lymphatic cells in response to a foreign substance called antigen. The newly formed protein is called an antibody and specifically combines with the antigen which triggered its synthesis.

Immunoglobulins are classified into three major classes called IgM, IgA, and IgG. Each class has many sub groups which are produced by specific cells by normal individuals. Each complete immunoglobulin is made up of two pairs of polypeptide chains, a pair of light (short) and a pair of heavy (long) chains.

Albumins

These constitute about 50% of the total plasma proteins and possibly are involved in fatty acid binding and anion transport. They serve to control the osmotic pressure of the blood as well as maintain the buffering capacity of the blood pH. Serum albumin is approximately 69,000 daltons in molecular weight and is a typical globular protein.

Fibrinogen

The third important protein in blood plasma is fibrinogen. Blood serum is devoid of it. Fibrinogen accounts for about 4% of the total plasma protein and it plays an unusually vital role in blood clotting.

The plasma proteins exert an osmotic pressure which influences the exchanges of fluid between blood and tissues. Plasma proteins also combine with many substances e.g. iron, thyroxine and steroid hormones to form transportable complexes from which active compounds are released at the appropriate sites.

Blood Sugar Content of Domestic Animals

Horse 72.7 mg/100 ml

Cattle 45.9 mg/100 ml

Dog 59.9 mg/100 ml

Blood Hb Concentration

Indian Cattle Hb 9.1 gm/100 ml (7-12 gm/100 ml)

European cattle 12 gm/100 ml (9.5-13.5 gm/100 ml)

Buffaloes 12.9 g/100 ml (7-15 gm/100 ml)

Specific Gravity of Blood

Plasma protein concentration is largely responsible for the specific gravity of plasma or serum.

Anticoagulants

Anticoagulants are chemical substances which delay or prevent the process of blood coagulation, prolonging the clotting time. Anticoagulants work by interrupting the process involved in the formation of blood clots. Common anticoagulants include warfarin and heparin.

Examples

- Heparin
- Antithrombin III
- Protein – C
- Sodium citrate
- Sodium, potassium and ammonium salts of oxalates and fluorides
- EDTA

Heparin, a conjugated polysaccharide, is a natural anticoagulant produced by basophilic mast cells present throughout the body especially in the connective tissue surrounding capillaries in lungs and other tissues. Heparin helps to maintain the normal fluidity of the blood. Heparin was first isolated from the liver (hence its name) but was subsequently demonstrated in extracts from many other organs eg lungs. Heparin is normally secreted by a group of connective tissue cells called mast cells present in the small vessels of the circulatory system. Chemically heparin is a polysaccharide derived from glucosamine and glucuronic acid. Heparin inhibits coagulation of blood both in vitro and in vivo. One mg of heparin will prevent coagulation of 10-20 ml of blood at room temperature (one unit of heparin is 0.01 mg of heparin sodium). Heparin is generally used as an anticoagulant to keep body fluid in vitro for the purposes of hematological analysis. Heparin is administered in cases of commencing or developed thrombosis. Heparin is rapidly destroyed by an enzyme heparinase in the liver. The basophils in blood also produce heparin but in insignificant quantities.

Sodium citrate in 0.2 to 0.4% of blood prevents coagulation by forming insoluble calcium salts by citrate and is normally used as anticoagulant for blood needed for transfusion. For analytical work, sodium, (4mg/5ml of blood) potassium and ammonium (6mg/5ml of Blood) salts of oxalates, ethylene diamino tetra acetic acid (EDTA) etc. are also used as anticoagulant.

Plasma volume is determined by injecting Evans Blue dye (T-1824) or radioactive iodine ^{131}I into the blood and then find out the dilution which these substances have undergone over a period of time using the formula. Amount injected/Concentration per ml of plasma.

Erythrocyte or red cell volume is similarly determined by injecting radioactive phosphorus (^{32}P) iron (^{58}Fe) chromium (^{51}Cr) or by injecting previously tagged erythrocytes with the above substances and find out the dilution which the tagged erythrocytes have undergone with time.

The packed cell volume (PCV) of venous blood is the venous PCV minus the trapped plasma which the packed cells contain. The correction factor for trapped plasma for arriving true PCV of elephant, man, dog, sheep and goat were 0.96, 0.99, 0.97, 0.96 and 0.91, respectively.

Mean Corpuscular volume (MCV)/Mean corpuscular haemoglobin (MCH)/Mean corpuscular haemoglobin conc. (MCHC). These values are of importance in diagnosing different anemias in animals. The cubical volume of the erythrocytes is taken into consideration while calculating MCV which is more realistic than the diameter of erythrocytes measures in dry smears.

Blood Lipids -Origin and Function

Because lipids are poorly soluble in water, they are transported in the blood as lipoproteins. The concentration of blood lipids depends on intake and excretion from the intestine, and uptake and secretion from cells. Most common types of lipids present in blood are triglycerides and cholesterol. Blood lipids are important in human health because the presence of elevated or abnormal levels of lipids and/or lipoproteins in the blood is a major risk factor for cardiovascular disease.

Cholesterol is a waxy substance found in the blood. Cholesterol is the most commonly occurring steroid. It is an important precursor of cholesterol esters, bile acids and steroid hormones. Body needs cholesterol to build healthy cells, but high levels of cholesterol can increase risk of heart disease. With high cholesterol, human beings can develop fatty deposits in blood vessels.

Total cholesterol levels less than 200 milligrams per deciliter (mg/dL) are considered desirable for human adults. A reading between 200 and 239 mg/dL is considered borderline high and a reading of 240 mg/dL and above is considered high.

Cholesterol is carried through blood, attached to proteins. This combination of proteins and cholesterol is called a lipoprotein. There are different types of cholesterol, based on what the lipoprotein carries. They are:

Low-density lipoprotein (LDL). LDL, or "bad" cholesterol, transports cholesterol particles throughout the body. LDL cholesterol builds up in the walls of arteries, making them hard and narrow.

High-density lipoprotein (HDL). HDL, or "good" cholesterol, picks up excess cholesterol and takes it back to your liver.

Cholesterol occurs in blood as part of all lipoproteins, but low density (LDL) and high density lipoprotein (HDL) fractions have the highest concentrations. LDLs are formed from very low density lipoproteins (VLDL) by endothelial lipoprotein lipase. They are responsible for transporting cholesterol to peripheral tissues, by binding to LDL receptors on these tissues, e.g. adrenal glands, ovary and testes. HDLs are synthesized in the liver and gastrointestinal tract and transport cholesterol from tissues to the liver (so-called "reverse" cholesterol transport, which is thought to be minimal in dogs due to the lack of some transferase enzymes). Once in the liver, cholesterol can be incorporated into VLDLs, synthesized into bile acids, esterified to long chain fatty acids or excreted into the bile. Bile is the main route of excretion of cholesterol. Measurement of cholesterol can give an indication of hepatic function, gastrointestinal disease, and metabolic disorders.

Triglycerides / Triacylglycerols: Triacylglycerols are highly concentrated stores of metabolic energy. The lipases digest the triacylglycerols into free fatty acids and monoacylglycerol. Triacylglycerols in blood are packaged in the form of chylomicrons. Chylomicrons also function in the transport of fat-soluble vitamins and cholesterol.

Lymph-Composition, Formation and Flow

The intracellular fluid diffuses and is filtered into blind ended ducts where it is called lymph. Lymph has the same concentration of salts as interstitial fluid and plasma, a lower concentration of proteins than plasma and a slightly higher concentration of proteins than interstitial fluid.

The distal lymphatics form a closed system of tubes, consisting of an endothelial lining supported by fibrous tissue. The larger vessels have muscle fibres in their walls. The lymphatic vessels possess numerous valves and the flow of lymph from the periphery to the thoracic duct is brought about by muscular and respiratory movements in the same way as the flow of blood in the veins. The lacteals of the intestine show rhythmic contractions ranging from 1 per min, which because of the numerous valves in these vessels, propel the lymph on to the thoracic duct.

In the sheep the lymph flow pressure may be as high as 25 mgHg.

Oedema : Complete obstruction of the lymphatic vessels draining a part of the body leads to oedema of the area. Oedema due to over-drinking is relatively uniform throughout all tissue compartments.

Coagulation Mechanisms

Haemostasis refers to the spontaneous arrest or prevention of bleeding from the injured/damaged vessels by the physiological process. It involves three main steps.

- Vasoconstriction,
- Formation of temporary haemostatic plug and
- Formation of the definitive haemostatic clot

Blood Coagulation, also known as blood clotting, is the process by which blood, when it leaves the blood vessels (such as after a cut) and comes in contact with external objects or air changes from a liquid to a gel, forming a blood clot. It potentially results in hemostasis, the cessation of blood loss from a damaged blood vessel, followed by repair. Such a process is useful in lessening the loss of blood when blood vessels are injured. This happens in the blood of all vertebrates which includes all domestic animals including dog, cat, buffalo, sheep, goat, camel and cattle. Coagulation and clotting involves a complex, interconnected sequence of chemical reactions called a coagulation cascade.

The process of blood clotting and then the subsequent dissolution of the clot, following repair of the injured tissue, is termed hemostasis. Hemostasis comprises four major events that occur in a set order following the loss of vascular integrity:

1. **Vascular constriction**: The initial phase of the process is vascular constriction. This limits the flow of blood to the area of injury. When the blood vessels rupture, the vessels contract by:1. Myogenic spasm 2. Local autacoid factors (local mediators) from traumatized tissue 3. Nervous reflexes by pain nerve impulses initiation 4. Vasoconstrictor substances from platelets eg. Thromboxane A2
2. **Formation of Platelet Plug** : Subsequently the platelets become activated by thrombin and aggregate at the site of injury, forming a temporary, loose

platelet plug. Platelets are key players in primary haemostasis. There are normally between 150 and 400 billion platelets per litre of blood in a healthy adult, produced by megakaryocytes in the bone marrow. The protein fibrinogen is primarily responsible for stimulating platelet clumping. Platelets clump by binding to collagen that becomes exposed following rupture of the endothelial lining of vessels. Upon activation, platelets release the nucleotide, ADP and the eicosanoid, TXA2 (both of which activate additional platelets), serotonin, phospholipids, lipoproteins, and other proteins important for the coagulation cascade. In addition to induced secretion, activated platelets change their shape to accommodate the formation of the plug.

3. **Clot formation :** To insure stability of the initially loose platelet plug, a fibrin mesh (also called the clot) forms and entraps the plug. If the plug contains only platelets it is termed a white thrombus; if red blood cells are present it is called a red thrombus
4. **Healing Process** : After clot formation in a ruptured blood vessel, the healing process begins. The clot is gradually dissolved, or fragmented, by the enzyme plasmin (a serine protease that circulates as the inactive proenzyme, plasminogen), and small portions are phagocytosed by leukocytes present in the blood. The clot may be invaded by fibroblasts (the formation and invasion is stimulated by platelet derived growth factor) within a few hours of its formation. The fibroblasts promote connective tissue formation within the clot and within 7-10 days the clot is organised into fibrous tissue.

When the hemorrhage occurs in large quantities and when the blood clot forms in the tissues, some special substances formed within the clot will dissolve the clot (lysis of clot). The plasma contains a glycoprotein called plasminogen or profibrinolysin. During the formation of a clot, this is trapped within the clot. This can be activated to plasmin or fibrinolysin by tissue plasminogen activator (tPA) released from the damaged tissues and vascular endothelium. The plasmin acts as a proteolytic enzyme and digests fibrin threads leading to dissolution of the clot.

Finally, the clot must be dissolved in order for normal blood flow to resume following tissue repair. The dissolution of the clot occurs through the action of plasmin a serine protease that circulates as the inactive proenzyme, plasminogen.Tissue plasminogen activator (tPA) and, to a lesser degree, urokinase are serine proteases which convert plasminogen to plasmin. Inactive tPA is released from vascular endothelial cells following injury; it binds to fibrin and is consequently activated. Urokinase is produced as the precursor, prourokinase by epithelial cells lining excretory ducts. The role of urokinase is to activate the dissolution of fibrin clots that may be deposited in these ducts.

Mechanism of tPA activation of fibrin clot breakdown: Release of tissue plasminogen activator (tPA) from vascular endothelial cells leads to the onset of the dissolution of fibrin clots. Low levels of circulating tPA are kept inactive by interaction with various inhibitors, where plasminogen activator inhibitor-1 and -2 (PAI-1 and PAI-2) are the most significant. tPA is also removed from the circulation by hepatic cell uptake. The clot dissolving enzyme, plasminogen, binds to the fibrin clot as the inactive zymogen. Once tPA interacts with plasminogen it hydrolyzes the protein releasing catalytically active plasmin. Plasmin then can hydrolyze the cross-linked fibrin polymers of the clot resulting in its dissolution (breakdown). Excess plasmin is controlled from over activity via interaction, in the plasma, with plasmin inhibitors such as α2-antiplasmin.

Streptokinase is a purified fraction of the filtrate from cultures of Streptokinase haemolyticus. Streptokinase (SK) is a thrombolytic medication and enzyme. Streptokinase interacts with plasminogen or plasmin to form a plasminogen activator in plasma. The activator complex in turn cleaves a bond in the plasminogen molecule to give rise to free plasmin. Streptokinase therefore results in systemic fibrinogenolysis as well as lysis of fibrin clot. As a medication it is used to break down clots in some cases of myocardial infarction (heart attack), pulmonary embolism, and arterial thromboembolism.

An enormous number of platelet receptors, signalling proteins, secreted factors, ligands, plasma factors, endothelial cell and leukocyte factors (including NETs) can all potentially play some part in the haemostatic response, as well as overlapping vascular functions.

Normally in the blood, anticoagulant activity predominates and blood does not coagulate. But, when a vessel is ruptured, the procoagulants activity in the damaged area becomes more and the blood clots.This clotting process is mediated by several blood clotting factors and calcium ions. Vitamin K, a fat soluble vitamin is also necessary for this process. Coumarol poisoning in cattle fed with hay made from sweet clover delays or prevents the blood clotting system of such animals.

Blood present in vessels of the body do not coagulate because of the presence of heparin, an anticoagulant produced from the liver. Heparin is a naturally occurring polysaccharide belonging to the family of glycosaminoglycans (GAG) ubiquitously present in mast cells. Mast cell is a cell filled with basophil granules, found in numbers in connective tissue and releasing histamine and other substances during inflammatory and allergic reactions in addition to Heparin.Heparin is a highly sulfated and polydisperse glycosaminoglycans (GAG) with molecular weights ranging between 5–40 kDa. Heparin exerts its anticoagulant properties indirectly by binding with antithrombin III (AT) and facilitating the subsequent inhibitory effect of AT on thrombin and activated factor X (factor Xa). Heparin released by mast cells and basophils, enhances the antithrombin action. The heparin-antithrombin complex removes other activated factors eg. XIIa, XIa, Xa, IXa . Heparin, the most widely used anticoagulant drug in the world today, remains an animal-derived product.

Phagocytes

The principal function of phagocytes is to defend against invading microorganisms by ingesting and destroying them, thus contributing to cellular inflammatory responses. There are 2 types of phagocytes: mononuclear phagocytes and granulocytes. Mononuclear phagocytes arise primarily from the marrow and are released into the blood as monocytes. They may circulate for hours to a few days before entering the tissues and differentiating to become macrophages. Granulocytes have a segmented nucleus and are classified according to their staining characteristics as neutrophils, eosinophils, or basophils. Neutrophils circulate for only a few hours before travelling to the tissues.

Phagocytosis : Five distinct stages in the process of phagocytosis have been identified: 1) attraction of phagocytes (chemotaxis) to microorganisms, antigen-antibody complexes, and other mediators of inflammation; 2) attachment to the organism; 3) ingestion; 4) fusion of cell lysosomes with ingested microorganisms and bacterial killing; and 5) digestion. In addition, many phagocytes have other specialized functions. Monocytes form a link to the specific immune system by processing antigen for presentation to lymphocytes and by producing substances like interleukin-1, which initiates fever and lymphocyte activation and stimulates early hematopoietic progenitors.

Eosinophils, while having a role as phagocytes, also have more specific functions that include providing a defense against metazoan parasites and modulating the inflammatory process. They respond chemotactically to histamine, immune complexes, and eosinophil chemotactic factor of anaphylaxis, a substance released by degranulating mast cells. Basophils are not true phagocytes but contain large amounts of histamine as well as other mediators of inflammation. Both eosinophilia and basophilia may be seen in response to systemic allergic reactions and invasion of tissues by parasites.

As with the RBC, the production and circulating numbers of phagocytes are tightly regulated and controlled by various humoral factors, including colony-stimulating factors and interleukins. Unlike the RBC, which remain circulating in the blood, the phagocytes use this compartment as a pathway to the tissues. Consequently, the number of phagocytes in the blood reflects circumstances in the tissues (eg, inflammation) as well as the proliferative function of the bone marrow. The sensitivity with which phagocytes reflect these conditions varies from species to species. Abnormal response, such as neutropenia from marrow failure, infections, drugs, or toxins, is likely to result in secondary bacterial infections. Finally, phagocyte precursors may undergo malignant transformation, which results in acute or chronic myelogenous leukemia.

Lymphocytes (White Blood Cells)

Lymphocytes are white blood cells that are also one of the body's main types of immune cells. They are made in the bone marrow and found in the blood and lymph tissue. The immune system is a complex network of cells known as immune cells that include lymphocytes.Lymphocytes are responsible for both humoral and cellular immunity. Cells of the 2 branches of the immune system cannot be differentiated morphologically, but they differ in their dynamics of production and circulation. Lymphocyte production in mammals originates in the bone marrow. Some of the lymphocytes destined to be involved in cellular immunity migrate to thee thymus and differentiate further under the influence of thymic hormones. These become T cells and are responsible for a variety of helper or cytotoxic immunologic functions. Most circulating lymphocytes are T cells, but T cells are also present in the spleen and lymph nodes. The B cells migrate directly to organs without undergoing modification in the thymus and are responsible for humoral immunity (antibody production).

Thus, lymphoid organs have populations of both B and T lymphocytes. In the lymph nodes, follicular centers are primarily B cells, and parafollicular zones are primarily T cells. In the spleen, most of the lymphocytes of the red pulp are B cells, whereas those of the periarteriolar lymphoid sheaths are T cells. Close association of T cells and B cells within lymphoid organs is essential to immune function.

Lymphocyte function in the cellular immune system features both afferent (receptor) and efferent (effector) components. Long-lived T cells of the peripheral blood are the receptors. In response to antigens to which they have been previously sensitized, they leave the circulation and undergo blast transformation to form activated T cells, which in turn cause other T cells to undergo blast transformation, both locally and systemically. Stimulated T cells produce lymphokines with a wide range of activities, such as attraction and activation of neutrophils, macrophages, and lymphocytes.

Lymphocytosis occurs in some species, especially the cat, as a response to epinephrine secretion. Atypical lymphocytes may be seen in the blood in response to antigenic stimulation (eg, vaccination). Persistent lymphocytosis in cattle infected with bovine leukemia virus is a benign polyclonal increase in lymphocyte numbers. Lymphoproliferative malignancies include lymphomas and acute lymphoblastic and chronic lymphocytic leukemias. Lymphopenia may occur most commonly as a response to glucocorticoid secretion.

Clot Retraction : When blood clot is allowed to stand for some time, the clot retracts to a smaller volume and presses out a clear fluid, the blood serum which will not clot any more.

The coagulation takes place most rapidly at body temperature and is generally slowed by cold. Thus if horse blood which always clots slowly is cooled to between 0°C and 1°C, it will remain fluid for an indefinite time. Similarly serum formation during summer is more quick as compared to winter, a common problem encountered by investigators working with serum. The remedy is to allow the clotting to occur at a higher temperature in an incubator.

Clotting time or Coagulation time: When blood is exposed to air, it clots within a short time. Coagulation time is the length of time required for coagulation to set in after the blood has been shed. The coagulation time is a measure of normality of blood. Clotting time is less than 5 min. in most of the domestic animals except cow and horse.

Bleeding time : The bleeding time is the time required for bleeding to stop after puncture of the skin. Bleeding time is a laboratory test to assess platelet function and the body's ability to form a clot. The test involves making a puncture wound in a superficial area of the skin and monitoring the time needed for bleeding to stop (ie, bleeding site turns "glassy"). The blood is blotted away every 30 seconds (ranges from 3- 6 min). Bleeding time is Two to four minutes in dogs. There are several different bleeding times, including the buccal mucosal bleeding time (BMBT), lip bleeding time (a still used test for primary hemostasis in large animals) and the cuticle bleeding time (a crude, outdated test of secondary hemostasis).

Mechanism of Blood Clotting

Blood clotting is essentially a series of enzymatic reactions involving a number of plasma proteins. Under normal conditions, these enzymes are present in the form of inactive precursors. However, when blood comes in contact with a wettable surface such as glass, a series of autocatalytic reactions are initiated.

In mammals, the blood clot consists of a matrix of an insoluble fibrous protein, called fibrin, in which the red blood corpuscles are entangled. Fibrin, is formed from another soluble protein present in blood called fibrinogen. The fibrinogen content of the blood approximates 0.3%. The transformation of fibrinogen to fibrin is catalysed by the enzyme, thrombin. Thrombin, too, is formed from an inactive precursor, prothrombin, present in the blood plasma. Clot is the meshwork of fibrin threads running in all directions to entrap the blood cells, platelets and plasma formed by two mechanisms.

- The intrinsic-In the intrinsic mechanism, injury to the blood alters the factor XII and the platelets of the blood. When the factor XII comes in contact with collagen or a wettable surface, it becomes a proteolytic enzyme called activated XII (XIIa).
- Extrinsic systems-The extrinsic mechanism is fast acting. The cascade reactions of the clotting process involving so many factors helps even a low amount of stimulus (damage) to produce large amounts of final end product (clot).

These are only the final steps in the complex sequence of biochemical events leading to the process of clotting of blood.

Blood pH

Blood pH usually refers to the pH of the blood plasma in an intact animal. The pH range of 7.2-7.3 is compatible with life and under normal circumstances it fluctuates within these narrow limits. Arterial blood is more alkaline than venous blood. The plasma is more alkaline than corpuscles.

A buffer solution is one that resists a change in pH on the addition of acid or alkali. Though large amounts of acids (carbonic, lactic, pyruvic, phosphoric, sulphuric, uric etc) and alkalis are produced as a result of body metabolism, the pH of the blood is maintained within the limits by buffer systems and by eliminating CO_2, ammonia and hydrogen ions through respiratory and renal mechanisms.Hb and HCO- are the important blood buffers. Proteins and organic phosphates provide intracellular buffering.

The **alkali reserve** is carbon dioxide combining capacity of blood. Around 95% of CO_2 unites with the bicarbonate in plasma and the remaining portion with plasma proteins and in physical solution. To maintain the acid base balance in turn the alkali reserve of the body, animals should ingest adequate quantities of electrolytes.

Blood Volume and their Determination

The volume of blood within the vascular system is referred to as blood volume. The blood volume varies with the capacity of the cardiovascular system and with alterations in the constituents of blood.

The total volume of blood is physiologically adjusted to meet the maximum circulatory requirement of the tissues which may arise under varying conditions.

Total blood volume is a measure of oxygen delivery capacity, and it is inherent to the individual. In a normal adult human being, about 5 to 6 litre of blood is present which is about 8 percent of the body weight. In domestic animals generally 5 to 8 percent of the body weight is blood (say 30-40 litre in a cow). Infants have a larger blood volume in proportion to their body weight as blood although there are exceptions. Thus an adult pig may have 4 to 5% of body weight as blood whereas the values may be as high as 10 % in case of thoroughbred horses. Animals that are more excitable and active usually have greater blood volumes. Blood volume varies with the age, weight, sex, breed, and physiological state of the animal. There is an increase in blood volume during pregnancy to assure an adequate blood supply to all the organs of the fetus and mother.

Blood volume helps in understanding and interpreting various hematological values and is important in blood transfusion and to differentiate anemias.

The fluid volume of blood is not changed when the animal drinks a large volume of water. The excess amount of water is got rid of by enhanced urine output. During haemorrhage, a large amount of blood is lost. The blood volume is soon restored to normal values, due to the influx of fluid from the tissues into the blood vessels. At the same time the urine output is also lowered considerably to make good of the losses. Apart from restoring the fluid volume of blood, the loss of erythrocytes is also compensated by their increased rate of production in the spleen and bone marrow. Haemorrhage is also accompanied by reduced cardiac output.

Methods for Determining Blood Volume

It is not feasible to bleed the animal completely to determine blood volume of the body. Indirect methods using dye dilution techniques are used to estimate blood volume. **Evans blue** is the most common inert dye used to estimate blood volume. Isotope methods using radioiodine 125 or 131 labelled human serum albumin methods have also been used in human medicine.

The assessment of blood volume is an important tool in clinical medicine for the evaluation of disorders ranging from polycythemia, anemia, blood loss and endocrine disorders to congestive heart failure and syncope.

1. **Bleeding through the artery:** The blood volume of an animal can be determined by collecting all the blood which flows from a cut artery. Bleeding by this method yields only a part of the total blood in the body. The blood remains in the tissues can be washed out by perfusing Locke's solution through the vessels. Although the fluid that emerges is blood diluted by lockers solution, the true

blood volume can be calculated by comparing the haemoglobin concentration of the animals undiluted blood with that diluted by the Locke's solution.

2. **Dilution method:** In this method a known volume of a nontoxic azo dye Evans blue is injected into the circulation. After mixing has occurred the extent of its dilution in the circulating plasma is found by measuring the concentration of the dye in the plasma. In order to calculate the blood volume, the calculated plasma volume is added to the calculated value of blood cells from haematocrit.

Blood Volume = Plasma volume + (Plasma volume × hematocrit/100)

Sometimes labelled serum albumin has been used instead of dye, as the dye tends to leave the circulation within a few minutes of injection.

Osmotic Fragility

The osmotic fragility test (OFT) is used to measure erythrocyte resistance to hemolysis while being exposed to varying levels of dilution of a saline solution. When erythrocytes are exposed to a hypotonic environment, water enters the cell and causes swelling and eventual lysis. The normal range for osmotic fragility of red blood cells had been estimated to include 5%--45% haemolysis at a salt concentration corresponding to 4.5 g NaCl/l.

This test is generally prescribed to diagnose hereditary spherocytosis and thalassemia. Hemolytic anemia due to iron deficiency may also show decreased osmotic fragility.

Erythrocyte Sedimentation Rate (ESR)

When the blood after the addition of a suitable anticoagulant is allowed to stand, the erythrocytes progressively settles at a certain rate to the bottom leaving clear plasma above, which is known as erythrocyte sedimentation rate. It is usually measured within one hour of collection of blood in standard tubes placed in vertical position by the distance in millimetres through which the upper most layer of erythrocytes pass in a given time. Plasma proteins (fibrinogen and/or globulin) may influence the degree of coagulation of erythrocytes which may be an important factor influencing ESR. The viscosity of plasma, specific gravity of the corpuscles or plasma or the size of erythrocytes had nothing to do with sedimentation rate.

Erythrocyte sedimentation rate helps to evaluate the health status of the animal. It is increased due to anemias, acute general infections, malignant tumours, inflammatory conditions, hypothyroidism, pregnancy etc. The sedimentation rate is much higher in horses whereas the erythrocytes of ruminants settle very slowly. The ESR of horse blood is also higher than in canine blood.

Haematocrit

Haematocrit is also called Packed Cell Volume (PCV). The haematocrit of blood is the percentage of cells in the blood. Thus if we say that an animal has an haematocrit of 40% it means that 40 percent of the blood volume is cells and the remainder is plasma. The haematocrit varies greatly with anaemia, degree of bodily activity and on the altitude of the place. More haematocrit means greater viscosity and hence greater force is required to pump the blood through the vessels.

The haematocrit or Packed Cell Volume is the ratio of red cell volume to whole blood volume and is expressed as a percentage. Normally it means the percent volume of packed blood cells present in whole blood after centrifugation at 3000 rpm for 30 minutes. The white blood cell and platelet fractions are usually ignored because they comprise a relatively small volume compared with the red cells and plasma. The term PCV is preferred over haematocrit to express packed cell volume.

Wintrobe Method : PCV is obtained by centrifuging blood sample containing suitable anticoagulant in graduated Wintrobe haematocrit tube using haematocrit centrifuge at 3000 rpm for 30 minutes (a layer of packed leukocytes is formed just above the packed erythrocytes). Wintrobe tubes have uniform 3 mm bore, calibrated by 10 cm scales with millimetre divisions. The wintrobe pipette with a long but narrow delivery tube is used to fill about 1 ml of blood into the wintrobe tube without air bubbles. Horse and dog blood require a relative centrifugal force of 2,260 G (generally 3000 rpm) for 30 minutes, while it is for 60 minutes in the case of cattle and pig blood. The blood of sheep and goat require higher relative centrifugal force than 2,260 G.

Micro-haematocrit method: Usage of micro-haematocrit technique where the heparinized blood samples are centrifuged at high speed for 3 to 5 minutes facilitates the determination of large number of samples in a short time, requiring very small amount of blood (one drop). PCV values in most domestic animals vary between 22 to 45%.

High temperature, muscular exercise, stress, pregnancy, hemorrhage, dehydration and burns, anemia, polycythemia and leukemia are some of the factors which affect PCV in domestic animals.

Hemolysis (Destruction of RBC)

Erythrocytes are the red blood cells, and they make up about 50% of blood volume, and 3 million cells are continuously produced per second from stem cells located in the bone marrow.Hemolysis refers to the destruction of RBCs.

Normal red blood cells (erythrocytes) have a lifespan of about 120 days. After they die they break down and are removed from the circulation by the spleen.

Hemolysis can occur due to different causes and leads to the release of hemoglobin into the bloodstream.

Hemolytic anemia is the term used to refer to anemia caused by the excess destruction of red blood cells.

Immune-mediated destruction of RBC is the most common cause in dogs, although infections, tumors, and other causes also occur.

Hemorrhagic Diseases

Haemophilia is a mostly inherited genetic disorder that impairs the body's ability to make blood clots. In such conditions, the coagulation time is unusually long with the result that a minor wound or cut will result in excessive loss of blood. Such a condition is transmitted from parents to offspring as a sex linked recessive character. This disease is found in several domestic animals and man.

The clotting mechanism works as a biochemical amplifier in a series of enzymatic steps, in which the enzymes formed in the first step serve as a catalyst or activator for the next step or so on. The enzymatic amplification allows clotting to take place rapidly, yet provides a considerable safety margin to prevent spontaneous coagulation within the vascular system.

Severe blood loss leads to a decrease in blood pressure and thus reduces the flow of blood to the damaged area. Damaged blood vessels constrict and thereby decrease blood flow.

During the winter of 1921, a new disease among cattle was reported in Canada and north-central United States, in which a cow might merely scratch herself on a barbed wire fence and bleed to death. The faulty clotting mechanism was related to the fact that the cattle had been eating mouldy sweet clover hay. It became known as sweet clover hay disease. Link and Campbell at the University of Wisconsin were able to extract the substance dicoumarol from mouldy hay. Later it was found that Dicoumarol acts on the liver, inhibiting the formation of prothrombin, so that within a few days the blood fails to clot. Now a days, after this discovery dicoumarol found extensive use as an anticoagulant.

Healing Process

Classification of Leucocytes

Leucocytes

Leucocyte- phagocytic and Immunogenic Functions

The white cells of blood, although normally fewer in number, are concerned with the body's response to injury and infection. Leucocytes or white blood corpuscles have phagocytic and immunogenic functions. White blood cells (WBCs) are cells of the immune system that defend the body against infectious disease and foreign material. Leucocytes are colorless blood corpuscles capable of amoeboid movement. The name "white blood cell" derives from the physical appearance of a blood sample after centrifugation. White cells are found in the buffy coat, a thin, typically white layer of nucleated cells between the sedimented red blood cells and the blood plasma. The scientific term leukocyte directly reflects its description. It is derived from the Greek roots leuk- meaning "white" and cyt- meaning "cell". Their chief function is to protect the body against microorganisms causing disease. The number leucocytes varies under different pathological conditions, physiological stages for example most bacterial infections are associated with income number of leucocyte (leukocytoines), whereas decrease in number of leucocytes (leukopeneta) is commonly seen in viral infections. The number of leucocytes was found to increase in swamp buffalo from 8.82 × 10^9/l a short time after parturition to 16.76 × 10^9/l at the age of six months. The number of WBC is less than the number of erythrocytes.

TLC- (Total leucocyte count): Normal TLC in an adult person is 6000-8000WBC/ mm^3 of blood.

DLC- (Differential leucocyte count): Number/ (%) of different type of leucocyte in per cubic mm. of blood.

Leucocytes in blood are classified into granulocytes, (Neutrophils, Eosinophils & Basophils) characterized by specific granules in their cytoplasm and agranulocytes (lymphocytes and monocytes). The granulocytes are further divided into neutrophils, eosinophils and basophils as per their staining reaction.

Granulocytes

Neutrophils

Formed from extravascular neutrophilic myeloblasts in bone marrow and enter blood circulation by amoeboid action and diapedesis. They are phagocytic, engulfing bacteria and small foreign bodies and appear in large numbers at the site of inflammation. They possess abundant fine granules in cytoplasm and are stained by neutral dyes. The nucleus of mature cells is divided into lobes or segments connected by filaments and is called as segmented cell. The nucleus of immature or young cells appear as curved or coiled band, rod like or deeply indented without segmentation and is called as band cell.

Eosinophils

Formed from eosinophilic myelocytes of bone marrow which are highly motile and phagocytic and occurs in small numbers in blood. Eosinophils in blood occur in more numbers during allergy, anaphylactic shock and parasitism. Eosinopenia is caused by ACTH and adrenaline administration. Eosinophils are large in size with less lobulated nuclei and large sized cytoplasmic granules which stain with acid dyes.

Basophils

Formed from basophilic myeloblasts of bone marrow occurring in small numbers in normal blood with slight phagocytic power. The cytoplasmic granules are water soluble and stain with alkaline dyes. The percentage of basophils in blood is very small e.g. around 1% in camels.

Agranulocytes

Lymphocytes

These cells originated from lymphoid tissue e.g. lymph nodes, spleen, tonsils, thymus etc. and found numerous in number in the blood of most of the domestic animals. They are highly motile and amoeboid in activity without phagocytosis. They produce antibodies by possessing gamma globulins. Administration of ACTH results in increased antibody production in blood through dissolution of lymphocytes and thus causing lymphopenia.

Monocytes

These cells formed from reticuloendothelial cells of the spleen and bone marrow occurring to a limited extent in blood which are motile and phagocytic. Possess large single nucleus and abundant and faintly granular cytoplasm.

The circulating blood transports leucocytes to the site of action where they function extravascularly and how long they live in these tissues (life span) is difficult to find out. The total leucocyte count is influenced by time of the day, meal, exercise, exo or endogenous adrenaline, anaesthesia and other stress conditions. The total count is made with the help of counting chambers of haemocytometer. Differential leucocyte count is expressed as either actual number per cu mm of blood or as percentage of total leucocyte count.

Macrophages- The Phagocytic Cells

Macrophages are phagocytic cells that engulf pathogens and cellular debris and play a major role in the innate immune response. Pathogens are taken up into specialized intracellular vesicles called phagosomes, where they are destroyed. Macrophages can also present antigens to lymphocytes. These cells are distributed widely in many different organs and tissues where they may further differentiate and acquire specialized functions. WBC upon infection by virus or bacteria respond by releasing large amounts of proinflammatory cytokines. If leukocytes are considered police officers, proinflammatory cytokines will be the bullets used to stop the perpetrator virus.

All white blood cells are produced and derived from multipotent cells in the bone marrow known as hematopoietic stem cells.

Natural killer cells (also known as NK cells, K cells, and killer cells) are a type of lymphocyte (a white blood cell) and a component of the innate immune system.

Natural Killer Cells

NK cells play a major role in the host-rejection of both tumours and virally infected cells.

These cells are cytotoxic and contain small granules in their cytoplasm with special proteins such as perforin and proteases known as granzymes.

When NK cells come in close contact with target cells, perforin forms pores in the cell membrane of the target cell through which the granzymes and associated molecules enter, inducing apoptosis or death of the cell.

NK cells are activated in response to interferons or macrophage-derived cytokines and control viral infections.

Immunity

Immunity is the ability of the body to resist the tissue damage by destroying the disease organisms or neutralising their toxins. Immune system is an elaborate defence system which combats the invading bacteria and virus which continuously attempts to make their way into the animal body. An animal that is immune to a pathogenic organism will not be affected by it.

The immune system attacks everything it considers foreign to the body. The immune system has the following functions.

1. To protect the body against pathogenic organisms.
2. To remove injured or dead cells and tissue
3. Attack and remove cancer cells.

Types of Immunity

Innate Immunity

- This type of immunity is present from birth. This type of immunity is non specific and acts on many organisms. It prevents first entry of microorganisms into the tissues or if the organisms has gained entry, eliminates them prior to the occurrence of the disease.
- This type of immunity is not effective on subsequent exposure to the same organisms. Non specific elimination of microorganisms is done by two methods:

  Phagocytosis: It is ingestion and killing of microorganisms by specialised cells such as neutrophils, monocytes, macrophages etc.

  Opsonisation: It is the process of coating the microorganisms with some of the proteins found in the plasma to make them more phagocytosable.
- Active immunity involves both the cell-mediated and humoral immunity as well as the innate immune system.
- Active immunity is induced in the host itself by the antigen, and lasts for a longer period of time.

Acquired Immunity

- The development of immunity against specific organisms, the bacteria, virus and foreign tissues or toxins is referred to as acquired immunity.
- This type of immunity is also known as adaptive or specific immunity. It is caused by a special immune system that forms antibodies or activated lymphocytes that attack and destroy the microorganisms.

Humoral Immunity or B Cell Immunity

Cell mediated Immunity or T Cell Immunity

In mammals, shortly before or after birth the stem cells or the committed lymphoid progenitor cells migrate either to thymus, liver and bone marrow (in mammals) or to bursa of Fabricius (in birds) where they are processed and differentiated.

The `T' lymphocytes are processed in the thymus and `B' lymphocytes are processed in bursa, liver and bone marrow. These lymphocytes then get into the circulation and localise in spleen and lymph nodes as clones of `T', and `B' lymphocytes.

Thymus plays a key role in the development of cellular immunity shortly before birth or few months after birth. The T-lymphocytes provide cellular immunity, and the B-lymphocytes provide humoral immunity, by producing specific antibodies. There are different types of B and T cells, each of which responds specifically to one particular antigen. All the different B and T cells capable of forming a specific antibody or activated T cells against a specific antigen which are called "clone of lymphocytes".

The invading organisms provide proteins, large polysaccharides and large lipoprotein complexes, which function as an antigen. The antigen stimulates a specific clone of lymphocytes.

Macrophages in lymphoid tissues stimulated by antigen releases interleukin I, and it promotes growth of specific lymphocytes. The helper T cells release interleukin II, which stimulate B cells to produce specific antibodies. Those B-lymphocytes specific for an antigen enlarge and form lymphoblasts, which differentiates to plasmablast and finally to plasma cells. The plasma cells produce antibodies very rapidly.

When these sensitised plasma cells are activated by an antigen, specific antibodies, the gamma globulins- IgG (75%), IgM, IgA, IgD and IgE (during allergy) are produced by them as primary response. However these antibodies have weak potency and short life.

Some of the lymphoblasts remain dormant and function as memory T and B cells, which on subsequent stimulation by the same antigen (booster) produce a more potent secondary response. On exposure to a specific antigen, the T cells of the specific clone proliferate and release large numbers of activated T cells, which neutralises the antigen. The memory T cells are retained in the lymphoid tissues.

Humoral immunity is developed as specific antibody (gamma globulin) by the "B"-lymphocytes, rarely persists for more than few months or utmost few years. On the other hand, the specific clones of "T" lymphocytes on stimulation by the very same antigens are converted into three major groups of "T" lymphocytes.

- Cytotoxic or killer "T" cells: These are the direct attack cells killing the micro-organisms. They have the lysosomal enzymes, the peroxidases, phosphatases and oxygenases and produce H_2O_2, which is lethal to the invading organisms.
- Helper `T' cells: These cells are very sensitive even to very small quantities of the specific antigen, release interleukin-2 (lymphokines), and activate the other two types of "T" cells, the cytotoxic and suppressor "T" cells and also the "B" lymphocytes. Helper "T" cells are not capable of secreting antibodies by themselves. It promotes the production of lymphokines.
- Lymphokines act as a macrophage migration inhibition factor, stop the chemotactically attracted macrophages and neutrophils in the infected area to effect more efficient phagocytosis, and thus limit the spread of the infection.
- Suppressor or regulatory "T" cells: Regulate the activities of both the helper and killer "T" cells. The activated "T" lymphocytes provide the cell-mediated immunity, which is far more persistent for many years than humoral immunity.

Naturally Acquired Active Immunity

Naturally acquired active immunity occurs when an individual is exposed to live pathogens, and develops antibodies against specific pathogens which leads to immunological memory.In some cases, the immunity may be life-long as in the case of smallpox, measles, chicken pox, yellow fever etc. while in some others the immunity may be lost after only a few years (e.g., diphtheria, tetanus) or even for lesser period (e.g., influenza, pneumonia).

Artificially Acquired Active Immunity

Artificially Acquired Active Immunity occurs when an antigen is intentionally introduced into a body to be immunized, the latter develops immunity .e.g., vaccine, toxoids.This immunity is artificial because the antigens are intentionally or purposely introduced, and it is active because the recipient's immune system synthesizes antibodies in response.**Vaccines** provide usually long-term immunity. Killed and attenuated strains of bacteria and viruses are widely used forms of immunization against many diseases

Passive Immunity

Passive immunity is the transfer of active immunity, in the form of readymade antibodies, from one individual to another. Passive immunity provides immediate protection to the individual, but the duration of passive immunization is relatively short, a few days to several weeks when compared to years for active immunity. This is due to the natural degradation of injected antibody from the circulation without internal replacement.Passive immunity can occur naturally, when maternal antibodies are transferred to the fetus through the placenta, and can also be induced artificially, when high levels of human (or horse) antibodies specific for a pathogen or toxin are transferred to non- immune individuals.

Platelets (Thrombocyte)

Platelets are colourless small round or rod shaped bodies in circulating blood in most domestic animals (3 μ in diameter) and are oval and nucleated in chicken (3-5 μ in width and 7-10 μ in length).

Platelets are formed in liver, spleen and bone marrow during prenatal life and in bone marrow in adults (pluripotent stem cells –to- megakaryoblast develops into thrombocyte or platelet via promegakaryocyte and megakaryocyte) under the influence of thrombopoietin. Bone marrow is the spongy center inside bones.

Bone marrow is the spongy tissue inside bones, such as your hip and thigh bones. It contains stem cells. The stem cells can develop into the red blood cells that carry oxygen through your body, the white blood cells that fight infections, and the platelets that help with blood clotting.

Platelets vary in number from species to species between venous and arterial blood and young and adults.

Normal platelet count in human beings is 2,50,000 (1,50,000 to 4,50,000) /cu mm of blood. A low platelet count may also be called thrombocytopenia. This condition can range from mild to severe, depending on its underlying cause.

Their life span is very short (8-11 days in circulating blood).

Their principal role is to prevent haemorrhage when blood vessels are injured in addition to numerous functions they perform in the animal body.

Platelets form the initial hemostatic plug whenever hemorrhage occurs. They provide platelet phospholipid for coagulation and carry several clotting factors on their surface.

Platelets form the initial hemostatic plug whenever hemorrhage occurs. They also are the source of phospholipid, which is needed for the interaction of coagulation factors to form a fibrin clot. Platelets are produced in the bone marrow from megakaryocytes, under the in fluence of thrombopoietin. Platelet production begins with invagination of the megakaryocyte cell membrane and the formation of cytoplasmic channels and islands. The cytoplasmic islands produce platelets by fragmentation from the megakaryocyte.

Platelet disorders are either quantitative (thrombocytopenia or thrombocytosis) or qualitative (thrombocytopathy). Thrombocytopenia is one of the most common bleeding disorders of animals. In general, platelet counts must fall to < 30,000/ µL before the risk of hemorrhage increases. Consumption, destruction, or sequestration of platelets causes thrombocytopenia associated with increased production by the bone marrow. Consumptive thrombocytopenia occurs with massive hemorrhage or with disseminated intravascular coagulation, secondary to a variety of diseases. Destruction occurs in immune-mediated thrombocytopenia, in which platelets become coated with antiplatelet antibodies and are removed from the circulation by the fixed phagocyte system. Excessive sequestration of platelets by an enlarged spleen (hypersplenism) may occur in conditions such as myeloproliferative diseases.

Thrombocytopathies comprise a poorly defined group of diseases in which platelet numbers are normal, but their function is impaired. Von Willebrand disease is characterized primarily by a defect in platelet adhesion to the endothelium. The platelets themselves are normal. Other hereditary disorders of platelet function have been described but are relatively rare. Probably the most common platelet function defect is the irreversible inhibition of thromboxane (which is necessary for platelet aggregation) caused by aspirin administration. When the cause of the reduction in platelet number is not known, the disorder is known as idiopathic thrombocytopenic purpura (ITP).

Summary

- Blood is a body fluid in animals and human beings that delivers necessary substances such as nutrients and oxygen to the cells and transports metabolic waste products away from those same cells.
- Homeostatic mechanisms keep substances in the blood at relatively constant levels.

- Haemostasis refers to the spontaneous arrest or prevention of bleeding from the injured/damaged vessels by the physiological process.
- Immunity refers to resistance of the body to pathogens and their toxic products.
- Anemia means a deficiency of red blood cells, which can be caused by either too rapid loss of blood or by too slow production of red blood cells or deficiency of haemoglobin in the red cells.
- Anemias may be classified according to number and size of cells and the haemoglobin content.
- Anticoagulants are chemical substances which delay or prevent the process of blood coagulation, prolonging the clotting time.
- The haematocrit or Packed Cell Volume is the ratio of red cell volume to whole blood volume and is expressed as a percentage. The haematocrit varies greatly with anaemia, degree of bodily activity and on the altitude of the place. More haematocrit means greater viscosity and hence greater force is required to pump the blood through the vessels.
- Haemophilia is a mostly inherited genetic disorder that impairs the body's ability to make blood clots. In such conditions, the coagulation time is unusually long with the result that a minor wound or cut will result in excessive loss of blood.

3

Heart

The circulatory system includes the heart, blood and lymph vessels, blood, lymph, cerebrospinal and tissue fluids.

The heart is a muscular structure that contracts in a rhythmic pattern to pump blood. The heart functions as a pump to provide a continuous circulation of blood throughout the body.The blood vessels that take blood from the heart to the various tissues are called arteries.Arterioles open into a network of capillaries which constitute the microcirculation. Circulation of blood in the body is important for the transport of nutrients to all parts of the body and for the transport of gases and waste products. The primary function of the heart is to transfer sufficient blood from the venous system to the arterial side of the circulation under sufficient pressure to maintain the circulatory needs of the body

Another important function of the cardiovascular system is regulation of body temperature. In the heat, blood vessels close to the surface of the skin enlarge. This process is called vasodilation. This allows more heat to be lost from the blood. In the cold, blood vessels at the skin's surface constrict. This process is called vasoconstriction and takes blood away from the surface of the skin to help prevent it from losing heat. When a person takes part in exercise their face can become pink due to vasodilation of the blood vessels close to the skin's surface.

In fact most of the functions of blood could not have been possible, if there were no circulation of blood. Thus the primary functions of the cardiovascular system is the distribution of nutrients and oxygen to all body cells and collection of waste products and carbon dioxide from different body cells , and to carry them to excretory organs for excretion. The secondary functions of cardiovascular system include thermoregulation, distribution of hormones to the target tissues and delivery of antibodies, platelets and leucocytes to aid body defence mechanism.

Heart- Morphological Characteristic

In order to constantly circulate the blood to all parts of the body and back, the body needs the services of an efficient pump. The pump or heart is based on the ability of muscle to contract or shorten. The blood is carried in a system of elastic tubes or pipes (arteries, capillaries and veins). The circulation of blood in the domestic animals or mammals is referred to as closed circulation because the blood returns to the heart without leaving this system of tubes.

The size of heart is a determinant of maximum heart capacity such as stroke volume or cardiac output and performance. In horses, heart mass approximates 0.9-1.0 % of body mass.Racing horses have larger hearts as compared to non racing horses.

The heart is a muscular organ covered by a double membrane called pericardium. Pericardium consists of two layers: outer fibrous and inner serous The pericardial fluid of the pericardium lubricates the heart to facilitate movement of the heart.

The heart is a two-sided, four-chambered structure with muscular walls, which act as two separate pump systems.The heart is divided into four chambers — two upper atria and two lower ventricles. The inter-atrial septum separates the two atria and the inter-ventricular septum separates the two ventricles. The atrium and the ventricle of each side are separated by the atrioventricular septum. Superior and inferior vena cavae open into the right atrium. The right ventricle opens into the pulmonary artery. Four pulmonary veins open into the left atrium.The left ventricle opens into the aorta. The opening between the right atrium and right ventricle is guarded by the tricuspid valve. The opening between the left atrium and left ventricle is guarded by the bicuspid (mitral) valve. The opening of the right ventricle into the pulmonary artery and the opening of the left ventricle into the aorta is guarded by the semilunar valves.

Oxygen-poor and carbon dioxide-rich blood flows into the right atrium from the body and is contained there momentarily until the opening of the tricuspid valve, which allows it to travel into the right ventricle. The right atrium receives blood from the upper and lower body through the superior vena cava and the inferior vena cava, respectively, and from the heart muscle itself through the coronary sinus. The right atrium is the larger of the two atria, having very thin walls. The right atrium opens into the right ventricle through the right atrioventricular valve(tricuspid), which only allows the blood to flow from the atria into the ventricle, but not in the reverse direction.

The right ventricle pumps the blood to the lungs to be reoxygenated. The left atrium receives blood from the lungs via the four pulmonary veins. It is smaller than the right atrium but has thicker walls. The valve between the left atrium and the left ventricle, the left atrioventricular valve(bicuspid), is smaller than the tricuspid. It opens into the left ventricle and again is a one-way valve. During systole, the second part of the cardiac cycle, the heart muscles contract. The atrium contracts first, producing an additional blood flow from the right atrium to the right ventricle. Once the right ventricle fills completely the ventricle contracts allowing for a rush of blood up through the pulmonary valve and into the pulmonary artery where the blood will be transported to the lungs in order to allow the carbon dioxide to exit the blood and allow for an intake of oxygen. The structure of the heart with its valves allows for the heart to work while preventing backflow into the chambers due to low pressure drops when certain chambers are empty or filled.

The left ventricle pumps the blood throughout the body through the dorsal aorta, which is the largest artery in the body. The walls of the left ventricle are the thickest among all the chambers.

The myocardium (muscular tissue of the heart) is the main tissue constituting the walls of the heart. It consists of three types of muscle fibres:

- Cardiac muscles forming the walls of the atria and ventricles.
- Muscle fibres forming the pacemaker, which is the site of origin of cardiac impulse.
- Muscle fibres forming the conducting system which transmits the impulse to the various parts of the heart.

Microcirculation and Lymphatic System

Arterioles divide 2-5 times and form capillaries.

Internal diameter of Arterioles is 10-15 μm and Capillaries is 5-9 μm. Metarterioles are the terminal arterioles. Thickness of the capillary wall is about 0.5 μm. Fluid filtration across capillaries is determined by hydrostatic and colloid osmotic pressure and capillary filtration coefficient.

Measurement of Capillary Hydrostatic Pressure

- Direct by micropipette method
- Indirect by iso gravimetric method

Note: Functional capillary pressure is always lower than capillary pressure measured by micropipette method.

Systemic Excitability Conduction & Transmission Processes

The heart has an inherent capacity to contract rhythmically without any stimulus. Even if the heart is completely removed from the body, it may continue to beat for a considerable time.

The sinus node, where the heart contraction originates is also known as the pacemaker of the heart. It starts the beat and sets the rate by its inherent rhythmicity. Two different mechanisms are involved in the control or the rate;

1. Nerve impulses to the pacemaker
2. Hormonal influences.

A branch of the vagus nerve, when stimulated slows the rate of heart beat. The nerve is of parasympathetic origin and acts by release of acetylcholine. Another nerve, the accelerans nerve is of sympathetic origin.When it is stimulated the heart accelerates because noradrenaline is released from the nerve endings of the pacemaker.

The volume of blood ejected in a single beat is known as stroke volume. Two major factors influence the stroke volume. One is the hormone adrenaline, which augments the force of the cardiac muscle contraction, thereby forcing a larger amount of blood out of the heart in a single stroke. The other is the amount of blood in the ventricles when contraction begins. The latter results from an inherent characteristic of heart muscle, which will contract with greater force if it is more distended at the moment contraction begins.

Atrioventricular conduction is dependent on distinct types of myocardial tissue and includes atrial inputs into the AV node, the various components of the AV node, and the His–Purkinje conduction system. The electrical conduction system of the heart transmits signals generated usually by the sinoatrial node to cause contraction of the heart muscle. The pacemaking signal generated in the sinoatrial node travels through the right atrium to the atrioventricular node, along the Bundle of His and through bundle branches to cause contraction of the heart muscle. This signal stimulates contraction first of the right and left atrium, and then the right and left ventricles. This process allows blood to be pumped throughout the body.

Heart; conduction system. 1. SA node. 2. AV node. 3. Bundle of His. 8. Septum

The conduction system consists of specialised heart muscle cells, and is situated within the myocardium. There is a skeleton of fibrous tissue that surrounds the conduction system.

Electrical signals arising in the SA node (located in the right atrium) stimulate the atria to contract. Then the signals travel to the atrioventricular node (AV node), which is located in the interatrial septum. After a delay, the electrical signal diverges and is conducted through the left and right bundle of His to the respective Purkinje fibers for each side of the heart, as well as to the endocardium at the apex of the heart, then finally to the ventricular epicardium; causing its contraction. These signals are generated rhythmically, which in turn results in the coordinated rhythmic contraction and relaxation of the heart.

Heart myocardial cells have a negative membrane potential when at rest. Stimulation above a threshold value induces the opening of voltage-gated ion channels and a flood of cations into the cell. The positively charged ions entering the cell cause the depolarization characteristic of an action potential. Like skeletal muscle, depolarization causes the opening of voltage-gated calcium channels and release of Ca2+ from the t-tubules. This influx of calcium causes calcium-induced calcium release from the sarcoplasmic reticulum, and free Ca^{2+} causes muscle contraction. After a delay, potassium channels reopen, and the resulting flow of K+ out of the cell causes repolarization to the resting state.

Cardiac Cycle:-Regulation of cardiac output

One complete series of events during heart activity constitutes one cardiac cycle. Since electrical activity precedes all other events in a cycle, the beginning of a cycle is taken as the generation of an impulse by the SA (Sino-atrial node) node. The events of a single cycle give information as to the electrical and mechanical events that occur as the heart beats.

The cardiac cycle can be described in terms of electrical disturbances which may be recorded as an **electrocardiogram**. The contraction of the heart chambers produces pressure and volume changes that cause the blood to flow. The working of the heart is accompanied by sounds known as heart sounds.

A single cycle of cardiac activity can be divided into two basic phases - **diastole** and **systole**.

Diastole represents the period of time when the ventricles are relaxed (not contracting). Throughout most of this period, blood is passively flowing from the left atrium (LA)

and right atrium (RA) into the left ventricle (LV) and right ventricle (RV), respectively (see figure at right). The blood flows through atrioventricular valves (mitral and tricuspid) that separate the atria from the ventricles. The RA receives venous blood from the body through the superior vena cava (SVC) and inferior vena cava (IVC). The LA receives oxygenated blood from lungs through four pulmonary veins that enter the LA. At the end of the diastole, both atria contract, which propels an additional amount of blood into the ventricles.

Systole represents the time during which the left and right ventricles contract and eject blood into the aorta and pulmonary artery, respectively. During systole, the aortic and pulmonic valves open to permit ejection into the aorta and pulmonary artery. The atrioventricular valves are closed during systole, therefore no blood is entering the ventricles; however, blood continues to enter the atria through the vena cavae and pulmonary veins.

Timing of the Cycle

Rate of heart beat varies with different species and also with age and other factors.

Cardiovascular Dynamics

The flow of blood through the cardiovascular system is governed by three factors.

1. Dynamics of the pumping action of the heart.
2. Characteristics of blood as a fluid.
3. Characteristics of the blood vessels through which the blood flows.

Aortic pressure is measured by inserting a pressure-measuring catheter into the aorta from a peripheral artery, and the left ventricular pressure is obtained by placing a catheter inside the left ventricle and measuring changes in intraventricular pressure as the heart beats. Left atrial pressure is not usually measured directly, except in investigational procedures; however, left atrial pressure can be estimated by recording the pulmonary capillary wedge pressure. Ventricular volume changes can be assessed in real time using echocardiography or radionuclide imaging, or by using a special volume conductance catheter placed within the ventricle.

Heart Sounds

Four heart sounds are produced during each cardiac cycle. The first and second heart sounds are more prominent and resemble the spoken words 'LUBB' and 'DUBB' respectively. These two heart sounds can be heard by using a **stethoscope**. The third heart sound is milk sound and the fourth heart sound is inaudible. The first heart sound coincides with the peak of "R"wave in ECG. The fourth heart sound coincides with the interval between the end of "P" wave and the onset of "Q"wave. In myocardial infarction the heart sound produced is like the sound produced during the galloping of the horse. So it is called "**galloping rhythm**".

The study of heart sounds has important diagnostic value in clinical practice because the heart sounds are altered during the cardiac diseases involving the valves of the heart.

Cardiac Output

Cardiac output is defined as the volume of blood ejected from the right or left ventricle and is usually expressed per minute. The volume of blood pumped by the left ventricle into the aorta per unit time is usually called the cardiac output or the cardiac minute volume. Cardiac output is an important indicator of muscle oxygen delivery capacity.

The determination of the cardiac output gives a direct indication of the ability of the heart to maintain the circulation. The cardiac output is increased during work or exercise. Cardiac output is the most important factor in the cardiovascular system because the rate of blood flow through different parts of the body depends upon the cardiac output.

Cardiac output (CO) is part of the measurement of cardiac performance and is the blood volume per minute supplied to the tissues. Cardiac output is the product of two factors; the rate of heart beat (Stroke Rate or SR) and the volume of blood ejected per beat (Stroke Volume or SV).

Cardiac output = Stroke rate (Beats/min) × Stroke volume (ml blood/beat)

A normal adult human being has a resting heart rate of 70-80 beat/min and a stroke volume of 60-70 ml of blood per beat. Thus a resting cardiac output may be calculated as lying between 4200-5600 ml of blood per minute. Normal Cardiac output range in the healthy human adult is about 4–6.5l/min.

Cardiac output of ox is about 34800 ml, Horse, 29000ml, Sheep 4000ml dog 1450ml, Buffalo calf (wt 100kg)-14300ml/min. The cardiac output is increased during exercise. Thoroughbred horses can have cardiac output values in excess of 350- litre per minute.

Regulation of Cardiac Output

The cardiac output varies with the physiological state of the animal. It increases tremendously with the increased excitement of the animal. The other factors which affect cardiac output is the volume of blood returned to the right atrium from the tissues. This is called **venous return**. During exercise, the volume of blood returned to the right atrium through the veins is increased by the massaging action of the active skeletal muscles. The right atrium and then the right ventricle are filled to a greater degree and as a result are stretched to a greater degree than normal. This involves the law of the heart and the contractions become stronger, ejecting more and more blood per beat; in short, stroke volume increases. More blood through the lungs increases venous return to the left atrium and ventricle and left ventricular output into the aorta is increased. Thus after a few beats, right heart inflow and left heart output are balanced. This mechanism is an example of auto regulation by the heart that is adjustment without the involvement of outside factors.

The other factor which affects cardiac output is peripheral resistance. The small arteries (arterioles) of the body have large amounts of circularly disposed smooth muscle around them. The vessels can thus change their diameter to a greater degree to their total diameter than any other vessel. A decrease in diameter (vasoconstriction) and an increase in diameter (vasodilation) increase and decrease peripheral resistance, respectively. Increased resistance calls for a greater pressure to maintain adequate flow through narrowed channels. The ventricles increase their strength of contraction, emptying the chamber more completely and thus raising the stroke volume, cardiac output and arterial blood pressure.

Temperature and Chemicals

Several chemicals like epinephrine liberated in response to exercise or stress on the body affect the cardiac output. Epinephrine acts by enhancing the SA node activity and also increasing the contractile strength.Moderate change in temperature does not affect cardiac output. Increase in temperature above 30ºC raises cardiac output.

Nervous Stimulation

Vagal stimulation results in a decreased rate of heart beat primarily due to the liberation of acetylcholine at the vagal termination. Nervous reflexes provide a continuous and critical control primarily over the stroke rate.

The maximum amount of blood that can be pumped by the heart above normal value is called cardiac reserve. Cardiac output is increased during exercise and this is made possible due to cardiac reserve.

Measurement of Cardiac Output

It is difficult to measure cardiac output accurately since heart action is influenced by many factors. There are many methods, invasive and non-invasive, for measuring cardiac output, such as lithium dilution, thermodilution, thoracic electrical impedance, pulse analysis, and Doppler echocardiography. Two of the common methods employed to measure cardiac output are the Fick and Dilution methods.

Fick Method: The Fick method compares the oxygen artery blood and knowing its rate of oxygen absorbed or carbon dioxide eliminated per minute by the lungs, we can calculate cardiac output by the following equation.

Cardiac out put (Litre blood/ min) = O_2 absorbed or CO_2 eliminated (ml/min)/AVO_2 or CO_2 difference (ml/L)

The Fick method is applicable to any organ that exhibits AV O_2 difference and is amenable to sampling of arterial and venous blood; it may be used to calculate blood flow through organs.

Dilution method : Injection of a known amount of material into the circulation is followed by measurement of the dilution of the material during a known period of time. A curve is obtained, the area of which may be calculated and related to cardiac output since the rapidity of dilution of the material, and thus the slope and height of the curve depends on the volume of blood flowing in a measured time span.

Doppler echocardiography is a non-invasive method that measures blood velocity in targeted areas of the heart and great vessels. If the average velocity is multiplied by the cross-sectional area of the vessel and heart rate, an estimate of cardiac output is obtained

Extrinsic and Intrinsic Regulation

Intrinsic regulation results from normal functional characteristics, not on neural or hormonal regulation –Frank-Starling's law of the heart. The Frank–Starling law of the heart represents the relationship between stroke volume and end diastolic volume. The law states that the stroke volume of the heart increases in response to an increase in the volume of blood in the ventricles, before contraction, when all other factors remain constant.

Extrinsic regulation: Involves neural and hormonal control –Parasympathetic stimulation Supplied by vagus nerve, decreases heart rate, acetylcholine secreted – Sympathetic stimulation Supplied by cardiac nerves, increases heart rate and force of contraction, epinephrine and norepinephrine released

Nervous Control of Heart

The vascular demands for blood vary with activity and stress. In an efficient vascular system, the heart accelerates or decelerates reflexly. The brain of most domestic or other mammals a vasomotor centre contains a vasomotor centre in the medulla which receives impulses from (i) Specific vascular receptors such as those in the carotid sinus and heart (ii) General somatic and visceral receptors (iii) Higher centres in the brain. The heart rate rises in compensation for a fall in blood pressure and heart slows when the pressure rises. The vagus nerve slows the heart and reduces its amplitude of contraction; the primary vagal fibres terminate in ganglia located in the heart, and secondary vagal neurons end in the heart musculature and nodal tissue. Secondary sympathetic fibres elicit cardio acceleration.

Stimulation of the cervical portion of the spinal cord causes quickening of the heart beat. This occurs even after the possibility of increase of blood pressure has been removed by section of the splanchnic nerves, and the tonic inhibition of the vagi has been cut off by their section. In the cervical portion of the spinal cord nerve channels must exist which are capable of stimulating the muscle fibres of the heart, so as to cause it to beat more quickly. These accelerator fibres pass from the cord through the communicating branches to the last cervical or first dorsal sympathetic ganglion, and thence to the heart. Stimulation of the ganglia, or of the branches passing thence to the heart, quickens its beat. Cardiac accelerator nerves consist of parasympathetic nerve fibers which extend from the medulla. Vagus nerve consists of sympathetic nerve fibers which extend from the cardiovascular center of the medulla to the spinal cord in the thoracic region and innervate the SA node and AV node. These fibers release norepinephrine causing an increased heart rate and increased strength of contraction.

Coronary Circulation

Coronary circulation is the circulation of blood in the blood vessels that supply the heart muscle (myocardium). Coronary arteries supply oxygenated blood to the heart muscle, and cardiac veins drain away the blood once it has been deoxygenated.

The major vessels of the coronary circulation are the left main coronary that divides into left anterior descending and circumflex branches, and the right main coronary artery. The left and right coronary arteries originate at the base of the aorta from openings called the coronary ostia located behind the aortic valve leaflets.

The heart muscle is far too thick to obtain its supplies of oxygen and nutrients directly from the blood passing through its chambers. The muscle has in fact, a copious blood flow supply brought to it from the aorta by the coronary arteries. These branch to form a capillary network in which the capillaries run parallel to the muscle fibres, with about one capillary to each fibre. The proper functioning of the heart is entirely dependent upon the integrity of this exceptionally rich blood supply, particularly because, unlike the skeletal muscle, heart muscle cannot incur an oxygen debt.

Properties of Pulse

The heartbeat frequency or pulse rate is usually given as the number of heart beats per minute. Heart rate (HR) is the number of times the heart beats (or the ventricles pump blood out) in one minute. The average resting HR is approximately 70 beats per minute (bpm) in human beings. The heart rate increases several times during exercise or thermal stress. However, in resting horses, a heart rate over 80 can be a sign of a serious problem. The normal pulse for a goat is 70 to 90 beats per minute. In order to take your goat's pulse: Make sure the goat is calm and resting.Find the goat's artery below and slightly inside the jaw with your fingers. Watching a clock and count the number of heartbeats in 15 seconds.

In medicine, a pulse represents the tactile arterial palpation of the heartbeat by trained fingertips. The pulse may be palpated in any place that allows an artery to be compressed near the surface of the body, such as at the neck (carotid artery), wrist (radial artery), at the groin (femoral artery), behind the knee (popliteal artery), near the ankle joint (posterior tibial artery), and on foot (dorsalis pedis artery). The normal heart rate in an adult human male is 70–80 beats/min.

The pulse of cattle and buffalo is taken at a point on the underside of the base of the tail, the normal rate is 40 - 80 per minute in the adult. In buffalo the pulse rate is 40 - 60 per minute. In sheep and goats, you can feel the pulse on the inside of the top of the back leg. The rate of the pulse is 70 - 90 per minute in the adult. The pulse of the horse is taken on the inside of the cheek. The normal rate is 35 - 40 per minute. The pulse of the camel is taken at a point on the underside of the root of the tail. The normal rate is 35 - 45 beats per minute.

Pulse (or the count of arterial pulse per minute) is equivalent to measuring the heart rate. The heart rate can also be measured by listening to the heart beat by auscultation, traditionally using a stethoscope and counting it for a minute.

The radial pulse is commonly measured using three fingers. This has a reason: the finger closest to the heart is used to occlude the pulse pressure, the middle finger is used get a crude estimate of the blood pressure, and the finger most distal to the heart (usually the ring finger) is used to nullify the effect of the ulnar pulse as the two arteries are connected via the palmar arches (superficial and deep). The study of the pulse is known as sphygmology. Pulse is generally higher in the young animal. In females the resting heart rate is comparatively higher than in males of the same age group. Heart rate increases with rise in body temperature.

Metabolism & Energetic of Working Myocardial Cell

Cardiac muscle possesses several unique characteristics which make it especially suited for the functions of the heart. The cardiac muscle forms a functional syncytium as opposed to an anatomical syncytium in that the individual cells, with single nucleus are demarcated by the intercalated discs. Thus when one cell is excited, the action potential spreads throughout the network.

The cardiac muscle fibres are striated and resemble quite a lot to the skeletal muscle fibres in structure. Cardiac muscle resemble skeletal muscle in its chemical composition and in its metabolic processes. The notable differences in cardiac muscle and skeletal muscles are as follows.

- Cardiac muscle cannot incur an oxygen debt i.e. they cannot contract after its oxygen supply has been consumed completely. Any disturbance in the coronary circulation is therefore a serious matter.
- Cardiac musclc unlike skeletal muscle can use lactate as well as glucose for the generation of energy.
- Cardiac muscle unlike the skeletal muscles, the cardiac muscles are involuntary

The cardiac muscle fibres are ribbon-like rather than cylindrical. These are branched and interdigitate freely with each other, but each fibre is a completely separate unit. The branches from the neighbouring fibres join together. At the point of contact of two muscle fibres,the membranes of both the muscle fibres are fused together and thrown into an extensive infolding forming the so-called intercalated disc. These discs form tight junctions between the muscle fibres and do not allow the ions to pass through. However, the intercalated discs provide a strong union between fibres and thus play an important role during the contraction of muscle fibres by transmitting pull of one contractile unit along its axis to the next, thereby increasing force of contraction.

Along the sides near the outer border of the intercalated disc, the two adjacent muscle fibres are connected with each other through the gap junctions. The action potential passes from one cardiac muscle cell to the other through gap junctions, which provide low-resistance bridges and thus the cardiac muscle acts as a functional syncytium of many cardiac cells. In this way, the cardiac impulse spreads throughout the muscle mass quickly resulting in a co-ordinated contraction of the whole tissue.

Cardiac muscle contraction is a strictly regulated process which conjugates a series of electrophysiological, biochemical and mechanical events, resulting in the pumping of blood to all bodily tissues. These phenomena require a very high energetic demand both for generating the necessary mechanical force, and for maintaining cellular homeostasis during the process. Cardiac muscle requires a continuous supply of oxygen and therefore myocardial cells under normal conditions, utilise aerobic metabolic system that provides a constant supply of high energy phosphate for mechanical and chemical working of the heart.

In the myocardium, fatty acids (FA) represent the main energy substrate, although other secondary substrates, such as glucose and ketone bodies (Acetoacetate and 3-hydroxybutyrate), may also be used. Heart muscle uses acetoacetate in preference to glucose. The major fuel required for cardiac metabolism is free fatty acids followed by glucose and lactate with a minor contribution from amino acids, ketones and pyruvates.

Myocardial Metabolism has Three Phases

Energy Liberation or Production: It is the stage during which energy is released from the carbon-hydrogen bonds of substrates including fatty acids, glucose, lactate and other compounds used by the heart.

Energy conservation or storage: It is the transfer of the energy into synthesis of high energy phosphate compounds such as ATP, creatine phosphate, AMP, ADP.

Energy Utilization: It is the release of this stored chemical energy into shortening or development of tension of cardiac contraction.

Cardiac muscle cells contain a larger number of mitochondria that are rich in enzymes of citric acid cycle and oxidative phosphorylation for muscle contraction. ATP is utilized by the myocardial cells for muscle contraction which is broken down to ADP and inorganic phosphate (Pi).

The increased amount of ADP and inorganic phosphate (Pi) formed stimulates oxidative phosphorylation, the citric acid cycle and glycolysis thereby increasing the high energy phosphate bond production. Creatine phosphate also provides an immediate source of high energy phosphate bonds.

Nevertheless, under certain conditions such as heart failure or myocardial ischemia, fatty acid metabolism may become deleterious via mechanisms such as oxidative stress and arrhythmogenesis. In an ischemic milieu, various metabolic changes occur as a consequence of hypoxia, favoring cell necrosis, ventricular arrhythmias, and death. Major events in this context include an increase in extracellular K^+, a decrease in pH, and accumulation of intracellular calcium.

Extrinsic and Intrinsic Regulation

The heart constantly requires high-energy turnover and has the highest oxygen consumption rate per weight of all organs. Cardiac cell homeostasis, and with this, contractility and cardiac output, relies on constant substrate availability. Changes in workload, substrate availability, hormones, and nutrients force the heart to adapt its metabolism in order to achieve energy homeostasis. The heart resorts to several mechanisms that affect metabolic fluxes by modulating the activity of key enzymes and transporters. The adaptive changes are immediate or delayed, depending on the type of mechanisms involved. They result from extrinsic control by hormones, nutrients, and nervous stimulation, which are mediated by signal transduction systems. The mechanisms include control of gene expression, control of enzyme activity by substrates and ligands, and by covalent modifications of enzymes. These mechanisms apply to the multisite coordinated control of metabolic pathways and allow for large changes in flux and minimal changes in the concentration of the metabolic intermediates.

Myocardial contractility is the ability of the cardiac muscle to contract, thereby generating force. Contractile functions of the myocardium are influenced by a number of intrinsic and extrinsic factors. The intrinsic factors, including the initial length of the muscle fibers, stimulation frequency and cardiac rhythm are modulated by neurohumoral mechanisms and extrinsic factors (ions and energy balance, temperature, pH, drugs, etc.).

By providing energy for contractile work, cellular building blocks and signaling molecules for regulatory processes, cardiac metabolism forms the basis of living cardiomyocytes. In the hypertrophied and failing heart, there are profound changes in the metabolic network. This metabolic remodeling is characterized by impaired cardiac substrate utilization and energetics, which may directly cause contractile dysfunction.

The link between energy production and energy utilization is predominantly met by the creatine kinase (CK) phosphagen system. CK catalyses the transfer of a high-energy phosphoryl group from ATP to creatine to form phosphocreatine (PCr). This reversible reaction facilitates energy transfer by obviating the need for ATP diffusion, while high PCr levels provide an energy buffer when demand outstrips supply. Compartmentalization of CK isoenzymes to the mitochondria and cytosol maintain favorable levels of local metabolites to maximize the energy available from ATP hydrolysis.

Cardiac ageing manifests as a decline in function leading to heart failure. At the cellular level, ageing entails decreased replicative capacity and dysregulation of cellular processes in myocardial and nonmyocyte cells. Various extrinsic parameters, such as lifestyle and environment, integrate important signalling pathways, such as those involving inflammation and oxidative stress, with intrinsic molecular mechanisms underlying resistance versus progression to cellular senescence. Cardiovascular ageing is inextricably tied to genetic predisposition and the complex interaction of hereditary influences.

ECG and Its Significance in Veterinary Sciences

As the heart undergoes depolarization and repolarization, the electrical currents that are generated spread not only within the heart, but also throughout the body. This electrical activity generated by the heart can be measured by an array of electrodes placed on the body surface. The recorded tracing is called an electrocardiogram (ECG, or EKG).

An electrocardiogram (ECG or EKG) is a recording of the electrical activity of the heart using electrodes placed on the skin. It is a safe, noninvasive procedure that uses clips (electrodes) placed on the skin over the chest and legs. The ECG is used commonly to evaluate the heart rhythm and identify abnormalities (arrhythmias) in the heartbeat. It may also help to identify enlargement of the heart, a common finding with many heart diseases. An electrocardiogram (ECG) is a medical test that detects cardiac (heart) abnormalities by measuring the electrical activity generated by the heart as it contracts. The machine that records the patient's ECG is called an electrocardiograph. With each heart beat, an electrical impulse (or "wave") travels through the heart. This wave causes the muscle to squeeze and pump blood from the heart.

Three electrodes are most frequently used in veterinary ECG: right arm (usually white), left arm (usually black), and left leg (usually red). In small animals these electrodes are most commonly placed on the 2 forelimbs and the left hindlimb. Hair should be clipped to improve contact between the ECG pad and the skin. Pads should be secured with tape and additional electrode gel or alcohol should be used to improve contact between the patient and electrodes. The electrodes are connected to the ECG machine by colour-coded cables.

Deflection of normal ECG are referred to as P, QRS and T waves. The different waves that comprise the ECG represent the sequence of depolarization and repolarization of the atria and ventricles. The ECG is recorded at a speed of 25 mm/sec (5 large squares/sec), and the voltages are calibrated so that 1 mV = 10 mm (2 large squares) in the vertical direction. Therefore, each small 1-mm square represents 0.04 sec (40 msec) in time and 0.10 mV in voltage. Because the recording speed is standardized, one can calculate the heart rate from the intervals between different waves.

P Wave (Atrial Depolarization)

It is a positive wave that indicates the sum of all the electrical potentials produced during the depolarisation of both atria and the spreading of the electrical activity from S.A node throughout the atrial musculature. It slightly precedes atrial systole and initiates the atrial contraction. There is a very brief interval between P wave and atrial systole, which is due to time lag between electrical and mechanical events.

The period of time from the onset of the P wave to the beginning of the QRS complex is termed the PR interval, which normally ranges from 0.12 to 0.20 seconds in duration. This interval represents the time between the onset of atrial depolarization and the onset of ventricular depolarization. If the PR interval is >0.20 sec, there is an AV conduction block, which is called a first-degree heart block

QRS Wave (Ventricular Depolarization)

The QRS complex represents ventricular depolarization. Ventricular rate can be calculated by determining the time interval between QRS complexes. QRS complex shows the spreading depolarization wave through the ventricular muscles, thus initiates ventricular systole (depolarization). QRS wave precedes isovolumetric contraction.

The duration of the QRS complex is normally 0.06 to 0.10 seconds. This relatively short duration indicates that ventricular depolarization normally occurs very rapidly. If the QRS complex is prolonged (> 0.10 sec), conduction is impaired within the ventricles. This can occur with bundle branch blocks or whenever a ventricular foci (abnormal pacemaker site) becomes the pacemaker driving the ventricle.

T wave (Ventricular Repolarization)

Generally, the T wave exhibits a positive deflection. The reason for this is that the last cells to depolarize in the ventricles are the first to repolarize. The positive (upward) deflection precedes ventricular diastole and indicates the initiation of ventricular repolarization (relaxation).

The T wave is longer in duration than the QRS complex that represents depolarization. The longer duration occurs because conduction of the repolarization wave is slower than the wave of depolarization. The reason for this is that the repolarization wave does not utilize the high-velocity bundle branch and purkinje system, and therefore primarily relies on cell-to-cell conduction.

ECG has no separate deflection or wave for atrial relaxation, which is due to the fusion of this deflection with QRS complex.

Nowdays electrocardiography (ECG) is gaining importance in the diagnosis of diseases of cardio-vascular system in dogs and cats. It is an important non-invasive tool being employed in routine health checkup and examination of heart in ailing canines. It has now started attracting the attention of veterinary medical specialists to detect electrical vectors, their magnitude and direction or diagnosing cardiac diseases as well as diseases that secondarily affect the heart, such as metabolic disorders. During these days electrocardiography is an important diagnostic intervention in canine medicine with a proven usefulness and utility.

The electrical current in the heart is created by positively charged ions moving through channels along the membranes of the muscle cells. When one cell reaches its maximum ionic charge, it depolarizes and the positive charge is conducted to the next cell. This cell conduction is extremely fast, and the cumulative effect of all these cells depolarizing is a muscle contraction. By investigating the time intervals, consistency, heart rate, and shape of these waves, we can locate which portion of the conduction system might be having a problem. On a normal ECG, each P wave is followed by a QRS complex at a species-specific normal interval. Specific measurements to obtain for thorough ECG interpretation include:

- P wave amplitude and duration
- P-R interval duration
- QRS complex duration
- R-wave amplitude
- QT segment duration.

Tachycardia is a condition that makes your heart beat more than 100 times per minute. There are three types of it: Supraventricular. This happens when the electrical signals in the organ's upper chambers misfire and cause the heart rate to speed up. It beats so fast that it can't fill with blood before it contracts. Ventricular. This is a rapid heart rate that starts in your heart's lower chambers. It happens when the electrical signals in these chambers fire the wrong way. Again, the heart beats so fast that it can't fill with blood or pump it through the rest of your body. Sinus tachycardia. This happens when your heart's natural pacemaker sends out electrical signals faster than normal.

Heart is made up of four chambers: the left and right atria and the left and right ventricles. One heartbeat, or one wave on the ECG, consists of the two atria depolarizing (which causes a contraction), followed by the ventricles depolarizing, and then the ventricles repolarizing. If the atrial depolarization wave exists without a corresponding ventricular wave, there is probably a problem in the conduction path between the atria and ventricles.

- It is a non-invasive method to evaluate cardiac function.
- To diagnose ventricular hypertrophy.
- To evaluate conduction system blocks, myocardial infarction and drug effects etc.'

ECG in veterinary science is generally carried out for dogs, cats, horses and goats. It is the most important test to perform in animals with an auscultable arrhythmia (other than sinus arrhythmia in dogs). The ECG may also yield useful information regarding chamber dilation and hypertrophy.

Echocardiography

Echocardiography refers to the ultrasonic evaluation of cardiac functions. It is a non-invasive technique that does not involve injections or insertion of a catheter. It involves B-scan ultrasound at a frequency of 2.25 MHz using a transducer, which also acts as a receiver of the reflected waves. This test allows to test the functioning of the heart and its valves. The images can help to spot blood clots in the heart.

A diagnostic echocardiogram can augment the understanding of dogs and cat heart disease by careful interrogation of the cardiac chamber sizes, great vessels, valvular anatomy, heart function and how the blood is flowing through the heart. Although a relatively new tool for the study of the heart in man it has already found wide acceptance in the area of cardiac research and in the study of clinical cardiac disease. Animals had often been used in the early experiments with cardiac ultrasound, but only recently has echocardiography been used as a research and clinical tool in veterinary medicine. Echocardiography is now an important adjunct to the field of veterinary cardiology.Different types of echocardiography include conventional 2-dimensional and doppler techniques, as well as advanced techniques such as tissue doppler, strain, 3-dimensional, transesophageal and contrast echocardiography.When combined with the Doppler techniques, echocardiography can be used to measure velocity and volume of flow through the valves.

Other advanced techniques include selective cardiac or peripheral angiography, CT angiography, CT imaging and MRI. CT imaging is often useful to diagnose coronary artery or vascular ring anomalies and for surgical planning for cardiac tumors, pericardial diseases and other congenital vascular abnormalities.

Haemorrhage and Haemostasis

Hemostasis is the physiological process by which bleeding is controlled. Haemostasis is the body's normal physiological response for the prevention and stopping of bleeding/haemorrhage. Generally speaking, it helps ensure blood fluidity and blood vessel integrity. Abnormalities in Haemostasis can result in bleeding (hemorrhage) or blood clots (thrombosis). Haemostasis consists of:

Primary Haemostasis

1) local vasoconstriction (to reduce blood flow to the injury site),
2) platelet plug formation.

Secondary Haemostasis or clotting of the plasma, involving interaction between numerous factors and inhibitors.

Fibrinolysis: a process which dissolves the clot once blood vessel integrity has been restored.

When there is a breach in a blood vessel, the first priority (primary Haemostasis) is to "plug" this breach. When a blood vessel is damaged, endothelial cells are separated, the underlying collagen is exposed, and the surface loses its smoothness. Platelets begin to contact the damaged surface initiating the adhesion process. Adhered platelets undergo a reaction releasing aggregating agents causing accumulation of more platelets. A loose plug is formed that is strengthened with the formation of a fibrin meshwork. The damaged vessel is then repaired by connective tissue and endothelial cell growth. The platelet-fibrin complex and cell debris is then removed by phagocytes. Vascular endothelium lines the entire cardiovascular system. Factors present in blood assist in coagulation.

Clotting factors: The process of coagulation involves a stepwise activation of certain substances mostly proteins present in blood and/ or tissue fluids, these are known as clotting factors. More than 12 clotting factors have been identified, using human patients with various deficiencies in clotting mechanisms. Most of the clotting factors are inactive proteolytic enzymes and when activated produce enzymatic activities leading to cascading reaction of the clotting process.

Many substances present in tissue and blood affect coagulation. Substances that promote coagulation are called as procoagulants, and those inhibiting coagulation are anticoagulants.

- Factor I (fibrinogen)
- Factor II (prothrombin)
- Factor III (thromboplastin)
- Factor IV (calcium)
- Factor V (labile factor or proaccelerin or accelerator globulin)
- Factor VI (non-existent)

- Factor VII (stable factor or proconvertin)
- Factor VIII [antihaemophilic factor A (AHF) or antihaemophilic globulin (AHG)]
- Factor IX [christmas factor or plasma thromboplastic component (PTC or antihaemophilic factor B)],
- Factor X (Stuart–Prower factor),
- Factor XI (plasma thromboplastin antecedent, i.e. PTA or antihaemophilic factor C)
- Factor XII (Hageman factor or glass factor or contact factor)
- Factor XIII (fibrin-stabilizing factor or fibrinase or LakiLorand factor)
- PL (platelet phospho**lipid)**

Vitamin K and Blood Clotting

Vitamin K is a fat-soluble vitamin essential for coagulation of blood. Vitamin K is a complex naphthoquinone derivative which is indispensable for the synthesis of prothrombin by the liver and for the post-translational processing of the prothrombin group of coagulation factors (Factors II, VII, IX, and X).

Vitamin K deficiency causes excessive bleeding due to failure of normal fibrin clot formation.The deficiency of vitamin K leads to a decrease in plasma prothrombin concentration and a corresponding prolongation of the coagulation time of the blood. Clinical signs of bleeding depend on duration and severity of vitamin K deficiency and include prolonged bleeding from minor wounds, spontaneous hematoma formation, intracavitary hemorrhage, and death due to blood loss and acute hemorrhagic shock. Anticoagulant rodenticide poisoning is the most common cause of severe, acute vitamin K deficiency in dogs and cats.

Vitamin K is widely distributed in nature; thus it is found in green vegetables, cereals and animal tissues generally. It is synthesized by bacteria in the rumen and bacteria present in the human intestine. Vitamin K deficiency from dietary abnormalities is very rare in man and domestic animals.

Dicoumarol preventing coagulation is actually a vitamin K antagonist. This substance is related to the naphthoquinone derivatives which have vitamin K activity. Because of chemical resemblance, dicoumarol acts as an anti vitamin K by the process of substrate competition. Dicoumarol replaces vitamin K in the liver, at the latter's normal site of action and thus prevents the vitamin from carrying out normal physiological function.

Prevention of Blood Clotting in Blood Vessels

The important factors that prevent the process of clotting within the vascular system are:

- Antithrombin III blocks the action of thrombin on fibrinogen and inactivates the thrombin it binds.
- Smooth endothelium, which prevents contact activation of intrinsic system

- Glycocalyx layer adsorbed to the inner surface of the endothelium that repels clotting factors and platelets
- Protein bound with endothelium which binds thrombin and removes its effect; this protein also activates a plasma protein called protein C which inactivates the activated factor V and VIII. Damage to endothelium causes loss of smoothness and the glycocalyx layer and thus initiates coagulation.
- Heparin produced by mast cells inhibits clotting.
- Fibrin threads formed during clotting
- A globulin known as antithrombin III, heparin and alpha2 macroglobulin.
- The thrombin formed during clotting becomes adsorbed to fibrin and thus prevents further spreading of the blood clotting. Thrombin not adsorbed to fibrin combines with antithrombin and gets inactivated. Heparin increases the effectiveness of antithrombin in removing thrombin. The heparin and antithrombin also inactivates the activated factors XII, XI, and X. The alpha2 macroglobulin acts similar to antithrombin.

Regulation of Haemostasis

- Regulation of normal haemostasis and blood flow involves complex interactions between plasma proteins and blood cells, including platelets, leukocytes and the endothelial lining of blood vessels. In normal wound healing the anticoagulant and fibrinolytic mechanisms are downregulated and the procoagulant and thrombotic mechanisms predominate with resultant generation of thrombin, fibrin clot formation and subsequent platelet adhesion and aggregation. Pro-inflammatory and prothrombotic cytokines downregulate the fibrinolytic and activated protein C pathways as well as inducing synthesis of specific procoagulant and prothrombotic mediators by platelets and leukocytes as well as endothelium.
- The kallikrein-kinin system comprises a complex of proteins that when activated leads to the release of vasoactive kinins. The kinins are released from both high molecular weight kininogen (HMWK) and low molecular weight kininogen (LMWK) as a result of activation of either tissue kallikrein or plasma kallikrein. The kallikreins themselves exist in inactive pre-forms. The kinins are involved in many physiological and pathological processes including regulation of blood pressure and flow (via modulation of the renin-angiotensin pathway), blood coagulation, cellular proliferation and growth, angiogenesis, apoptosis, and inflammation.

Fibrinolysis

Fibrinolysis is a process that prevents blood clots from growing and becoming problematic. This process has two types: primary fibrinolysis and secondary fibrinolysis. Fibrinolysis is a highly regulated enzymatic process that prevents unnecessary accumulation of intravascular fibrin.

Fibrin plays an essential role in hemostasis as both the primary product of the coagulation cascade and the ultimate substrate for fibrinolysis. Fibrinolysis efficiency is greatly influenced by clot structure, fibrinogen isoforms and polymorphisms, the rate of thrombin generation, the reactivity of thrombus-associated cells such as platelets, and the overall biochemical environment. Regulation of the fibrinolytic system, like that of the coagulation cascade, is accomplished by a wide array of cofactors, receptors, and inhibitors.

Anticoagulation Mechanism

Anticoagulants are medicines that help prevent blood clots. They're given to people at a high risk of getting clots, to reduce their chances of developing serious conditions such as strokes and heart attacks. A blood clot is a seal created by the blood to stop bleeding from wounds. Many people with congenital heart defects need to take anticoagulants (*blood thinners). Common reasons for this type of treatment include heart valve replacements, heart rhythm disorders or prior complicated surgeries such as the Fontan operation. Blood-thinning medicines slow blood clotting, preventing complications like blood clots forming on artificial valves, valve obstruction and blood clots traveling to the brain and causing stroke. Bleeding may be a complication of taking these medications.

The common anticoagulants include Aspirin, Clopidogrel and warfarin. Aspirin tends to cause fewer bleeding complications. Heparin and low molecular weight heparin are also used as blood –thinning medications.

Thromboembolic agents are indicated for a variety of conditions, ranging from disseminated intravascular coagulation to pulmonary thromboembolism in both dogs and cats. Thromboembolism is formation of a clot (thrombus)in a blood vessel that breaks loose and is carried by the blood stream to plug another vessel. The clot may plug a vessel in the lungs (pulmonary embolism), brain (stroke), gastrointestinal tract, kidneys, or leg.

Summary

- The cardiovascular system (CVS) consists of the heart and the blood vessels.
- The heart acts as a system of two pumps working in series and forms the driving force for blood flow.
- The blood vessels that take blood from the heart to various tissues are called arteries. The smallest arteries are called arterioles. Arterioles open into a network of capillaries which constitute the microcirculation.
- The most important function of blood vessels, i.e. the rapid exchange of materials between the blood and extracellular fluid bathing the tissue cells is served by the capillaries.

4

Hemodynamics of Circulation

Transport systems are crucial to survival. Unicellular organisms rely on simple diffusion for transport of nutrients and removal of waste. Multicellular organisms have developed more complex circulatory systems. The circulatory system is responsible for the transport of the various essential compounds and other factors around the body, as well as the removal of the metabolic wastes that accumulate in the tissues from body activities to places of elimination. The compounds and other factors transported around the body are blood, nutrients, medications and antibodies to fight infection, the residue of worn out cells and the wastes of metabolism. There are times when undesirable compounds and factors are found in the system as well - compounds such as poisons or toxins and disease causing organisms.

The main components of the circulatory system are the heart, arteries, capillaries, and veins. The cardiovascular system consists of the heart (cardio) and the vessels required for transport of blood (vascular). The vascular system consists of arteries, veins and capillaries. The circulatory system delivers food and oxygen to the cells of the body and eliminates waste products. It contains blood, which consists of red blood cells, white blood cells, and platelets. Red blood cells carry oxygen while white blood cells help the body fight disease.

There are two major sub divisions of circulation of blood in the body : the systemic circulation and the pulmonary circulation. Blood flows with almost no resistance in all the larger vessels, but this is not the case in the arteries and capillaries, where considerable resistance does occur. To cause blood to flow through these small resistance vessels the heart pumps blood into the arteries under high pressure.

Type of Blood Vessels

1. Distensible vessels **(Windkessel)** e.g. aorta, pulmonary artery and their branches
2. Resistance vessels e.g. arterioles, metarterioles, precapillary sphincter
3. Exchange vessels e.g. capillaries
4. Capacitance vessels e.g. venules and venous compartment
5. Shunt (thoroughfare) vessels e.g. most notably present in skin.

Hemodynamics of Circulation

The study of physical principles of blood flow through the vessels especially the interrelationship between pressure, flow and resistance and other basic physical principles of blood circulation is called haemodynamics.The haemodynamic response continuously monitors and adjusts to conditions in the body and its environment. At a fundamental level, the study of hemodynamics is concerned with the distribution of pressures and flows in the circulatory system. The main factors involved are the pulsatile driving pressure generated by the heart, the flow characteristics of blood, and the geometric structure and mechanical properties of the vessels. Consideration of hemodynamics is essential for a comprehensive understanding of the functioning of the circulatory system.

The quantitative reasoning of William Harvey (1578–1657) led in 1628 to the concept that blood continuously circulates.

Hemodynamics ultimately begins with the heart which supplies the driving force for all blood flow in the body. Cardiac output propels blood through the arteries and veins as a function of ventricular contraction.

Poiseuille's Law

Poiseuille's law expressing the relation between the flow (Q) and pressure gradient (P) in a long narrow tube of length (L), the viscosity of fluid (η) and the radius (r) of the tube is as:

$Q = Pr^4/8nl$

According to the Poiseuille's law, the flow (Q) of a fluid through a rigid tube is determined by the following-Pressure gradient, Radius of the tube and Viscosity of fluid and length of the tube. The Poiseuille's law is valid for straight rigid tubes with Newtonian fluid flowing through them. Since, the blood vessels are not rigid and the blood is not a Newtonian fluid, therefore, strictly speaking the Poiseuille's law does not apply to flow of blood through the vascular system. Nevertheless, the important principles relating flow, pressure gradient and resistance remain applicable, so they are discussed in relation to blood flow as:

Blood flow and pressure gradient relationship and

Blood flow and resistance relationship.

From the Poiseuille's law, it can be derived that the flow is inversely proportional to the resistance. The major factors that determine the resistance to flood flow are:

I. The viscosity of blood and
II. The radius of vessels.

Reflex Regulation of the Circulation

In addition to the many ways in which signals transmitted from the brain to the blood vessels and heart can alter circulatory function, a system of specific circulatory reflexes can also regulates the circulation. Most of these reflexes are concerned with the regulation of arterial pressure or with the regulation of blood flow to specific local areas of the body.

Arterial pressure reflexes: The most important of the arterial pressure reflexes is the baroreceptor reflex. An increase in arterial pressure stretches the walls of the major arteries in the chest and this in turn excites stretch receptors located in the vessel walls, especially stretch receptors located in the carotid sinuses and in the aortic arch. (*The carotid sinus is the reflex area of the carotid artery, consisting of various nerve receptors for baroregulation (pressure regulation of the body) in sync to external conditions. The carotid sinus contains numerous baroreceptors which function as a "sampling area" for many homeostatic mechanisms for maintaining blood pressure.* Signals are transmitted from these receptors to the vasomotor center of the brain stem, and reflex signals are transmitted back to the heart and to the blood vessels to slow the heart and to dilate the vessels, thereby reducing the arterial pressure towards normal. A decrease in arterial pressure causes exactly the opposite effects.

Circulatory

Reflexes for Control of Blood Volume

When the blood volume increases, the volume of blood in the central veins and in the right and left atria usually also increases. This stretches the walls of the atria and large veins, again exciting stretch receptors. These stretch receptors also transmit signals to the vasomotor center and reflex signals are then transmitted to the kidneys to increase the urinary output of fluid. Also, signals are transmitted to the hypothalamus to decrease the rate of secretion of antidiuretic hormone, thereby also increasing the output of fluid by the kidneys. Thus this reflex mechanism helps to control the total body fluid and blood volume.

Reflexes for Control of Body Temperature

When the body temperature rises too high, special neurons in the anterior hypothalamus become excited: these in turn send signals through the sympathetic nervous system to dilate the skin blood vessels: thereby allowing transfer of major amounts of internal body heat to the skin. This heat then passes through the skin to the surroundings. As a result, the body temperature falls back toward normal. This reflex is also associated with sweating reflex and with other aspects of body temperature control.

The Functional Parts of the Systemic Circulation

The different parts of the systemic circulation include the arteries, arterioles, capillaries, venules and veins. The function of the arteries is to transport blood under high pressure to the tissues. For this reason the arteries have strong vascular walls and blood flows rapidly in the arteries to the tissues.

The arterioles are the last small branches of the arterial system and they act as central valves through which blood is released into the capillaries. The arterioles has a strong muscular wall that is capable of closing or of allowing it to be dilated several fold, thereby vastly altering blood flow to the capillaries.

The function of the capillaries is to exchange fluid and nutrients between the blood and the interstitial spaces. For this role, the capillary walls are very thin and permeable to small molecular substances.

The venules collect blood from the capillaries. They gradually coalesce into progressively larger veins.

The veins function as conduits for transport of blood from the tissues back to the heart. Since the pressure in the venous system is very low, the venous walls are thin. Even so, they are muscular, and this allows them to contract or expand and thereby to store either a small or large amount of blood depending upon the needs of the body.

Resistance to Flow, Vasoconstriction

Resistance is a force that opposes the flow of a fluid. Resistance to blood flow within a vascular network is determined by the size of individual vessels (length and diameter), the organization of the vascular network (series and parallel arrangements), physical characteristics of the blood (viscosity, laminar flow versus turbulent flow), and extravascular mechanical forces acting upon the vasculature.In blood vessels, most of the resistance is due to vessel diameter. As vessel diameter decreases, the resistance increases and blood flow decreases. Very little pressure remains by the time blood leaves the capillaries and enters the venules.

Changes in vessel diameter, particularly in small arteries and arterioles, enable organs to adjust their own blood flow to meet the metabolic requirements of the tissue. Therefore, if an organ needs to adjust its blood flow (and therefore, oxygen delivery), cells surrounding these blood vessels release vasoactive substances that can either constrict or dilate the resistance vessels.

The ability of an organ to regulate its own blood flow is termed local regulation of blood flow and is mediated by vasoconstrictor and vasodilator substances released by the tissue surrounding blood vessels (vasoactive metabolites) and by the vascular endothelium. There is also a mechanism intrinsic to the vascular smooth muscle (myogenic mechanism) that is involved in local blood flow regulation.

In organs such as the heart and skeletal muscle, mechanical activity (contraction and relaxation) produces compressive forces that can effectively decrease vessel diameters and increase resistance to flow during muscle contraction.

Besides local regulatory mechanisms, there are extrinsic mechanisms acting on the vasculature to regulate vessel diameter. One important extrinsic mechanism regulating vascular diameter operates through the autonomic innervation of blood vessels. In general, sympathetic adrenergic influences acting through vascular alpha-adrenoceptors cause resistance vessels as well as veins to be partially constricted under basal conditions. This is termed "sympathetic vascular tone." Therefore, removal of sympathetic adrenergic influences (for example, by administration of an alpha-adrenoceptor antagonist or by sympathectomy) leads to vasodilation and an increase in organ blood flow. A second type of extrinsic influence on the vasculature is circulating vasoactive hormones such as angiotensin II, epinephrine and norepinephrine, vasopressin (antidiuretic hormone, ADH), atrial natriuretic peptide (ANP), and endothelin. Both the neural and humoral factors, while affecting organ blood flow, primarily serve the function of regulating arterial pressure by altering systemic vascular resistance.

Nervous and Circulating Fluid Volume Controls of Blood Pressure

Blood pressure is almost always measured in terms of millimetre of mercury (mm Hg) because the mercury manometer has been used as the standard reference for measuring blood pressure throughout the history of physiology. Actually blood pressure means the force exerted by the blood against any unit area of the vessel wall. The pressure of the circulating blood decreases as blood moves through arteries, arterioles, capillaries, and veins; the term blood pressure generally refers to arterial blood pressure, i.e., the pressure in the larger arteries. When one says that the pressure in a vessel is 50 mm Hg, this means that the force exerted is sufficient to push a column of mercury upto a level of 50 mm. If the pressure is 100 mm Hg it will push the column of mercury upto 100 mm. Systolic blood pressure refers to the force with heart pumps blood around the body. Diastolic pressure refers to the resistance to blood flow in blood vessels. Normal blood pressure in human beings is considered to be a reading between 90/60 mmHg and 120/80 mmHg.

Slight change in diameter of a vessel causes tremendous change in its ability to conduct blood flow.

Poiseuille's Law

$Q = Pr^4/8nl$

where

Q = Blood flow

P = Pressure difference r = Radius

n = Blood viscosity l = Length

Thus the rate of blood flow is directly proportional to the fourth power of the radius of the vessel.

The diameter of the blood vessel unlike that of metal pipes and glass tubes, increases as the internal pressure increases, because *blood vessels are distensible.* However, the vascular distensibility differ greatly in different segments of the circulation.

Arterial Blood Pressure (ABP)

Arterial blood pressure (ABP) is a basic hemodynamic index often utilized to guide therapeutic interventions, especially in critically ill animals and human beings.

Difference in Distensibility of the Arteries and the Veins

Anatomically the walls of the arteries are far stronger than those of the veins. Consequently the veins on the average are about 6 to 10 times as distensible as the arteries. That is, a given rise in pressure will cause about 6 to 10 times as much extra blood to fill a vein as an artery of comparable size.

Vascular Compliance or Capacitance

In haemodynamic studies it is important to know the total quantity of blood that can be stored in a given portion of the circulation for each mm Hg rise in pressure than to know the distensibility of the individual vessel. This value is called compliance or

capacitance, which are physical terms measuring the increase in volume caused by a given increase in pressure as follows.

Vascular compliance = Increase in volume/ Increase in pressure

Compliance and distensibility are quite different. A highly distensible vessel which has a very slight volume may have far less compliance than a much less distensible vessel which has a very large volume, for compliance is equal to distensibility x volume. The compliance of a vein is about 24 times that of its corresponding artery because it is about 8 times as distensible and it has a volume about 3 times as great ($8 \times 3 = 24$).

Blood Pressure

The blood pressure is the lateral pressure exerted on the walls of the vessels by the contained blood. Systolic arterial pressure: Systolic arterial pressure is the maximum pressure in the arteries during systole.Diastolic pressure: It is the lowest pressure during diastole. Pulse pressure: The pulse pressure is the difference between diastolic and systolic pressure.

Pulse, Origin and Maintenance of Blood Pressure

Since the heart is a pulsatile pump, blood enters arterial intermittently causing pressure pulses in the arterial system. In the normal young adult the pressure at the height of a pulse, the systolic pressure, is about 120 mm. Hg and at its lowest point, the diastolic pressure is about 80 mm Hg. The difference between these two pressures, about 40 mm Hg is called the pulse pressure.

Systolic value – blood pressure while the heart is squeezing

Diastolic value – blood pressure while the heart is relaxing

The average blood pressure for an adult is 120/80 mmHg. The first number is the systolic value and the second number is the diastolic value.

Blood pressure is determined by Q (cardiac output) and the resistance to the blood flow (R). Resistance to blood flow is caused both by the diameter of the blood vessels and by the thickness of the blood. Furthermore, if a person has a condition called atherosclerosis (plaque in the arteries), their resistance to blood flow will increase and so will blood pressure.

With age there is a loss of the normal endothelial compliance in the blood vessels. This change causes blood vessels to act stiffer and less distensible with the pressures of systole. The main result of this seemingly minor change is an increase in blood pressure with age. By increasing the blood pressure, more load is placed on the heart, predisposing it to further compromise in the form of hypertrophy (i.e., the heart gets thicker in an attempted push against this greater vascular resistance) or direct vascular damage from the increased pressure (e.g., hemorrhagic stroke)

There are two major factors that affect the pulse pressure (i) The stroke volume output of the heart and (ii) The compliance of the arterial tree.

In general, the greater the stroke volume output, the greater the amount of blood that must be accommodated in the arterial tree with each heartbeat and therefore, the greater is the pressure rise during systole and pressure fall during diastole, thus causing a greater pulse pressure.

On the other hand, the greater the compliance of the arterial system, the less will be the rise in pressure for a given stroke volume of blood pumped into the arteries. In effect, then, the pulse pressure is determined approximately by the ratio of stroke volume output to compliance of the arterial tree. Therefore any condition of the circulation that affects either of these two factors will affect the pulse pressure.

Nervous and Humoral Control of Blood Flow by the Tissues

The circulatory system is provided with a complex system for control of blood flow to the different parts of the body. In general, these are of three major types as follows.

1. Local control of blood flow in each individual tissue, the flow being controlled mainly in proportion to that tissues need for blood perfusion.
2. Nervous control of blood flow which often affects blood flow in large segments of the systemic circulation, such as shifting blood flow from non muscular vascular beds to the muscles during exercise or altering the blood flow in the skin to control body temperature.
3. Humoral control, in which various substances dissolved in the blood such as hormones, ions or other chemicals can cause either local increase or decrease in tissue flow or widespread generalized changes in flow.

Neurohormonal Control of Vascular Smooth Muscle

The term '**humoral regulation**' means regulation by substances in the body fluids such as **hormones**, **ions** etc.

Stress and anxiety also can contribute to elevated blood pressure. This effect takes place in the form of excess catecholamines (e.g., norepinephrine and epinephrine), which increase cardiac contractility, which increases flow and selectively constrict blood vessels, which increases vascular resistance. Adrenal medulla secrete both epinephrine and norepinephrine. Norepinephrine has vasoconstrictor effects in almost all vascular beds of the body and epinephrine has similar effects in some, but not all beds. For instance, epinephrine causes vasodilation in both skeletal and cardiac muscle.

Renin-Angiotensin-Aldosterone System (RAAS)

Angiotensin(I and II) : Angiotensin is the most powerful **vasoconstrictor** substance known. As little as one ten millionth of a gram can increase the arterial pressure of a human being as much as 10-20 mmHg under some conditions. A decrease in arterial pressure or a decrease in the quantity of sodium in the body fluids will cause the kidneys to secrete the substance renin. The renin in turn acts on one of the plasma proteins, renin substrate, to split away the vasoactive peptide angiotensin (I and II). The angiotensin in turn causes marked constriction of the peripheral arterioles. It also causes constriction of the renal tubules, thereby causing the kidneys to retain both water and salt, thus increasing the body fluid volume, which helps to raise the arterial pressure. Hence, an initial decrease in arterial pressure or decrease in sodium causes a compensatory build up of body fluid and sodium as well as an increase in arterial pressure, thereby compensating for the original deficit. Aldosterone is the end effector of this pathway, and in addition to vasoconstriction, causes reabsorption of sodium in the distal tubule of the kidney, which increases blood volume and blood pressure.

Histamine *:* Histamine is released by essentially every tissue of the body that becomes damaged. Most of the histamine is probably derived from eosinophils and mast cells in the damaged tissues.Histamine has a powerful vasodilator effect on the arterioles and also has a very potent effect to increase capillary porosity, allowing leakage of both fluid and plasma proteins into the tissues. Though the role of histamine in normal regulation of circulation is unknown, in many physiological conditions the intense arteriolar dilation and increased capillary porosity caused by histamine cause tremendous quantities of fluid to leak out of the circulation into the tissues to cause oedema.

Circulatory Controls- Shock Stresses

Emotional stress has been recognized as a modifiable risk factor for cardiovascular diseases. The impact of stress on physiological and psychological processes is determined by characteristics of the stress stimulus. Imbalance during intense stress might lead to failure of circulatory homeostasis and to shock. Cardiovascular responses to stress are exquisitely coordinated and functional up to a point.

Stress contributes to diverse pathophysiological changes including sudden death, myocardial infarction, myocardial ischemia etc.

The heart and blood vessels comprise the two elements of the cardiovascular system that work together in providing nourishment and oxygen to the organs of the body. The activity of these two elements is also coordinated in the body's response to stress. Acute stress —causes an increase in heart rate and stronger contractions of the heart muscle, with the stress hormones — adrenaline, noradrenaline and cortisol — acting as messengers for these effects. In addition, the blood vessels that direct blood to the large muscles and the heart dilate, thereby increasing the amount of blood pumped to these parts of the body and elevating blood pressure. This is also known as the fight or flight response. Once the acute stress episode has passed, the body returns to its normal state.

Chronic stress contributes to long-term problems for heart and blood vessels. The consistent and ongoing increase in heart rate, and the elevated levels of stress hormones and of blood pressure, can take a toll on the body. This long-term ongoing stress can increase the risk for hypertension, heart attack or stroke.

The number one cause of heart failure is coronary artery disease (CAD). CAD reduces coronary blood flow and oxygen delivery to the myocardium. This leads to myocardial hypoxia and impaired function. Another common cause of heart failure is myocardial infarction (infarction- obstruction of the blood supply to an organ or region of tissue, typically by a thrombus or embolus, causing local death of the tissue), which is the final and often fatal culmination of CAD. Infarcted tissue does not contribute to the generation of mechanical activity so overall cardiac performance is diminished. Furthermore, non-infarcted regions must compensate for the loss of function and this extra burden can precipitate changes that lead to failure.

Regional and Fetal Circulations

Coronary Circulation

The heart needs to pump blood to all parts of the body at high pressure and in the process performs a large amount of work. For this, the heart needs a large supply of oxygen as well as means for the removal of large amounts of waste products of metabolism. This large supply of blood for the heart is supplied by coronary arteries.

The total coronary artery blood flow averages approximately 5 percent of the total cardiac output. During stress, the coronary blood flow may increase substantially. The blood flow to the heart is controlled by autonomic nervous system.

Ruminal Circulation

Blood flow to the rumen is greatly influenced by rumen volume and products of rumen fermentation. Feeding is followed by an increase in blood flow to the rumen. The increase in ruminal blood flow after feeding does not depend solely upon the mechanical effect due to the volume of rumen digesta increases in rumen contraction rate but upon stimulation provided via contact between mucosa and constituents of the normal rumen contents. Volatile fatty acids, the product of rumen fermentation, increase the ruminal blood flow. This increased blood to the rumen after feeding is important to increase the process of digestion and also to increase the removal of products of ruminal fermentation.

Fetal Circulation

The lungs finish their development after birth. Before this, the lung's function is taken over by the placenta, which is the oxygen-transfer organ during fetal life. During pregnancy the placenta does the work of exchanging oxygen and carbon dioxide. The fetus is connected by the umbilical cord to the placenta, the organ that develops and implants in the mother's uterus during pregnancy. Through the blood vessels in the umbilical cord, the fetus receives all the necessary nutrition, oxygen, and life support from the mother through the placenta. Waste products and carbon dioxide from the fetus are sent back through the umbilical cord and placenta to the mother's circulation to be eliminated.

Fetal circulation differs from the adult circulation due to the presence of certain vessels and **shunts**. These shunts close after birth, and most of the fetal vessels are visible as remnants in the adult circulation. The function of these shunts is to direct oxygen-rich venous blood to the systemic circulation and to ensure oxygen-deplete venous blood bypasses the underdeveloped pulmonary circulation.

Capillary Exchange

Capillary exchange refers to the exchange of material from the blood into the tissues in the capillary. Exchange of materials between the circulating blood and the organs and tissues of the body takes place in the capillaries and postcapillary venules. These are often designated exchange vessels. In these vessels:

- Blood velocity is slowest
- Surface area per unit mass of tissue is highest
- Blood-to-cell distances are generally very short

All these factors favor rapid exchange.

Order of size of pore in capillaries: Liver > GIT > Muscles > Brain

Configurations of microvascular networks vary according to the structures of specific organs and tissues. In skeletal muscles, the exchange vessels tend to run parallel to the muscle fibers, in the interstices between them. In glandular organs, acini and tubules are surrounded by basket-like networks. In the lungs, the capillaries are sandwiched between the walls of adjacent alveoli. Exchange vessels are distributed more densely in organs and tissues of high metabolic rate (heart, brain) or specialized transport function (lungs, kidneys). Total exchange vessel blood flow depends mainly on arteriolar resistance, because the capillaries and venules contribute only a small fraction of total vascular resistance. Lymphatic system is a *scavenger system* that removes excess fluid, excess protein molecules and other matter from the tissue space. Permeability of renal glomerular membrane for water and electrolytes is about 500 times the permeability of muscle capillaries.

There are 3 Types of Capillaries, namely *Continuous capillaries, Discontinuous capillaries (*Also known as 'sinusoids') and *Fenestrated capillaries,* which perform capillary function with different efficiencies in different organs. Arteriovenous Shunts. In most organs and tissues, all the blood passes through exchange vessels. Arteriovenous shunts, specialized thick-walled muscular vessels connecting arterioles directly to muscular venules and bypassing local exchange vessels, are found mainly in the skin, particularly in hairless, exposed regions (fingers and toes; face, ears, and nose). Their function is related to control of skin temperature and heat loss.

The walls of capillaries and postcapillary venules consist of a single layer of thin endothelial cells supported on their collagenous basement membrane (basal lamina). Permeation of water and solutes may take place through the cells, around the cells, or through the junctional spaces between them.

Fluid, electrolytes, gases, small and large molecular weight substances can transverse the capillary endothelium by several different mechanisms: diffusion, bulk flow, vesicular transport, and active transport.

Small molecules can cross into and out of capillaries via simple or facilitated diffusion. Diffusion is particularly important for gases (O_2 and CO_2) and lipid-soluble substances; fluid and electrolytes are also exchanged, in part, by diffusion forces. Glucose, amino acids, and ions—including sodium, potassium, calcium, and chloride—use transporters to move through specific channels in the membrane by facilitated diffusion. Some large proteins in blood plasma can move into and out of the endothelial cells packaged within vesicles by endocytosis and exocytosis. Water moves by osmosis.

Control of Blood Pressure

Blood pressure is a measure of how well the cardiovascular system is working. Blood pressure (BP) is the pressure exerted by circulating blood upon the walls of blood vessels and is one of the principal vital signs. The pressure of the circulating blood decreases as blood moves through arteries, arterioles, capillaries, and veins; the term blood pressure generally refers to arterial blood pressure, i.e., the pressure in the larger arteries. Regulation of blood pressure is through renal, baro-receptor and chemoreceptors mechanisms.

The cardiovascular center can alter heart rate and stroke volume to increase blood pressure and flow. The cardiovascular center is a part of the human brain found in the medulla oblongata, responsible for regulation of cardiac output. The cardiovascular center contains three distinct components: the cardioaccelerator center, the cardioinhibitor center, and the vasomotor center.Numerous receptors in the circulatory system can detect changes in pH or stretch and signal these changes to the cardiovascular center.The cardiovascular center can alter heart rate and stroke volume to increase blood pressure and flow.

The cardioaccelerator center stimulates cardiac function by regulating heart rate and stroke volume via sympathetic stimulation from the cardiac accelerator nerve. The cardioinhibitor center slows cardiac function by decreasing heart rate and stroke volume via parasympathetic stimulation from the vagus nerve. The vasomotor center controls vessel tone or contraction of the smooth muscle in the tunica media. Changes in diameter affect peripheral resistance, pressure, and flow, which in turn affect cardiac output. The majority of these neurons act via the release of the neurotransmitter norepinephrine from sympathetic neurons. Although each center functions independently, they are not anatomically distinct.

The kidneys provide a hormonal mechanism for the regulation of blood pressure by managing blood volume. The renin-angiotensin-aldosterone system of the kidneys regulates blood volume. In response to rising blood pressure, the juxtaglomerular cells in the kidneys secrete renin into the blood.

Blood pressure is controlled chemically through dilation or constriction of the blood vessels by vasodilators and vasoconstrictors. Generalized vasoconstriction usually results in an increase in systemic blood pressure, but it may also occur in specific tissues, causing a localized reduction in blood flow. Vasoconstriction results from increased concentration of calcium (Ca^{2+}) ions within vascular smooth muscle.

When blood vessels dilate, the flow of blood is increased due to a decrease in vascular resistance. Therefore, dilation of arterial blood vessels (mainly the arterioles) causes a decrease in blood pressure. Localized tissues increase blood flow in multiple ways, including releasing vasodilators, primarily adenosine, into the local interstitial fluid, which diffuses to capillary beds provoking local vasodilation.

Many physical factors that influence arterial pressure. Each may in turn be influenced by physiological factors such as diet, exercise, disease, drugs or alcohol, stress, and obesity.

Adjustments of Circulation During Exercise

Understanding of the physiology of exercise is important for anyone involved in the care, handling, training, feeding, breeding, or use of horses and several draught animals like ox,camel and buffalo etc .

Oxidation of substrate during exercise is dependent upon a nearly constant supply of oxygen. Oxygen delivery to the muscle is dependent upon optimal functioning of the respiratory and cardiovascular systems. Increased oxygen delivery to muscle is achieved through increases in minute ventilation, alveolar ventilation, oxygen-carrying capacity of blood, and cardiac output.

The integrated response to severe exercise involves fourfold to fivefold increases in cardiac output, which are due primarily to increases in cardiac rate and to a lesser extent to augmentation of stroke volume.

Exercise increases the sympathetic activity and reduces parasympathetic activity, leading to increased contractility and increased stroke volume. The increased stroke volume and heart rate cause an increase in cardiac output, which is necessary to deliver more oxygen to exercising skeletal muscle.

During exercise the mechanoreceptors present in the muscles detect changes in the tension of the muscle and send afferent sensory information to the brain, thereby activating the cardiovascular control centre in the medulla.

The cardiovascular control centre reduces the activity of the parasympathetic nervous system and increases the activity of sympathetic nervous system, changing the efferent signals going to the heart and the arteriolar smooth muscle.

This change in parasympathetic and sympathetic activity has greater effect on cardiac output. Cardiac output can be increased 4-8 times the value at rest in humans where as in a trained thoroughbred horse a ten fold increase occurs during maximum exercise.

At the onset, parasympathetic activity decreases causing an increase in heart rate. At the same time, increase in muscular activity and breathing improves the function of respiratory and skeletal muscle pumps causing an increase in venous return to the heart, resulting in increased stroke volume. Therefore, during initial stages of exercise, the cardiac output increase is due to increase in heart rate and stroke volume.

Next, sympathetic stimulation of the heart increases, causing an increase in both heart rate and contractility. During the later stage of exercise, increase in heart rate, increases cardiac output rather than increase in stroke volume.

In addition to changes in cardiac output, blood flow pattern also changes during exercise. During rest, skeletal muscle receive only about 20% of cardiac output, whereas during exercise they receive 88% of total cardiac output i.e., blood flow to skeletal muscles is increased from 1.2 l/min at rest to 2.2 l/min during exercise. These changes in blood flow are as a result of vasodilation of the arterioles of skeletal muscle and heart. The increase in activity causes a generalised vasoconstriction of the arterioles of other organs.

In skeletal muscle, local release of paracrine factors causes vascular smooth muscle to release by opposing vasoconstrictive effects of α-adrenergic receptor stimulation. These factors together cause an intense local vasodilatation thereby increasing the blood flow to the muscles.

Vasodilatation of the arterioles of skeletal muscles and vasoconstriction of arterioles of other organs causes a decrease in the total peripheral resistance.

As a result blood pressure increases slightly during exercise. This stimulates the baroreceptor reflex and brings back the BP to the normal by decreasing cardiac output or total peripheral resistance. The afferent signal from the muscle mechanoreceptors also changes the set point of the baroreceptor reflex allowing BP to increase slightly during exercise. However, in the presence of circulatory impairment, where oxygen delivery to the exercising muscles is impaired as occurs to complete heart block where normal heart rate increases during exercise are prevented, or in congestive right heart failure, where normal stroke volume increases during exercise are impaired, or in the presence of severe anemia, where oxygen-carrying capacity of the blood is limited, visceral blood flows are reduced drastically and blood is diverted to the exercising musculature.

Aerobic metabolism and anaerobic glycolysis result in the production of waste products, principal among which are carbon dioxide and lactate. The blood lactate is the biochemical index of muscular fatigue.

Horses develop a capacity to store some extra oxygenated blood in their spleen. When the horse runs, its spleen contracts and forces a fresh supply of oxygen-rich red blood cells into its blood stream, effectively pumping extra oxygen into its cardiovascular system virtually on demand.

Identification of performance genes in race horses has been carried out recently.

Training imparts the animal with the physiologic adaptations necessary to perform at a high level with minimal risk of injury.Training results in a multitude of changes in the body at cellular, tissue, organ,and whole organism levels. At an organ level training results in an increase in function, usually associated with increases in organ size.

Performance testing of draught animals and horses requires measurement of heart rate and or muscle lactate measurement. Fitness tests increasingly use treadmills for performance testing.

Summary

- The circulatory system is responsible for the transport of the various essential compounds and other factors around the body, as well as the removal of the metabolic wastes that accumulate in the tissues from body activities to places of elimination.
- The main components of the circulatory system are the heart, arteries, capillaries, and veins.
- The ability of an organ to regulate its own blood flow is termed local regulation of blood flow and is mediated by vasoconstrictor and vasodilator substances released by the tissue surrounding blood vessels (vasoactive metabolites) and by the vascular endothelium.
- Blood pressure means the force exerted by the blood against any unit area of the vessel's wall.

5

Muscle Physiology

The muscular system allows movement and necessary functions such as circulation, digestion, and breathing. It is made up of muscles and connective tissue, such as tendons. The muscular system also helps provide support and shape. In the body, muscles have primary functions to provide motion, maintain posture, and generate heat

Muscle cells are excitable cells which produce an action potential along their cell membrane on being excited electrically, chemically or mechanically. Muscle cells contain contractile proteins which get activated by the generated action potential and produce a contractile action.

Muscles consist largely of protein and are the lean meat of an animal that is used as food for human consumption. Muscles can be voluntary or involuntary. Voluntary muscles are those that can be controlled. When an animal walks or chews, it is using voluntary muscles. Involuntary muscles are automatic and operate without any thought on the part of an animal. Muscles that operate the heart, intestines, and lungs are involuntary.

Thus muscles are endowed with the following characteristics.

- Excitability
- Contractility
- Extensibility
- Elasticity

The muscular system performs the following functions in the body

- Movement
- Maintain posture
- Stabilize joints
- Generate heat
- Movement of substances within the body

Muscle converts chemical energy into mechanical energy. The energy source of muscles is energy rich phosphate compound phosphorylcreatine which is hydrolysed to creatine and phosphate groups, a process wherein considerable energy is released.

Muscle Physiology-Muscles and Movement

Movement is one of the basic characteristics of all living things. All animals can move and one of the important attributes of the movement is contractility which may occur in various ways. The movement of the body parts or as a whole is due to the unique property of specialized tissues called the muscle tissue. Muscles are excitable tissues or effector organs which may respond to various stimuli, such as pressure changes, heat, light etc. The functions of various systems such as digestion, reproduction, respiration, circulation, excretion and the like, are also due to movements of muscles . Muscles are therefore the tissues which accomplish the movements in an organism.

Muscles have the property of contractility, extensibility and elasticity. In most vertebrates, muscles have two kinds of arrangements.

- Those muscles which move the appendages find their origins as well as insertions on the endoskeletal structures are called phasic muscles. Phasic muscles function on a lever system and always occur in antagonistic pairs.
- Besides this, muscles occurring in soft organs like heart, urinary bladder, digestive tract and the body wall are called tonic muscles. These muscles do not have origins and insertions comparable to phasic muscles.

The function of the muscles is closely related to the structure, and therefore a detailed structure of the different types of muscles is necessary. In vertebrates, there are three distinct types of muscles which constitute about 60-75 percent of the total body weight. They are : (1) Skeletal muscles (2) Smooths muscles and (3) Cardiac muscles.

Muscle is covered in a layer of connective muscle tissue known as the Epimysium. The epimysium is composed of irregular connective tissue. The Epimysium protects the muscle from friction against other muscles and bones. The next layer is the perimysium. The perimysium surrounds groups of 10 to 200 muscle fibers separating them into bundles called fascicles.The deepest layer is the endomysium. It surrounds each muscle fiber separating one from another. It is composed of loose connective tissue.

Skeletal Muscle (striated muscle)

Skeletal muscle is controlled by the conscious mind and moves the bones of the skeleton so that the animal can move around. It is called skeletal muscle because it moves the bones of the skeleton, which in turn move the animal around. The function of skeletal muscles in the body is movement and heat production. Skeletal Muscles are those which attach to bones and have the main function of contracting to facilitate movement of our skeletons. They are also sometimes known as striated muscles due to their appearance. Even under low-power magnification, skeletal muscle cells are obviously striped. The cause of this 'stripy' appearance is the bands of Actin and Myosin which form the Sarcomere, found within the Myofibrils. A whole muscle consists of a large number of muscle Fibers (cells), plus connective tissue wrappings, blood vessels, and nerve fibers. Fascia separates the skin from skeletal muscle.

Skeletal muscles are also sometimes called voluntary muscles because we have direct control over them through nervous impulses from our brains sending messages to the muscle. Contractions can vary to produce powerful, fast movements or small precision actions. Skeletal muscles also have the ability to stretch or contract and still return to their original shape.

Skeletal muscle comprises the great mass of the somatic musculature. The voluntary muscle of the body is called skeletal muscle because attachments are made with bone. Skeletal muscle has well developed cross striations and does not contract in the absence of nervous stimulation.Myofibrils account for about 80 % of the cellular volume of a skeletal muscle fiber. Myofibrils are the contractile elements of skeletal muscle fibers.Within the myofibril are thick and thin myofilaments. These myofilaments are arranged in a regular pattern, which produces a repeating series of dark and light bands.

The muscles are made up of a large number of parallel fibres, which are between 0.1 and 0.01 mm in diameter, but may be several centimetres long. These fibres in turn are made up of thinner fibrils. These fibrils have characteristic cross striations : the so called Z lines, which are repeated at completely regular intervals. The region between two Z lines is called a sarcomere. In vertebrate muscles the distance between the 2 Z lines, the sarcomere length, tends to be very uniform, about 2.5 μm in a relaxed muscle.

A sarcomere is the functional contractile unit of skeletal muscle. It consists of several proteins. Actin and myosin are two contractile proteins. There are two regulatory proteins present which help to control the contraction process.The two regulatory proteins are tropomyosin and troponin. The myofibrils are made up of several structural proteins such as myomesin, connectin and titin etc. These proteins are responsible for the alignment, stability, elasticity and extensibility of myofibrils.

From the narrow Z line very thin filaments extend in both directions and in the center, these thin filaments are interspersed with somewhat thicker filaments. The result is a number of less conspicuous bands located between the Z lines, the appearance of these bands changes with the state of contraction of the muscle. The thin filaments are about 0.005 μm in diameter and thick filaments are about twice that size, about 0.01 μm in diameter. The length of the thick filament is about 1.5 μm. The thin filament in different muscles differ somewhat more in length. They are often between 2 and 2.6 μm from tip to tip (or about half this length measured from Z line to the tip). The arrangement of the filaments is extremely regular and well ordered. In striated muscles the thick filament consists of myosin and thin filament of the actin. The thick and thin filaments are linked together by a system of molecular cross linkages and when the muscle contracts and shortens, these cross linkages are rearranged so that the thick filaments slide in between the thin filaments, reducing the distance between the Z lines.

This model of muscle structure is well supported by electron micrographs of the filaments in various stages of contraction. Neither the thick filaments, nor the thin filaments change in length during contraction, but it can clearly be seen that they move relative to each other.

What is even more important in support of the sliding filament model is that the force developed by a muscle is related to the amount of overlap of the filaments.

The immediate source of energy for muscle contraction is adenosine triphosphate (ATP

) a high energy compound formed in the mitochondria of the cell. ATP is the only substance in the muscle proteins can use directly. However the amount of ATP present in the muscles is very small. The total quantity may be sufficient for no more than ten rapid contractions. It follows, therefore, that ATP must be restored again very rapidly, for otherwise the muscles would soon be exhausted.The restoration is brought about by creatine phosphate, which is present in larger amounts. The creatinine phosphate must, however, eventually be replenished and the ultimate energy source is the oxidation of carbohydrates or fatty acids. Carbohydrates are stored in the muscle in the form of glycogen, which is often present in an amount of between 0.5 and 2% of the wet weight of the muscles. In the absence of oxygen, the glycogen can still yield energy by being split into lactic acid, but the amount of energy is then only a small fraction, about 7% of that available from complete oxidation.

Smooth Muscle

Smooth muscle carries out most of the unconscious, internal movements that the body needs to maintain itself.The general function of smooth muscle is to propulsion of food and urine. In contrast to the striated muscle (the skeletal and heart muscle), the muscles of internal organs are smooth (also called unstriated, non striated, plain or involuntary muscle). This type of muscle occurs in the stomach, intestine, bladder, ureters, uterus, bronchi, blood vessels and so on. Smooth muscle is also known as Involuntary muscle due to our inability to control its movements, or unstriated as it does not have the stripy appearance of Skeletal muscle. Smooth muscle is found in the walls of hollow organs such as the Stomach, Oesophagus, Bronchi and in the walls of blood vessels. This muscle type is stimulated by involuntary neurogenic impulses and has slow, rhythmical contractions used in controlling internal organs, for example, moving food along the Oesophagus or constricting blood vessels during Vasoconstriction.

Vertebrate smooth muscle is innervated from the autonomic nervous system by two sets of nerves. One set is stimulatory and the other is inhibitory (i.e. the two sets act in an antagonistic manner). Smooth muscle differs from voluntary muscle in that the muscle layers, mostly located in the walls of the hollow organs contain numerous nerve fibres and nerve cells.

Smooth muscles need not to be stimulated in order to contract. It shows spontaneous rhythmic contractions that can vary greatly in both frequency and intensity. The internal neurons and nerve fibres in the muscle may have considerable influence on this activity.

The reason that no striations are visible in smooth muscle is that the filaments, which presumably are present, are not regularly aligned to form visible bands.

Cardiac Muscle

Cardiac muscle as the name indicates is found only in the heart.The general function of cardiac muscle is pumping blood to the heart, lungs and body. This type of muscle is found solely in the walls of the heart. Cardiac muscle starts the entire heart beating long before an animal is born and keeps it going until the animal dies. It has similarities with skeletal muscles in that it is striated and with smooth muscles in that its contractions are not under conscious control. Cardiac muscle has a well-developed system of T-tubules and sarcoplasmic reticulum.In contrast to skeletal muscle, cardiac muscle consists of short, branched muscle fibers, bound tightly together in a meshwork. The contact regions between the muscle fibers contain gap junctions that couple the cells electrically, allowing the action potential to spread from cell to cell throughout the cardiac muscle. Action potentials in cardiac muscle tissue spread from fiber to fiber, which allows depolarization to spread through the entire heart, leading to coordinated virtually simultaneous contraction of all the cardiac muscle fibers in a heart chamber and permitting the movement of large volumes of blood through the cardiovascular system. This is why cardiac muscle tissue is considered to be a functional syncytium.

Properties of Cardiac Muscles

Cardiac muscle (also called heart muscle or myocardium) is one of three types of vertebrate muscles, with the other two being skeletal and smooth muscles. It is an involuntary, striated muscle that constitutes the main tissue of the walls of the heart.

1. Conductivity **2. Contractility**

1. Conductivity

Impulse can pass from cell to cell through the specialized gap junctions in the intercalated discs.

Force velocity curve

Curve against total load and initial velocity of contraction

When load is zero ———— Velocity is maximum

When load is maximum ———— Velocity is zero

2. Contractility

Myocardial cells have many features and properties of red skeletal muscle cells.

In cardiac muscle, Ca^{2+} influx during action potentials induces Ca^{2+} release from sarcoplasmic reticulum. The depolarization phase of the action potentials in cardiac muscle cells lasts 200-300ms in large mammals which is in contract to few milli seconds in case of neurons and skeletal muscle cells.

Cardiac muscle is highly specialised. It is under the control of the autonomic nervous system, however, even without a nervous input contraction can occur due to cells called pacemaker cells. Cardiac muscle is highly resistant to fatigue due to the presence of a large number of mitochondria, myoglobin and a good blood supply allowing continuous aerobic metabolism. Cardiac muscle requires a continuous supply of oxygen to regenerate ATP by oxidative metabolism. The cardiac muscle cells contain many more mitochondria which equip them for high rate of continuous aerobic phosphorylation.

Basic Muscle Unit Characteristic-Electrical Phenomenon in Muscle Cell

Each muscle fibre itself contains cylindrical organelles known as Myofibrils. Each muscle fiber contains hundreds to thousands of Myofibrils. These are bundles of Actin and Myosin proteins which run the length of the muscle fiber and are important in muscle contraction.

In muscle cells, for example, an action potential is the first step in the chain of events leading to contraction. In neurons, action potentials play a central role in cell-to-cell communication. Action potentials in neurons are also known as "nerve impulses" or "spikes". Nearly all cell membranes in animals maintain a voltage difference between the exterior and interior of the cell, called the membrane potential. A typical voltage across an animal cell membrane is −70 mV. This means that the interior of the cell has a negative voltage relative to the exterior. In most types of cells, the membrane potential usually stays fairly constant. Some types of cells, however, are electrically active in the sense that their voltages fluctuate over time. In some types of electrically active cells, including neurons and muscle cells, the voltage fluctuations frequently take the form of a rapid upward spike followed by a rapid fall. These up-and-down cycles are known as action potentials. Waveform analysis plays an important role in the assessment of nerve and muscle action potentials. Electromyography can distinguish primary nerve and muscle disorders.

Membrane Potential- ionic Basis of Resting Membrane Potential

Nerves are responsible for controlling the contraction of muscles, determining the number, sequence and force of muscular contraction.

The action potential that is conducted along the length of the muscle cell originates in a depolarization of the postsynaptic membrane of the neuromuscular junction caused by the release of acetylcholine from the presynaptic nerve terminal. The synapse is thus potentially a key control point in the chain of command for muscular contraction.

A resting (non-signaling) neuron has a voltage across its membrane called the resting membrane potential, or simply the resting potential. The resting potential is determined by concentration gradients of ions across the membrane and by membrane permeability to each type of ion. In a resting neuron, there are concentration gradients across the membrane for Na^+ and K^+. Ions move down their gradients via channels, leading to a separation of charge that creates the resting potential. The membrane is much more permeable to K^+ than to Na^+ ions , so the resting potential is close to the equilibrium potential of K^+ (the potential that would be generated by K^+ if it were the only ion in the system).

Muscle Action Potential

Action potential, the brief reversal of electric polarization of the membrane of a muscle cell. In the muscle cell it produces the contraction required for all movement. Before stimulation, a muscle cell has a slightly negative electric polarization; that is, its interior has a negative charge compared with the extracellular fluid. This polarized state is created by a high concentration of positively charged sodium ions outside the cell and a high concentration of negatively charged chloride ions (as well as a lower concentration of positively charged potassium) inside. The resulting resting potential usually measures about −75 millivolts (mV), or −0.075 volt, the minus sign indicating a negative charge inside.

In the generation of the action potential, stimulation of the cell by sensory muscle receptor cells partially opens channel-shaped protein molecules in the membrane. Sodium diffuses into the cell, shifting that part of the membrane toward a less-negative polarization. If this local potential reaches a critical state called the threshold potential (measuring about −60 mV), then sodium channels open completely. Sodium floods that part of the cell, which instantly depolarizes to an action potential of about +55 mV. Depolarization activates sodium channels in adjacent parts of the membrane, so that the impulse moves along the fibre.

If the entry of sodium into the fibre were not balanced by the exit of another ion of positive charge, an action potential could not decline from its peak value and return to the resting potential. The declining phase of the action potential is caused by the closing of sodium channels and the opening of potassium channels, which allows a charge approximately equal to that brought into the cell to leave in the form of potassium ions. Subsequently, protein transport molecules pump sodium ions out of the cell and potassium ions in. This restores the original ion concentrations and readies the cell for a new action potential.

Thus the muscle contraction cycle can be divided into

- **Latent period of muscle:** The delay / gap between the receipt of a stimulus by a sensory nerve and the response to it is called latent period.
- **Contraction period:** During this period the muscle undergoes depolarization and it starts contracting.
- **Relaxation period:** It is the period during which the muscle relaxes as the stimuli is stopped or moves away.
- **Refractory period:** It is the period that follows stimulation during which the muscle becomes unresponsive to the further stimulation. An important characteristic of the action potential is the refractory period, which is the time after initiation of an action potential when it is impossible or more difficult to generate a second action potential. The absolute refractory period is the time from initial depolarization to when repolarization is almost complete. The basis for the absolute refractory period is Na+ channel inactivation, when it is impossible to recruit a sufficient number of Na+ channels to generate a second depolarizing stimulus until the previously activated Na+ channels have recovered from inactivation, which takes several milliseconds.

Excitation and Propagation of Impulse Characteristics-latent Period Refractiveness, Threshold Level-all & None Characteristics

Excitability is defined as the reaction or response of a tissue to irritation or stimulation. It is a physicochemical change. Stimulus is the change in environment. It is defined as an agent or influence or act, which causes the response in an excitable tissue.

The myelinated nerve fibres have a wrapping of myelin sheath with gaps at regular intervals which are devoid of myelin sheath (nodes of Ranvier). The myelin sheath acts as an insulator and does not allow the current flow. Therefore, in myelinated nerve fibres the local circuit of current flow only occurs from one node of Ranvier to the adjacent node. That is, the impulse (action potential) jumps from one node of Ranvier to next. This is known as saltatory conduction. Since the impulse jumps from one node to other, the speed of conduction in the myelinated fibres is much rapid (50–100 times faster) than the unmyelinated fibre.

In transmission across neuromuscular junction, an end plate potential (EPP) is developed at the motor end plate by the nerve impulse travelling across the innervating axon. The End Plate Potential is localized and non-propagated. However, when EPP reaches a threshold level it produces an action potential which propagates over muscle fibre surface and into the muscle fibre along the transverse tubules.

The muscle action potential lasts roughly 2–4 ms and the absolute refractory period is roughly 1–3 ms, shorter than other cells.

The all-or-none law is a principle that states that the strength of a response of a nerve cell or muscle fiber is not dependent upon the strength of the stimulus. If a stimulus is above a certain threshold, a nerve or muscle fiber will fire. Essentially, there will either be a full response or there will be no response at all for an individual neuron or muscle fiber. If a stimulus is strong enough, an action potential occurs and a neuron sends information down an axon away from the cell body and toward the synapse.

In electrophysiology, the threshold potential is the critical level to which a membrane potential must be depolarized to initiate an action potential. Changes in cell polarization result in the signal being propagated down the length of the axon.

While the all-or-none law was initially applied to the muscles of the heart, it was later found that neurons and other muscles also respond to stimuli according to this principle.

Contractile Mechanism

Each muscle fibre is made up of smaller fibres called myofibrils. These contain even smaller structures called actin and myosin filaments. These filaments slide in and out between each other to form a muscle contraction hence called the sliding filament **theory**.

- A nervous impulse arrives at the neuromuscular junction, which causes a release of a chemical called Acetylcholine. The presence of Acetylcholine causes the depolarisation of the motor end plate which travels throughout the muscle by the transverse tubules, causing Calcium (Ca+) to be released from the sarcoplasmic reticulum.

- In the presence of high concentrations of Ca+, the Ca+ binds to Troponin, changing its shape and so moving Tropomyosin from the active site of the Actin. The Myosin filaments can now attach to the Actin, forming a cross-bridge.
- The breakdown of ATP releases energy which enables the Myosin to pull the Actin filaments inwards and so shorten the muscle. This occurs along the entire length of every myofibril in the muscle cell.
- The Myosin detaches from the Actin and the cross-bridge is broken when an ATP molecule binds to the Myosin head. When the ATP is then broken down the Myosin head can again attach to an Actin binding site further along the Actin filament and repeat the 'power stroke'. This repeated pulling of the Actin over the myosin is often known as the ratchet mechanism.
- This process of muscular contraction can last for as long as there are adequate ATP and Ca+ stores. Once the impulse stops the Ca+ is pumped back to the Sarcoplasmic Reticulum and the Actin returns to its resting position causing the muscle to lengthen and relax.

Substrates within the muscle serve to power muscular contractions. They include molecules such as adenosine triphosphate (ATP), glycogen and creatine phosphate. Metabolites are the substances (generally waste products) produced as a result of muscular contraction. They include chloride, potassium, lactic acid, ADP, magnesium (Mg^{2+}), reactive oxygen species, and inorganic phosphate. Accumulation of metabolites can directly or indirectly produce metabolic fatigue within muscle fibers through interference with the release of calcium (Ca^{2+}) from the sarcoplasmic reticulum or reduction of the sensitivity of contractile molecules actin and myosin to calcium.

Anaerobic metabolism is less efficient than aerobic metabolism and results in rapid buildup of lactate. Lactate decreases the pH of the blood and tissues and is metabolized slowly.

Excitation-contraction Coupling

Excitation–contraction coupling is the physiological process of converting an electrical stimulus to a mechanical response. It is the link (transduction) between the action potential generated in the sarcolemma and the start of a muscle contraction. The muscle receives a neural signal and converts that signal into mechanical force after synapsing at the neuromuscular junction.

1. The spread of depolarization
2. The binding of calcium to troponin
3. The generation of force

Muscle action potentials produced by the excitation-contraction coupling initiate calcium signals. The calcium signals activate a contraction-relaxation cycle. Contraction refers to activation of the cross-bridge cycle. Ca^{2+} activates the attractive forces between the filaments of actin and myosin by binding to troponin. However, the process of contraction will only continue if there is energy; this energy is derived from the high-energy bonds of adenosine triphosphate (ATP), which are degraded to adenosine diphosphate (ADP). In the presence of Ca2+ and ATP, the heads of the myosin molecules form cross-bridges with active sites on the thin filaments of actin. The resulting energy produces a conformational change in the myosin head region that exerts a directional force on the actin filament. As a result, the actin filaments are drawn toward the center of the sarcomere, overlapping the myosin filament. The net result is shortening of the sarcomere, or contraction of the muscle.

After cross-bridge formation during the contraction phase of excitation-contraction coupling, relaxation occurs. Ca-ATPase pumps the calcium back into the SR, lowering the calcium levels and producing muscle relaxation. The concentration of calcium must drop to allow the unbinding of Ca2+ from troponin. The filaments slide back to their initial position assisted by elastic connective tissues within the muscle and titin.

EC coupling can be modulated in response to different demands of muscle use.

Neuro-muscular Rransmission

Neuromuscular transmission is a process that permits the central nervous system to control the movement of muscles in the body. Neuromuscular junction refers to the intimate contact of the nerve endings with the muscle fibre to which they innervate. Neuromuscular junctions are specific chemical synapses. Neuromuscular transmission is a process that permits the central nervous system to control the movement of muscles in the body. Signals from the motor neuron cross a chemical synapse, the neuromuscular junction, to the muscle fiber to produce muscle contraction. This complex process involves action potentials, numerous ion channels, the neurotransmitter acetylcholine (ACh), and receptors.

- The axon of a neuron supplying a skeletal muscle loses its myelin sheath and divides into a number of fine branches which end in small swellings (knobs) called terminal buttons or end feet which form a neuromuscular junction at the centre of muscle fibre. The nerve terminal or the so-called synaptic knob contains a large number of vesicles containing acetylcholine and mitochondria. The acetylcholine is synthesized by the mitochondria and is stored in the vesicles.
- Presynaptic membrane refers to the axonal membrane lining the terminal buttons of the nerve endings. Muscle fibre membrane (sarcolemma) in the region of neuromuscular junction is called postsynaptic membrane. The muscle membrane in this region is thickened and is called motor end plate. Postsynaptic membrane is thrown into large number of folds called subneural clefts which increase the surface area. The postsynaptic membrane near the junction folds contains receptor sites for acetylcholine. The matrix of subneural cleft contains the enzyme cholinesterase which can degrade acetylcholine.
- The motor neuron's axon receives an action potential leading to depolarization of the presynaptic terminal. "Active zones" of the presynaptic terminal contain

high concentrations of voltage-dependent Ca2+ channels, mitochondria, and presynaptic vesicles containing ACh. Upon depolarization, these voltage-gated Ca2+ channels open, causing an influx of calcium into the nerve terminal. Ca2+ influx induces the cascade that begins with phosphorylation of proteins called synapsins, which keep vesicles containing ACh in a presynaptic actin network. Once this cascade starts, presynaptic vesicle release from the actin network begins, allowing presynaptic membrane fusion. Vesicle contents, which include ACh, are subsequently released into the synaptic cleft via exocytosis.

Sequence of events which causes transmission of impulse through the neuromuscular junction are

- Release of acetylcholine by the nerve terminals,
- Effect of acetylcholine on the postsynaptic membrane,
- Development of end plate potential,
- Miniature end plate potential,
- Removal of acetylcholine by cholinesterase and
- Nerve impulses cause the release of a neurotransmitter, acetylcholine (ACh), into the junction between the nerve cell and the muscle cell.Acetylcholine diffuses across the 30-50 nm synaptic cleft to reach its target, nicotinic receptors, on the postjunctional muscle fiber. Some of the neurotransmitter is lost and some is inactivated before reaching the postjunctional membrane.
- Once ACh reaches the postjunctional membrane, it binds to nicotinic ACh receptors, which are permeable to Na+ and Ca2+. Binding of ACh to these receptors causes a conformational change, allowing Na+ and Ca2+ influx into the cell. These receptors are also permeable to K+ (although to a lesser extent), which flows out of the cell. Acetylcholine binding cation influx causes a miniature end-plate potential (MEPP) in which the cell starts to become depolarized. If several vesicles are released, the MEPPs summate to generate an end-plate potential of the muscle fiber that leads to an action potential if large enough. This action potential spreads among the plasma membrane and T-tubule system, causing release of Ca2+ from the sarcoplasmic reticulum and ultimately muscle contraction.

Acetylcholine is rapidly degraded by acetylcholinesterase to prevent re excitation of muscle. Acetylcholine is hydrolyzed by acetylcholinesterase to acetate and choline. The ion channels on the postsynaptic membrane close following ACh reduction, thus repolarizing the cell and causing muscle relaxation.

Neuromuscular blockers (e.g. Curare , Succinylcholine and Carbamylcholine) are the drugs that block transmission at the neuromuscular junction. Muscle relaxant function by blocking neuromuscular transmission. In clinical use, neuromuscular block is used adjunctively to anesthesia to produce paralysis, and causing relaxation of skeletal muscles. Dogs or cats with a neuromuscular disorder present with varying degree of muscle weakness and muscle wastage. This muscle weakness may affect the limbs so that animals are unable to stand or exercise normally but also can affect other muscles in the body. The most common diseases affecting the neuromuscular junction are botulism, tick paralysis and myasthenia gravis.

Types of Muscle Contraction

Muscle contractions are defined by the changes in the length of the muscle during contraction. Muscle fiber generates tension through the action of actin and myosin cross-bridge cycling. While under tension, the muscle may lengthen, shorten, or remain the same. Although the term contraction implies shortening, when referring to the muscular system, it means muscle fibers generating tension with the help of motor neurons. Several types of muscle contractions occur and they are defined by the changes in the length of the muscle during contraction. Muscle contractions during exercise can be divided into three categories; isotonic (meaning same tension throughout the contraction), isometric (meaning same tension), also known as a static contraction and isokinetic muscle contractions which are performed with a constant speed throughout the movement. There are different types of muscle contractions:

Isometric Contraction

Isometric contractions occur when there is no change in the length of the contracting muscle. If I hold the weight still, the muscle is engaged but doesn't change length. This occurs when carrying an object in front of you as the weight of the object is pulling your arms down but your muscles are contracting to hold the object at the same level. Another example is when you grip something, such as a tennis racket. There is no movement in the joints of the hand, but the muscles are contracting to provide a force sufficient enough to keep a steady hold on the racket.

Isotonic Contraction

Isotonic contractions are those which cause the muscle to change length as it contracts and causes movement of a body part. There are two types of Isotonic contraction:

Concentric

Concentric contractions are those which cause the muscle to shorten as it contracts. An example is bending the elbow from straight to fully flexed, causing a concentric contraction of the Biceps Brachii muscle. Concentric contractions are the most common type of muscle contraction and occur frequently in daily and sporting activities

Eccentric Contractions

Eccentric contractions are the opposite of concentric and occur when the muscle lengthens as it contracts. This occurs when lowering the dumbbell down in a bicep curl exercise. The muscle is still contracting to hold the weight all the way down but the bicep muscle is lengthening.

Isokinetic Contractions

Isokinetic contractions are similar to Isotonic in that the muscle changes length during the contraction, where they differ is that Isokinetic contractions produce movements of a constant speed. The best is breaststroke in swimming, where the water provides a constant, even resistance to the movement of adduction.

Phenomenon of Fatigue

Fatigue is defined as the decrease in muscular activity due to repeated stimuli. When stimuli are applied repeatedly, after some time, the muscle does not show any response to the stimulus. This condition is called fatigue.Fatigue may also be defined as physical and/or mental weariness resulting from exertion, that is, an inability to continue exercise at the same intensity with a resultant deterioration in performance. Fatigue may result from a number of causes, including loss of muscle mass, muscle deconditioning, nutritional deficiencies, oxygen delivery, and anemia. Fatigue is a failure of the muscle to sustain force in a prolonged contraction or to reattain force in repeated contractions. Fatigue is a reversible phenomenon. Fatigued muscle recovers if given rest and nutrition.

There are two main causes of muscle fatigue:

- the limitations of a nerve's ability to generate a sustained signal (neural fatigue);
- and the reduced ability of the muscle fiber to contract (metabolic fatigue)

Muscle fatigue is the decline in ability of a muscle to generate force.There is a relationship between the development of fatigue and the depletion of energy stores in exercising muscle. In prolonged exercise, such as marathon running, fatigue is associated with glycogen depletion due to oxidative glycolysis. Intense exercise that lasts only a few minutes is associated with the accumulation of lactate and an intracellular acidosis due to anaerobic (nonoxidative) glycolysis. In both types of exercise there is a reduction of phosphocreatine, although no appreciable depletion of adenosine triphosphate (ATP).

Repeated bouts of high-intensity activity can also result in depletion of the intracellular substrate, glycogen. Since glycogen is the fundamental fuel used to sustain both glycolysis and oxidative phosphorylation, fatigue is readily apparent as cellular resources are exhausted.

Cardiac muscle is highly resistant to fatigue due to the presence of a large number of mitochondria, myoglobin and a good blood supply allowing continuous aerobic metabolism.

Rigor Mortis

The rigidity of a body after death is called rigor mortis. Rigor mortis is due to a biochemical change in the muscles that occurs several hours after death. When muscle fibers are completely depleted of ATP and phosphorylcreatine, they develop a state of extreme rigidity called rigor. When this occurs after death, the condition is called rigor mortis.

When the animal dies, lack of oxygen to the cells causes normal activities and barriers within the cells to break down. After death, most of the Ca2+ spills out of the sarcoplasmic reticulum which causes contraction of skeletal muscle fibers, fueled by the last of the ATP molecules in the sarcoplasm. As all the ATP is used up in the contraction and no more is being made; therefore no energy source is available to relax the muscles. So muscles get stuck in the contracted position.

Rigor mortis is not a permanent condition because as soon as the muscle fibers begin to decompose, the cross-bridges between the myosin and actin filaments break down and the muscles become relaxed. The time of death of the animal can be established on the basis of onset of rigor mortis and the subsequent muscle relaxation.

The energy required for muscle activity in the live animal is obtained from sugars (glycogen) in the muscle. In the healthy and well-rested animal, the glycogen content of the muscle is high. After the animal has been slaughtered, the glycogen in the muscle is converted into lactic acid, and the muscle and carcass becomes firm (rigor mortis). Rigor Mortis or postmortem rigidity, is the third stage of death. It is one of the recognizable signs of death, characterized by stiffening of the limbs of the corpse caused by chemical changes in the muscles post-mortem. After death, respiration in an organism ceases, depleting the source of oxygen used in the making of adenosine triphosphate (ATP). ATP is required to cause separation of the actin-myosin cross-bridges during relaxation of muscle. When oxygen is no longer present, the body may continue to produce ATP via anaerobic glycolysis. When the body's glycogen is depleted, the ATP concentration diminishes, and the body enters rigor mortis because it is unable to break those bridges. Rigor is usually complete by 6 to 8 hours after death and may last 1 to 2 days. The times are variable depending on environmental conditions and carcass conditions. During rigor mortis calcium ions of the proteins embedded in the muscle fibers are released, causing the muscle fibers to contract and become stiff.

At the time of death, a condition called "primary flaccidity" occurs. Following this, the muscles stiffen in rigor mortis. All muscles in the body are affected. Starting between two and six hours following death, rigor mortis begins with the eyelids, neck, and jaw. The sequence may be due to different lactic acid levels among different muscles, which is directly related to the difference in glycogen levels and different types of muscle fibers.

Rigor mortis is very important in meat technology. The onset of rigor mortis and its resolution partially determine the tenderness of meat. If the post-slaughter meat is immediately chilled to 15 °C (59 °F), a phenomenon known as cold shortening occurs, whereby the muscle sarcomeres shrink to a third of their original length. Cold shortening is caused by the release of stored calcium ions from the sarcoplasmic reticulum of muscle fibers, in response to the cold stimulus. The calcium ions trigger powerful muscle contraction aided by ATP molecules. To prevent cold shortening, a process known as electrical stimulation is carried out, especially in beef carcasses, immediately after slaughter and skinning. In this process, the carcass is stimulated with alternating current, causing it to contract and relax, which depletes the ATP reserve from the carcass and prevents cold shortening.

Rigor mortis then spreads to the other muscles, including the internal organs, within the next four to six hours. The onset of rigor mortis is affected by the individual's age, sex, physical condition, and muscular build. Rigor mortis may not be perceivable in many young animal corpses due to their smaller muscle mass.

Several factors also affect the progression of rigor mortis. One must take these into account when estimating the time of death. One such factor is the ambient temperature. In warm environments, the onset and pace of rigor mortis are sped up by providing a conducive environment for the metabolic processes that cause decay. Low temperatures, however, slow them down. Therefore, an animal which dies outside in frozen conditions rigor mortis may last several days more than normal.

Summary

- Muscles are excitable tissues or effector organs which may respond to various stimuli, such as pressure changes, heat, light etc.
- Muscles are characterized by the fact that a mechanical contraction follows an action potential.
- Function of the muscles is closely related to the structure.
- There are three types of muscles in the body ie- (1) Skeletal muscles (2) Smooths muscles and (3) Cardiac muscles.
- The cross-bridges of the sarcomere in skeletal muscles are made up of myosin.
- In muscle cells, an action potential, is the first step in the chain of events leading to contraction.
- Smooth muscles are largely under the control of autonomic nervous system.
- The rigidity of a body after death is called rigor mortis. Rigor mortis is due to a biochemical change in the muscles that occurs several hours after death.

6

Nervous System

A neuron is the basic unit of nervous tissue. It is specialized for the function of reception, integration and transmission of information in the body. The nerve cells are excitable, i.e. capable of generation of electrical impulses at their membranes. The electrical impulses generated in the excitable tissues, in most instances, can be used to transmit signals along the membranes.

To understand the physiological aspects it is imperative to have a knowledge about the functional anatomy and physiological properties of the nerve.

Organization of Nervous system- Mechanism of Information Processing, Hierarchical Control

Nervous system is the body's incredible information processing system. The nervous system is a complex network of nerves and cells that carry messages to and from the brain and spinal cord to various parts of the body. The mammalian nervous system has two major subdivisions: the central nervous system and the peripheral nervous system. The central nervous system comprises the brain and the spinal cord. The brain lies within the skull. The central nervous system is distinguished from the peripheral nervous system in that it is made up of a concentration of tracts, ganglia and nuclei. Thus nervous system is a structural and functional mechanism involved in the coordination of an animal's responses to internal and external environment. The Peripheral nervous system is made up of the Somatic and the Autonomic nervous systems.

The brain is surrounded by the skull to protect it from shock and external injury. The brain is precious, and evolution has gone to great lengths to protect it from damage. The most obvious is our 7mm thick skull, but the brain is also surrounded by protective fluid (cerebrospinal fluid– of the brain and spine) and a protective membrane called the meninges. Both provide further defense against physical injury. The nervous system collects and integrates sensory information, formulates a response plan and produces a motor response or output.

There are a few differences between the human and cow brain. The human brain is larger in size and shape when compared to the cow's brain. The cow brain does not have as many gyri and sulci when compared to human brain. The human brain of an adult weighs about 1200–1500 g, and 10–20 cm in length. A cow's brain is elongated in shape, whereas a human brain is rounded. The human brain is not only larger, but also heavier than a cow's brain, because it is only 400–600 g compared to 1200-1500 g of the human brain. Human brain represents 2% of weight, the largest brain in the animal world compared to the body size.

Domesticated animals have smaller brains than those of their wild forebears. At a similar body weight, the brain of the domestic cat (with an average value of 30 grams) is 23.9 % lighter than that of the wild cat, the brain of the dog is 29 % lighter than that of the wolf, and the brain of the pig is 34 % lighter than that of the wild boar.

All animals, including domestic animals and humans, depend entirely on their sense organs and nervous system for information about external environment and the internal status of their bodies. Sensory inputs, together with the genetically inherited organization and properties of the nervous system is responsible for all knowledge and determines how each animal behaves.

Nervous system specializes in Irritability and conduction.

Irritability is the ability to receive and respond to the messages from the external and internal environments.

Conduction is the ability to transmit messages to and from the coordinating centers.

The brain and nervous system are made of nerve cells called neurons. Neurons send electrochemical signals to one another, forming the basis of the brain's complex, essential functions: to form memories and thoughts, to produce actions, and to interpret the world around us. The brain contains around 100 billion neurons. But neurons don't work alone. In fact, there are as many non-neuronal cells, called glia, in the brain as there are neurons. Neurons show basic nervous system functions, such as responding to stimuli and conducting impulses from one part of the cell to another. Nerves are concerned with the quick control of bodily functions and coordination.

Nervous system may be viewed as an anatomical arrangement of neurons with a large number of different kinds of synapses through which sensory information from the periphery of the body is transmitted through numerous sensory neurons to a set of neurons in a central region of the body, where the information is integrated and from which impulses are then directed out through numerous motor neurons to effectors.

The functional arrangement of the nervous system is hierarchical. The hierarchy consists of effectors (sensory and motor) and different levels of information processing and integration in the spinal cord, brainstem and forebrain.

Glucose is virtually the sole fuel for the animal as well as human brain, except during prolonged starvation. The brain lacks fuel stores and hence requires a continuous supply of glucose. Glucose is the primary substrate for fetal metabolism. In the absence of fetal gluconeogenesis , the maternal circulation is the only source of supply and thus the mechanisms for placental uptake and transfer of glucose are of major importance. Glucose transport across the syncytiotrophoblast, the transporting epithelial layer in the placenta, occurs via sodium-independent facilitated diffusion down a concentration gradient through glucose transporters (the GLUT family). GLUT proteins have several isomers. GLUT3 has a higher affinity for glucose compared to the ubiquitous GLUT1. Glucose is transported into brain cells by the glucose transporter GLUT3. Since its discovery in 1988, GLUT3 has been the subject of numerous studies regarding tissue expression and was originally designated the neuronal glucose transporter.

Fatty acids do not serve as fuel for the brain, because they are bound to albumin in plasma and so do not traverse the blood-brain barrier. In starvation, ketone bodies generated by the liver partly replace glucose as fuel for the brain. A rise in ketone bodies also occurs in diabetes. The lack of insulin prevents the liver to absorb glucose and curtails fatty acid mobilization by adipose tissue, resulting in severe acidosis as ketone bodies are moderately strong acids. The decrease in pH impairs functioning of central nervous system adversely.

Human brain accounts for only 2% of the body's mass; it demands a large portion of the body's total energy budget, some 20%. Most of this energy is derived from the oxidation of glucose supplied to the cerebral tissue through the blood. High metabolic demands of nervous tissue are associated with complex cognitive processing by the brain tissue. The main function of energy in the brain is to fuel neural signaling and information processing. Conscious perception of sensory stimuli increases energy consumption in brain. There is a direct connection between energy in the brain and consciousness.

The brain is one of the largest and most complex organs in the human body. It is made up of more than 100 billion nerves neurons that communicate in trillions of connections called synapses. The brain integrates sensory information and directs motor responses; in higher vertebrates. It is also the centre of learning.

The brain is also divided into several lobes:

- The frontal lobes are responsible for problem solving and judgment and motor function.
- The parietal lobes(relating to the wall or outer surface of a body part) manage sensation, handwriting, and body position.
- The temporal lobes (each of the paired lobes of the brain lying beneath the temples duiVh) are involved with memory and hearing.
- The occipital lobes (the lower back part of the head) contain the brain's visual processing system.

The forebrain includes the *cerebral hemispheres* and, under these, the *brainstem,* which contains the *thalamus and hypothalamus.*

The cerebral hemispheres are separated by a deep groove, the longitudinal cerebral fissure. At the base of this fissure lies a thick bundle of nerve fibres, called the corpus callosum, which provides a communication link between the hemispheres. The left hemisphere controls the right half of the body, and vice versa, because of a crossing of the nerve fibres in the medulla or, less commonly, in the spinal cord. Although the right and left hemispheres are mirror images of one another in many ways, there are important functional distinctions. In most people, for example, the areas that control speech are located in the left hemisphere, while areas that control spatial perceptions are located in the right hemisphere.

- The *thalamus* is the main relay centre between the medulla and the cerebrum;
- The hypothalamus is an important control centre for sex drive, pleasure, pain, hunger, thirst, blood pressure, body temperature, and other visceral functions.

The hypothalamus produces hormones that control the secretions of the anterior pituitary gland, and it also produces oxytocin and antidiuretic hormone, which are stored in and released by the posterior pituitary gland.

The spinal cord is protected by a series of cervical, thoracic or lumbar vertebrae and ligaments.

Major Functional System-sensory, Consciousness, Emotion, Motor and Visceral Control

The sensory nervous system is a part of the nervous system responsible for processing sensory information. A sensory system consists of sensory neurons (including the sensory receptor cells), neural pathways, and parts of the brain involved in sensory perception. Commonly recognized sensory systems are those for vision, hearing, touch, taste, smell, and balance.

Consciousness

Consciousness serves a basic function in the nervous system that is intimately related to the actions of the skeletal muscle system. Consciousness serves as a frame that constrains and directs skeletal muscle output, thereby yielding adaptive behavior. Human brain accounts for only 2% of the body's mass; it demands a large portion of the body's total energy budget, some 20%. Most of this energy is derived from the oxidation of glucose supplied to the cerebral tissue through the blood. High metabolic demands of nervous tissue are associated with complex cognitive processing by the brain tissue. The main function of energy in the brain is to fuel neural signaling and information processing. Conscious perception of sensory stimuli increases energy consumption in brain. There is a direct connection between energy in the brain and consciousness.

Motor and Visceral Control

Many of the subconscious activities of the body are controlled in the lower areas of the brain in the medulla, pons, mesencephalon, hypothalamus, thalamus, cerebellum and basal ganglia. Subconscious control of arterial blood pressure and respiration is achieved primarily in the reticular substance of the medulla and pons. Control of equilibrium is a combined function of the older portions of the cerebellum and the reticular substance of the medulla, pons and mesencephalon. The coordinated turning movements of the head, of the entire body and of the eyes are controlled by specific centres located in the mesencephalon, paleocerebellum and lower basal ganglia. Feeding reflexes, such as salivation in response to taste of food and licking of the lips, are controlled by areas in the medulla, pons, mesencephalon, amygdala and hypothalamus. Many emotional patterns, such as anger, excitement, sexual activities, reaction to pain or reaction of pleasure can occur in animals, without a cerebral cortex.

In short, the lower brain level coordinate functions of the body as well as many of the life processes themselves -arterial pressure and respiration, for instance are controlled by lower regions of the brain, regions that usually, but not always, operate below the conscious level.

Basic Functional Unit - Neuron Structure, Type- Functional Characteristics of Sub-Units of Neuron

Neurons : The central and peripheral portion of the nervous system are comprised of nerve cells (neurons) and supporting tissues. The neuron is the major functional unit of the nervous system.

The supportive tissues of the peripheral nervous elements consist primarily of connective tissue and specialized cells called neurolemma or Schwann cells. The supportive tissues of central nervous system are glia cells or neuroglia. These cells have functional and nutritive roles in addition to their roles as supportive tissue. The glial cells surround neurons and provide support for and insulation between them. Glial cells are the most abundant cell types in the central nervous system. Types of glial cells include oligodendrocytes, astrocytes, ependymal cells, Schwann cells, microglia, and satellite cells.

Spinal and cranial nerves form the peripheral nervous system and they carry electrical signals in the form of action potentials. The action potentials can be away from the central nervous system or towards it.

Neuron is defined as the basic structural and functional unit of the nervous system.The neuron is composed of the neuron cell and long cytoplasmic extensions referred to as axons and dendrites of neurons. Each neuron usually possesses many dendrites but only one axon. The dendrites collect information from other nerve cells or receptors organs. The axons transfer this information to other neurons or cells of the body. Neurons does not have a centrosome so it cannot undergo division. The cytoplasm of nerve cells is in a constant flow called axoplasmic flow, so as to ensure transfer of nutrients from the cell body to the terminals of long nerve fibres. Neurons belong to the category of excitable cells. Excitable cells can generate and propagate a bioelectrical potential change called action potential in their limiting membranes. Neurons have a very high requirement for oxygen. Brain cells or neurons suffer permanent damage if oxygen supply to the brain is impaired for more than a few minutes. Adult neurons cells do not have the ability to reproduce. Their inability to reproduce is the reason for long lasting effects of nervous system damage due to head injuries or strokes.

Neurons can be divided into unipolar, bipolar and multipolar neurons on the basis of number of poles. Functionally the neurons can be divided into Sensory Neurons and Motor Neurons.

The neuron consist of three parts. Nerve cell body, dendrites and axon.

The dendrite and axon together form the processes. The dendrites are short processes and axons are long processes. Each neuron has only one axon but variable number of dendrites. The axon is the longer process of the cell. The length of the longest axon is about one meter. Most of the axons are insulated by a myelin sheath and are called a myelinated axons. The myelin sheath does not form a continuous sheath and is absent at regular intervals and such area where myelin sheath is absent are called nodes of Ranvier. Myelin sheath is responsible for white colour of the nerve fibers.

The nerve fibers which are without myelin sheath are called nonmyelinated nerve fibers.Myelin sheath is formed by concentric layers of proteins alternating with lipids. The lipids are cholesterol, lecithin and sphingomyelin. Myelin sheath is responsible for faster conduction of impulse through the nerve fibers.Myelin sheath also has a high insulating capacity. Because of this, the myelin sheath restricts the nerve impulse within the single nerve fiber and prevents the stimulation of neighbouring nerve fibers. Surrounding the myelin sheath, there is a thin membrane called neurilemma. Neurilemma (also known as neurolemma, sheath of Schwann, or Schwann's sheath) is the outermost nucleated cytoplasmic layer of Schwann cells (also called neurolemmocytes) that surrounds the axon of the neuron. It forms the outermost layer of the nerve fiber in the peripheral nervous system.Neurilemma is absent in central nervous system. Neurilemma is essential for the formation of myelin sheath.

The nerve cell body is irregular in shape and constituted by a mass of cytoplasm called neuroplasm covered by a cell membrane. The nerve cell contains Nissl bodies which are granules of basophilic nature.The presence of neurofibrils is another characteristic feature of the neurons. The neurofibrils consist of microfilaments and microtubules.

Neurotrophins

Neurotrophins are substances which facilitate the growth, survival and repair of the nerve cells. Chemically the neurotrophins are proteins. Nerve growth factor is one such neurotrophin which is a peptide with 118 amino acids. Nerve growth factor promotes the growth of cholinergic neurons in central nervous system. It is extracted from snake venom and is used for treatment of sympathetic neuron diseases. There are several other neutrotrophins such as Brain derived Neurotrophic growth factor, ciliary neurotrophic factor, fibroblast growth factor, Neurophin 3 and glial cell line derived neurotrophic factor.

Synapse

The cell membranes of two fibres from different nerve cells organized to form a junction called as **synapse**.Gray classified two types of synapses within the brain based on the ultrastructural characteristics of the presynaptic (vesicle-bearing) and postsynaptic partners (length of apposed membrane, membrane thickenings and synaptic cleft):Type 1 and Type 2. Type 1 synapses were found on dendritic spines and dendrite shafts, whereas Type 2 synapses occurred primarily on dendrite shafts and neuronal cell bodies.

Receptors: To transmit information through the neurons, the body relies on special cells called **receptors**. Receptors receive information from both external and internal environments and play an important role in converting this information into electrical impulses. The receptors are of two types. **Exteroceptive** sensors and **interoceptive** sensors. Interoceptive sensors receive signals from inside the body and convey information about internal conditions to the brain.

Membrane Potential-ionic Basis of Resting Membrane Potential (RMP) Nerve Action Potential

Excitable tissues are characterised by their ability to produce and propagate action potentials. Action potentials are changes in the resting membrane potential which are actively propagated along the membrane of the cell.

The synapse is the site of both neuronal integration and the interneural transfer of information. The release of a specific chemical transmitter by the presynaptic axon transfers neuronal activity across the synapse. The transmitter interacts with the post synaptic dendrites and soma, producing brief changes in their membrane potentials, called synaptic potentials.

Electric (voltage) potential difference across cell membranes of a resting cell : can be determined by inserting a very fine electrode into the cell, another into the extracellular fluid surrounding the cell and connecting the two to a voltmeter. It has been found by such measurements that all cells of the body exhibit a membrane potential oriented so that the inside of the cell is negatively charged with respect to the outside. This potential is called the resting membrane potential. The normal ionic composition of the fluid bathing the cells (the extra cellular fluid) is approximately.

Excitation and Propagation of Impulse Characteristics- Latent period-refractiveness, Threshold Level-all & None Characteristics

Transmission of Impulses with the Help of Ions

There are several other substances in the extracellular fluid but sodium and potassium play the most important role in the generation of the resting membrane potential. Now it is clear that the potassium concentration is much greater inside the cell than out and the sodium concentration gradient is the opposite and secondly the cell membrane is about 50 to 75 times more permeable to potassium than to sodium. A diffusion potential will be generated across the membrane largely because of the movement of potassium down its concentration gradient so that the inside of the cell is negative with respect of outside.

The outside of the cell membrane of a resting neuron is positively charged whereas the inside is negatively charged. This potential difference is maintained with the help of a Sodium pump, which actively pumps out sodium ions (Na^+) from the inside of the nerve fibre by using energy. This potential difference is usually –70 mV. When a stimulus excites a nerve fibre, the sodium pump at that region immediately becomes inactive. As a result, the cell membrane becomes more permeable to sodium ions and sodium ions get into the neuron. This causes a depolarization of the cell membrane so that the inside becomes positive and outside becomes negative. The sodium pump immediately resumes activity and sodium ions are once again pumped out of the neuron using energy from ATP. The cell membrane becomes impermeable to these ions. Thus the potential difference once again becomes –70 mV and the membrane reaches the resting stage. This is called repolarization. In accordance with the inward and outward movement of sodium ions, movement of potassium ions also takes place. When one region of the axon undergoes repolarization, the succeeding region is excited and is depolarized. This process continues and thus impulse travels through the membrane in the form of a wave of depolarization.

The transmission of nerve signals across synapses is through acetylcholine receptors. The acetylcholine channel opens in response to the binding of acetylcholine receptor with acetylcholine. Thus it is a sort of gated channel which opens in response to binding to a ligand i.e. ligand-gated channel.

In contrast, the sodium and potassium channels, which mediate action potentials in neuron axon membranes , are opened by membrane depolarization. Therefore, these channels are called voltage- gated channels instead of ligand-gated as explained above in acetylcholine receptors.

There is a third type of channel which allows the transport of ions and metabolites between cells directly and these cell-to-cell channels are called gap junction. Gap junctions allow ions and small molecules to flow between communicating cells.Thus inorganic ions and most metabolites such as sugars, amino acids and nucleotides can flow between the interior of cells joined by gap junctions.Gap junctions are important for intercellular communication.Gap junctions are essential for the nourishment of cells that are distant from blood vessels , as in eye lens and bone.

Free energy required for active transport is obtained in the cell in the form of hydrolysis of high energy-rich molecules called ATP to ADP and AMP. Membrane proteins use ATP hydrolysis to pump ions and molecules across membranes.

The channels for transport of ions across membranes are highly selective. The ionic selectivity partly depends on steric factors(three dimensional structure).

Fluid Filled Spaces in the Brain

Within the brain there are four interconnected fluid filled spaces known as cerebral ventricles. The ventricles are continuous with the central canal of the spinal cord. Within each ventricle there is a highly vascular structure known as choroid plexus. The choroid plexuses are responsible for the production of cerebrospinal fluid which fills the ventricles. Cerebrospinal fluid is isotonic with blood plasma, but is not merely produced by a process of filtration since it differs from plasma in several ways. It contains only a small amount of protein and less potassium and calcium than plasma. The concentrations of sodium and chloride, on the other hand, are greater than those in plasma. Choroid plexuses form approximately 300ml of cerebrospinal fluid per day in man.

Cerebrospinal fluid apparently provides mechanical support to the CNS, acts as a buffer against mechanical shock, controls the chemical environment of the brain (together with blood circulation) and exchanges nutrients and waste materials with the brain tissue.

The Three Major Levels of Nervous System Function

In animals there are three major levels of nervous system functions.

1. The spinal cord level
2. The lower brain level
3. The higher brain or cortical level.

Each of the levels cited above has special functional significance.

Spinal Cord Level

Sensory signals are transmitted through the spinal nerves into each segment of the spinal cord and these signals can cause localized motor responses either in the segment of the body from which the sensory information is received or in adjacent segments. Essentially all the spinal cord motor responses are automatic and occur almost instantaneously in response to the sensory signal. In addition, they occur in specific patterns of responses called reflexes.

Muscle Stretch Reflex

If a muscle suddenly becomes stretched, a sensory nerve receptor in the muscle called muscle spindle becomes stimulated and transmits nerve impulses through a sensory nerve fibre into the spinal cord. This fibre synapses directly with a motor neuron in the anterior horn of the cord grey matter and the motor-neuron in turn transmits impulses back to the muscle to cause the effector muscle to contract. The muscle contraction opposes the original muscle stretch. Thus, this reflex acts as a feedback mechanism operating from a receptor to an effector, to prevent sudden change in length of the muscle. This allows an animal to maintain his limbs and other parts of the body in desired positions despite sudden outside forces that tend to move the part out of position.

Withdrawal reflex : This is a protective reflex that causes withdrawal of any part of the body from an object that is causing pain. For instance let us assume that the hand is placed on a sharp object. Pain signals are transmitted into the gray matter of the spinal cord and after appropriate selection of information by the synapses, signals are channelled to the appropriate motoneurons to cause flexion of the biceps muscle. This obviously lifts the hand away from the sharp object.

The withdrawal reflex is much more complex than the stretch reflex, for it involves many neurons in the gray matter of the cord and signals are transmitted to many adjacent segments of the cord to cause contraction of the appropriate muscles.

Cord Function After the Brain is Removed

The following list of important cord functions that occur even after the brain is removed illustrates the many capabilities of the spinal cord.

1. The animal can under certain conditions be made to stand up.

   This is caused primarily by reflexes initiated from the pads of the feet. Sensory signals from the pads cause the extensor muscles of the limb to tighten, which in turn allows the limbs to support the animal's body.

2. A spinal animal held in a sling so that its feet hang downward often begins walking or galloping movements, involving one, two or all its legs. This illustrates that the basic pattern of causing the limb movements of the locomotion are present in the spinal cord.
3. A flea crawling on the skin of a spinal animal causes reflex to and for scratching by the paw, and the paw can actually localize the flea on the surface of the body.
4. Cord reflexes exist to cause emptying of the urinary bladder and of the rectum.

This list of some of the segmental and multisegmental reflexes of the spinal cord demonstrates that many of our day to day and movement by movement activities are controlled locally by the respective segmental levels of the spinal cord and brain plays only a modifying role in these local controls.

Brain

Brain is regarded to be made up of three parts.

Cerebrum

Cerebellum

The brain stem

Diencephalon - Thalamus & Hypothalamus

Mesencephalon

Metencephalon

Myelencephalon

The brainstem may be regarded as a much modified prolongation of the spinal cord; the cerebellum are developed as two large expansions of the stem. Phylogenetically, brainstem and cerebellum are called as old brain. Cerebrum - the new brain.

In the lower vertebrates, the fishes, the brain stem and cerebellum are fairly well developed, but the cerebrum is altogether lacking or but poorly developed. With advance in the scale of animal life, through the amphibians, reptiles, birds and mammals, the cerebrum gradually not only becomes anatomically larger in size, as compared with the rest of the brain, but acquires, especially in the highest mammals and more particularly in man, a functionally dominant place. We may therefore consider the brain stem and cerebellum as being phylogenetically the old brain, the cerebrum is of much later origin.

The brain is made up of many specialized areas that work together:

- The cortex is the outermost layer of brain cells. Thinking and voluntary movements begin in the cortex.
- The brain stem is between the spinal cord and the rest of the brain. Basic functions like breathing and sleep are controlled here.
- The basal ganglia are a cluster of structures in the center of the brain. The basal ganglia coordinate messages between multiple other brain areas.
- The cerebellum is at the base and the back of the brain. The cerebellum is responsible for coordination and balance.

The Brain is also Divided into Several Lobes

- The frontal lobes are responsible for problem solving and judgment and motor function.
- The parietal lobes(relating to the wall or outer surface of a body part) manage sensation, handwriting, and body position.
- The temporal lobes (each of the paired lobes of the brain lying beneath the temples) are involved with memory and hearing.
- The occipital lobes (the lower back part of the head) contain the brain's visual processing system.

The forebrain includes the cerebral hemispheres and, under these, the brainstem, which contains the thalamus and hypothalamus.

The thalamus is the main relay centre between the medulla and the cerebrum;

The hypothalamus is an important control centre for sex drive, pleasure, pain, hunger, thirst, blood pressure, body temperature, and other visceral functions. The hypothalamus produces hormones that control the secretions of the anterior pituitary gland, and it also produces oxytocin and antidiuretic hormone, which are stored in and released by the posterior pituitary gland.

Brainstem

The central grey matter in the brain stem does not form a solid, continuous column as in the spinal cord. Instead, it is broken up into a number of separate masses of various sizes known as ganglia and nuclei. The fibres constituting the white matter describe devious pathways, winding over, under and between the ganglia and nuclei. This makes the anatomy of the brain stem complicated.

Reticular Formation

The cells and nuclei scattered throughout the brain stem together constitute reticular formation. Although this region is not well defined, anatomically it has an important role in both visceral and somatic functions. It occupies a large part of the medulla oblongata the upper termination.The reticular formation occupies the mid ventral portion of the medulla and midbrain.

The vestibular nuclei are included within the fomation these are the cell groups serving the special visceral afferent system, that is, the autonomic nerves.

The reticular formation receives impulses from the spinal cord by way of collateral fibres from the ascending sensory pathways. It also has input from the cerebellum and cerebral hemisphere and sends impulses to these structures. The diffuse connections with the cortex are made through a number of relays in subcortical nuclei.The reticular formation contains many of the areas concerned with the regulation of heart rate, blood pressure and respiration.

Hypothalamus

The hypothalamus occupies the ventral portion of the rostral extremity of the brain stem. Hypothalamus forms a part of the diencephalon part of the fore brain i.e. the structures bounding the third ventricle. Thus the ventral and inferior parts of the lateral walls and the floor of the third ventricle forms the hypothalamus.

The hypothalamus is a portion of the brain that contains a number of small nuclei with a variety of functions. One of the most important functions of the hypothalamus is to link the nervous system to the endocrine system via the pituitary gland.

The hypothalamus is composed of several specialized functional regions or nuclei. The hypothalamus serves as a major central control of visceral motor activity, systemic metabolism and so called consummatory motor behaviour such as feeding, drinking, sexual activity, aggressiveness, sleep, fear and rage. From a physiologists point of view the nuclei of the hypothalamus can be divided into four groups.

1. Anterior (including the paraventricular and supra-optic nuclei).
2. Middle (including the tuberal, dorsomedial and ventro medial hypothalamic nuclei)
3. Posterior (including the posterior hypothalamic nuclei and the mammillary nuclei)
4. Lateral.

Functions

The hypothalamus is richly supplied with blood vessels. The hypothalamus receives and sends impulses from and to many parts of the brain.

1. The supraoptico-hypophyseal tract sends a large number of non- myelinated nerve fibres to the posterior lobe of the pituitary gland. It is now well established that the efferent connections of the neurons of the supra-optic and paraventricular nuclei of the hypothalamus serves as endocrine cells for the production of secretions of the neurohypophysis (posterior pituitary). The antidiuretic hormone (vasopressin) and oxytocin so synthesized are transported to the neurohypophysis by way of axons of these neurons.
2. The hypothalamus through the hypophyseal portal system controls the production and release of endocrine secretions by the anterior hypothalamus. This control is mediated through the synthesis and release of a group of hypophysial release and release inhibiting factors. The synthesis and release of these factors is further under the feedback control of the hormones of the target organs of anterior pituitary.
3. Electrical stimulation and ablation of regions of the hypothalamus has indicated the presence of feeding and satiety centres in the hypothalamus. Lesions or destruction of ventro medial hypothalamic nuclei causes the animal to become obese. Similarly feeding centres are present in the lateral hypothalamus, lesions in which nuclei cause an animal to stop eating or to reduce its food intake.

   Ventro-medial nucleus- Feeding Center

   Lateral nucleus - Satiety Center

The two centers are interrelated in their activity.

4. The hypothalamus contains centres which elicit or stop drinking behaviour. The administration of small amounts of hypertonic solution directly into the hypothalamus of goats, elicits excessive drinking. The drinking centre is closely related anatomically to the ventromedial feeding center and is neurally connected to the supra-optic and paraventricular nuclei of the hypothalamus. Thus, an increase in osmotic pressure of the blood stimulates the drinking centre and at the same time elicits the release of ADH so that water is retained by the kidney tubules.

5. The heat production and heat loss from the body is regulated by centres in the hypothalamus. Thus heat loss centre is situated in the rostral hypothalamus (medial preoptic area) which when stimulated causes the animal to behave as if it were exposed to a high environment temperature. These receptors receive neural connections from peripheral thermoreceptors situated on the body skin.

   The heat gain centre is situated in the caudal hypothalamus, dorsolateral to the mamillary bodies which when stimulated causes the animal to behave as if exposed to cold stress. Both the heat loss and heat production centres are under the control of central and peripheral thermoreceptors with a high degree of integration among them. The two centres are also closely interrelated to each other and the activity of the one modifies the activity of the other.

6. Stimulation of various areas of caudal hypothalamus also affect a number of body reactions such as blood pressure, heart rate, respiration rate and augmentation of somatomotor reflex activities. Thus the posterior hypothalamus appears not only to play a significant role in the regulation of specific activity of the autonomic and somatic motor systems and in the regulation of the production of hormones of the hypophysis but it also has a key role in the functions of the ascending reticular formation.

Cerebral Hemispheres

Cerebral hemispheres constitute a part of the central nervous system. It is composed of the following parts.

1. *Olfactory system:* collectively referred to as rhinencephalon. The rhinencephalon at the base of the brain is so named because of its supposed connection with the sense of smell (Rhinos, smell). The rhinencephalon is much larger in animals in which the sense of smell is well developed. It is from an evolutionary point of view, one of the oldest parts of the cerebrum.

2. *Cerebral cortex :* The pallium or cerebral cortex is divided into a small archipallium (part of rhinencephalon) and the neopallium, which is the most highly developed part of the brain in man.

3. *Corpus striatum :* The corpus striatum consists of large nuclei of nerve cells situated within the substance of the hemispheres.

Cerebral Cortex

The superficial layer of cortex of the hemispheres consists of grey matter containing numerous nerve cells, while the deeper part or the white matter is made up of fibres connecting the various parts of the hemispheres with one another and with lower parts of the central nervous system such as the brainstem and spinal cord.

The surface of the cerebral cortex is marked by furrows called sulci, the areas between sulci being called gyri or convolutions.

The highest functions of the nervous system - the power to reason and construct ideas, to be aware of one's sensory environment, to create abstract thoughts, and to store experiences - are to a large extent centred in the cerebral cortex. The total awareness of the relationship between oneself and the surrounding environment depends on excitation of the neural networks in the cerebral cortex. It is the site of both consciousness and **intellect**. Conscious awareness is closely associated with the cerebral cortex, an intricately folded and connected sheet of nervous tissue. Each experience corresponds to a specific set of neural activities, called the neuronal correlates of consciousness, in a posterior hot zone of the brain that consists of parietal, occipital and temporal lobes of the cerebral cortex. Posterior hot zone is most active during a conscious experience.

Organization of The Cerebral Cortex

The cerebral cortex contains several billions of neurons (10 billion in the man). Most of these neurons are arranged into six layers of cells to form the neocortex. The neocortex is the highest integrative center in the somatic nervous system. It is concerned with both the processing and interpretation of sensory information (auditory, gustatory, somatesthetic and visual) and the control of complex movements generated by the skeletal muscles. It contains centres involved in the abstraction of ideas, speech and the storage of experiences. Most of its functions are under voluntary control.

The allocortex forms the second major subdivision of the cerebral cortex. In contrast to the neocortex, it has a simpler three layered neural structure and is under voluntary control. It includes the cortical structures associated with the limbic system (limbic cortex). It contains the highest centres of visceral control.

The neocortex is divided into four lobes.

Limbic System

The term limbic system is often applied to the region of the cerebral cortex which lies on the median side of the hemisphere adjacent to the corpus callosum and the attachment of the brain stem.

In man and some animals the cortical areas have been extensively mapped to localize specific sensory and motor functions. The highest types of mental activities, such as voluntary muscle control, interpretation of sensations and reasoning, involve the cells of the cerebral cortex, thus leading to the use of the term 'grey matter' as synonymous with mental ability.

The corpus striatum of each cerebral hemispheres consists of a mixture of white and gray matter thus giving a striated appearance, as the name implies. The gray matter of the corpus striatum is represented by a number of nuclear masses sometimes called the *basal ganglia* or *basal nuclei*, even though the term ganglion usually refers to an accumulation of cell bodies outside the central nervous system. The white matter of the corpus striatum consists, to a large extent, of projection fibres that connect the cerebral cortex with other parts of the central nervous system and indirectly with the peripheral nervous system.

The two main sulci are the lateral and the central sulcus. The area in front of (rostral to) the central sulcus is the frontal lobe, the area immediately behind the central sulcus is the parietal lobe. The most caudal (posterior) part of the cerebral hemispheres is the occipital lobe. The area below the posterior ramus of the lateral sulcus is the temporal lobe. Smaller sulci divide up each lobe into numerous gyri. The specific regions of the cortex receive their principal inputs from either the specific sensory nuclei of the thalamus or specific motor nuclei of the thalamus.

Diencephalon

The thalamus, the epithalamus, the hypothalamus and most part of the third ventricles are included in the diencephalon.

The thalamus is essentially a relay center for nerve fibres, connecting the cerebral hemispheres with the brainstem and spinal cord.

The epithalamus includes the habenuclear nuclei (associated with smell), white matter tracts and the pineal body.

The hypothalamus includes the pituitary gland and the structures closely associated with it. These structures include the tuber cinereum, which attaches the stalk of the pituitary gland to the brain; the optic chiasma, or crossing the optic nerves just cranial to the pituitary gland; and the mammillary bodies located immediately caudal to the pituitary gland.

Mesencephalon

The mesencephalon, or midbrain, is that portion of the brain that does not subdivide during the development from the embryo to the adult. The two cerebral peduncles and four quadrigeminal bodies are the largest structures of the mesencephalon or midbrain.

The cerebral peduncles also called crura cerebri are essentially continuation of the left halves of the spinal cord and brain stem into the respective cerebral hemispheres. They contain fibre tracts and nuclei. The quadrigeminal body (corpora quadrigemina) consists of a right and left anterior (cranial or superior) colliculus and a right and left (caudal or inferior) colliculus. The anterior colliculi are associated with vision. The posterior are associated with hearing.

Cerebellum

The cerebellum consists of two lateral hemispheres and a medium ridge called the vermis, because of its resemblance to a worm. The surface of the cerebellum consists of many laminae, called the folia. When cut in the medium line, the cerebellum gives the appearance of foliage, thus leading to the ancient term 'arbor vitae' or 'tree of life' for this view of cerebellum. In the cerebellum the white matter is chiefly centrally located and the gray matter peripherally located, as they are in the cerebrum.

In the white matter of the interior of the cerebellum are found masses of grey matter (deep nuclei) one of them is the dentate nucleus.

Medulla oblongata-Myelencephalon

The myelencephalon forms the medulla oblongata. It is the cranial continuation of the spinal cord, from which it is arbitrarily separated at the foramen magnum, the largest foramen in the skull.

The myelencephalon houses several vital nerve centres; the center for respiration, phonation, vasoconstriction, vasodilation, cardiac inhibition and acceleration, mastication, deglutition, salivary, and gastric secretions and perspiration.

The medulla oblongata is related dorsally with the fourth cerebral ventricle and cerebellum and is continued as pons. The caudal boundary of the medulla is rostral (*Ro*stral refers to the anterior (front)) to the most cranial rootlets of the first cervical nerve.

The pons is located ventral to the cerebellum and appears to form a bridge of fibres from one hemisphere of the cerebellum to the other.

Many other fibre tracts and nuclei make up the remainder of the pons. The fourth ventricle is located ventral to the cerebellum and dorsal to the pons and brainstem.

Functionally the medulla and pons are not basically different from the spinal cord. These structures are predominantly **reflex centers** with controls imposed from higher centres of the brain and from the spinal cord.

Accessory Functions of Nervous System

The accessory functions of the nervous system include **sleep** and **memory**.

Functions of Nervous System-reflexes-control of Posture and Movements

Postural control is a term used to describe the way our central nervous system (CNS) regulates sensory information from other systems in order to produce adequate motor output to maintain a controlled posture. This involves two processes

1. **Posture** based on the distribution of tonic muscle activity. Postural orientation control the body's alignment and tone with respect to gravity, support surface, visual environment, and internal references
2. **Equilibrium** –compensation for internal or external perturbations. The coordination of sensorimotor strategies to stabilize the body's centre of mass during both self-initiated and externally triggered stimuli constitutes postural equilibrium. Peripheral regulation of posture is dependent on the unique structure, specialization and properties of skeletal muscles.

Initial studies pointed out that lesions of the central nervous system resulted in pronounced changes in posture.

The visual, vestibular, and somatosensory systems are the main sensory systems involved in postural control and balance

- The visual system is the primary receiver of sensory information to maintain postural balance, and as such our postural stability increases with the improvement of the visual environment.
- The vestibular system orientates the trunk to vertical using sensory orientation and weighting appropriate sensory cues under different sensory environments.
- The somatosensory system is a complex system of sensory neurons and pathways that responds to changes at the surface or inside the body. It is also involved in maintaining postural balance by relaying information about body position to the brain, allowing it to activate the appropriate motor response or movement.
- Mechanoreceptors are specific sensory receptors located in the muscle spindles. They provide the nervous system with information about the muscle's length and velocity of contraction, thus contributing to the individual's ability to discern joint movement and position sense.
- The vestibular system, somatosensory system and visual system do not act in isolation but are a complex postural control system that work together to achieve balance.

The autonomic nervous system together with neural centres in the medulla, hypothalamus and limbic system regulates the motor functions. Somatic motor activity depends ultimately on the pattern and rate of discharge of the spinal motor neurons and homologous neurons in the motor nuclei of the cranial nerves.

The inputs converging on motor neurons have three functions: they bring about voluntary activity, they adjust body posture to provide a stable background for movement, and they coordinate the action of the various muscles to make movements smooth and precise.

Degeneration and Regeneration of Nerve Fibre

Nerve damage can be caused by physical injury or swelling (autoimmune disease), infection, diabetes, or failure of the blood vessels surrounding the nerve. When a nerve fiber is injured, various changes occur in the nerve fiber and nerve cell body. All these changes are together called the degenerative changes.

Causes for Injury : Injury to nerve fiber occurs due to following causes:

1. Obstruction of blood flow
2. Local injection of toxic substances
3. Crushing of nerve fiber
4. Transection of nerve fiber.

First Degree of Injury is the most common type of injury. It is caused by applying pressure over a nerve for a short period leading to occlusion of blood flow and hypoxia. First degree of injury is called Seddon neuropraxia. There are no or little changes in the muscles. Second Degree of Injury is due to the prolonged severe pressure which causes Wallerian degeneration. The endoneurium is intact. Second degree of injury is called axonotmesis. The axonotmesis lesions are divided into three further subtypes, depending on what component of the surrounding nerve stroma is affected.

Nerves can be easily damaged in a traumatic event, but can regenerate if the soma and a small portion of the neurilemma remain. Neuroregeneration refers to the regrowth or repair of nervous tissues, cells, or cell products. Such mechanisms may include generation of new neurons, glia, axons, myelin, or synapses. When an axon is damaged, the distal segment undergoes Wallerian degeneration, losing its myelin sheath. The proximal segment can either die by apoptosis or undergo the chromatolytic reaction, an attempt at repair.Peripheral Nervous System PNS has an intrinsic ability for repair and regeneration, the Central Nervous System is for the most part incapable of self-repair and regeneration. Axonal sprouts form at the proximal stump and grow until they enter the distal stump. The growth of the sprouts are governed by chemotactic factors secreted from Schwann cells (neurolemmocytes). Axon regeneration has three phases: sprouting, elongation, and maturation. Neurotrophins are expressed by both Schwann cells and invading macrophages after peripheral nervous system PNS injury which help in regeneration. At the same time that neurotrophin levels increase, Schwann cells upregulate expression of the low-affinity neurotrophin receptor p75 on their cell surface. Axon growth and regeneration is controlled by various transcriptional factors.

Unlike PNS injury, injury to the CNS including spinal cord injury is not followed by extensive regeneration. It is limited by the inhibitory influences of the glial and extracellular environment. The injured CNS environment does not support regeneration because it contains relatively low levels of growth factors and because inhibitory molecules are present in the glial scar formed at the injury site and in the rostral and caudal spinal cord. The hostile, a non-permissible growth environment is in part created by the migration of myelin-associated inhibitors, astrocytes, oligodendrocytes, oligodendrocyte precursors, and microglia. The environment within the CNS, especially following trauma, counteracts the repair of myelin and neurons.

Synaptic and Junctional Transmission

Impulses are transmitted over chemical or electrical synapses linking one neuron (presynaptic cell) with another neuron, muscle, or gland (postsynaptic cell). At electrical synapses, the membranes of the presynaptic and postsynaptic neurons are close together, and gap junctions form low-resistance bridges through which ions pass with relative ease from one neuron to the next. At chemical synapses, an impulse in the presynaptic axon causes secretion of a chemical that diffuses across the 30-nm-wide (approximately) synaptic cleft and binds to receptors on the surface of the postsynaptic cell. This triggers events that open or close channels in the membrane of the postsynaptic cell, mediating excitation or inhibition. At electrical synapses, the membranes of the presynaptic and postsynaptic neurons are close together, and gap junctions form low-resistance bridges through which ions pass with relative ease from one neuron to the next. Most synaptic transmission is chemical,.

Functions of Nervous System-reflexes Control of Posture and Movements

Posture is the body segments configuration at any given time. Posture is maintained by tonic muscle contractions acting against gravity and stabilizing the positions of body segments . During the execution of voluntary movements, many aspects of the same task are coordinated and performed simultaneously. Coordination between posture and limb movement is an excellent example of coordinated function of the nervous system. In such a situation there is need for an accurate performance of a goal-directed movement on the one hand, and the maintenance of equilibrium and an appropriate posture, or set of postures, on the other hand. The elaboration of a locomotor gait requires coordination between a postural function (support of the body segments against gravity and forward acceleration of the center of mass and the rhythmic movements of locomotion. Body's orientation with respect to gravity is determined by a group of reflexes that sets the body segments' collective orientation and stabilizes this orientation against external disturbances. Equilibrium control is often considered part of postural control.

Center of pressure (CoP) oscillations is as important measure of postural stability whereas a Center of Mass (CoM) is an important for maintaining equilibrium. In Horse and Camel the centre of Mass is very high making them little unstable. Under standard conditions, the higher the CoM location, the larger the CoP oscillations. However, in actual situations, the centre of pressure oscillations are never very high due to nervous control in animals such as horse or camel. One of the important factors in postural control is tonic muscle activity which provides anti gravity support. Integration of several sensory and motor areas has developed through millions of years of life evolution with the purpose of providing accurate regulation of body orientation in the gravity field.

Upright posture depends on sensory (vision, vestibular, and somatosensory) input to provide postural equilibrium and a proper alignment of body segments with respect to gravity. When jumping, the horse raises his center of gravity to the point where his haunches(a hindquarter of an animal) can propel him over the obstacle. The horse must be free to raise his head and neck to facilitate the displacement of his center of gravity.When riding a horse, the rider must always be seeking to drop their centre of gravity towards that of the horse, so that a unification of the two body masses can be achieved.

Somatic motor activity depends ultimately on the pattern and rate of discharge of the spinal motor neurons and homologous neurons in the motor nuclei of the cranial nerves. These neurons, the final common paths to skeletal muscle, are bombarded by impulses from an immense array of descending pathways, other spinal neurons, and peripheral afferents. Some of these inputs end directly on α-motor neurons, but many exert their effects via interneurons or via γ-motor neurons to the muscle spindles and back through the Ia afferent fibers to the spinal cord. It is the integrated activity of these multiple inputs from spinal, medullary, midbrain, and cortical levels that regulates the posture of the body and makes coordinated movement possible.

The inputs converging on motor neurons have three functions: they bring about voluntary activity, they adjust body posture to provide a stable background for movement, and they coordinate the action of the various muscles to make movements smooth and precise.

Autonomic Nervous System and Visceral Control

The autonomic nervous system together with neural centres in the medulla, hypothalamus and limbic system regulates the visceral functions. These visceral control centres are concerned with the maintenance of a constant internal environment. All of the visceral systems - cardiovascular, endocrine, gastrointestinal, metabolic, renal, reproductive and respiratory are affected by the activity of these neural control centres.

The visceral nervous system regulates both the contraction of the visceral muscles (cardiac and smooth) and the secretion of the gland cells. Its activity is under involuntary control. The involuntary visceral nervous system is often contrasted with the voluntary somatic nervous system, which controls the contraction of the skeletal muscles. The activities of the somatic nervous system are under voluntary control. The somatic nervous system includes the major sensory motor pathways, their nuclei, the cerebral cortex, the basal ganglia, and the cerebellum.

Each subdivision of the visceral nervous system, such as limbic system, hypothalamus, medulla and autonomic nervous system is concerned with a different level of visceral control. The limbic system, formed by the interconnection of several neural centres in the forebrain, is concerned with the control of complex behaviour patterns, e.g. feeding, maternal sexual and territorial. The hypothalamus the major homeostatic regulator, contains centres for the regulation of body temperature, water balance, feeding, sexual and emotional behaviour. It is also an important endocrine regulator because it controls the activity of the anterior and posterior pituitary glands. The medulla contains centres for the regulation of the cardiovascular and respiratory systems.

The visceral effector neurons originate in the autonomic nervous system the primary function of which is to provide the neural pathways connecting the central nervous system with the viscera.

The anatomical peculiarities of the visceral efferent nerves have important effects on the physiology and pharmacology of this part of the nervous system. One important characteristic is that instead of there being one neuron to transmit an impulse from the spinal cord to the muscle effector, an autonomic pathway has a relay ganglion between the cord and the effector. There are therefore two components to a visceral efferent pathway, a preganglionic fibre (which is myelinated) and a post ganglion and each of these structures is able to discriminate in its relaying. The transmission of impulses in the ganglia is always by acetylcholine release, but the post ganglionic fibres stimulate the visceral effectors by either norepinephrine or acetylcholine release.

The cell bodies of the preganglionic fibres are within the spinal cord but the course of their axons are different at various levels. The axons rising from the thoracic and lumbar segments of the cord pass to lateral ganglia or to collateral ganglia.

The lateral or vertebral ganglia lie in a chain down each side of the spinal cord and fairly close to it. The chain is frequently called the sympathetic trunk. The collateral or prevertebral ganglia lie further from the cord within the abdomen and thorax.

These thoracolumbar fibres are part of the sympathetic division of the autonomic nervous system.

Fibres arising from the cranial and sacral portions of the cord go to the terminal ganglia within the viscera. These are part of the parasympathetic division. The terminal ganglia lie actually within the visceral organs the fibres they serve and it is apparent that these postganglionic fibres are very short.

Most visceral organs are innervated by both parasympathetic and sympathetic divisions. The effects of sympathetic and parasympathetic activity are usually antagonistic; a visceral muscle or gland cell that is excited by parasympathetic excitation is usually inhibited by sympathetic activity.

Sympathetic Nervous System

The sympathetic system is not essential to life and in human beings large part of it have been removed without serious impairment of function. Cats which have undergone as complete a removal as possible of the sympathetic system appear to live normally if they are kept in a protected environment but they do not survive long if exposed to adverse conditions such as cold, loss of blood or general anaesthesia, the adjustments to which involves complex reactions within the body.

The preganglionic fibres of the sympathetic division emerge from the cord in the ventral roots . They branch off as white rami communicantes and lead to the lateral ganglia down each side of the cord. Here, some fibres synapse with their postganglionic fibres which emerge as the grey rami communicantes and rejoin the spinal nerves for distribution to vasomotor and pilomotor muscles. Other fibres pass uninterrupted through the lateral ganglia to the collateral ganglia, which are near the bifurcations of important blood vessels in the abdomen.

From these ganglia, post ganglionic fibres called the splanchnic nerves are distributed to the abdominal viscera. Each lateral ganglia is joined to those above and below it; an arrangement partly responsible for the widespread response by sympathetic discharges. Furthermore, there are more than ten times as many postganglionic fibres as preganglionic. Therefore, a visceral efferent impulse arising from the hypothalamus has a more diffuse effect than a comparable somatic motor impulse.

The sympathetic stimulation of effector organs such as the smooth muscle of visceral blood vessels, is by norepinephrine release at the ends of postganglionic fibres. An injection of non epinephrine has a similar effect to sympathetic stimulation.

The adrenal medulla is exceptional in that it receives preganglionic sympathetic fibres directly from the spinal cord; the cells of the adrenal gland which produce epinephrine (adrenaline) and norepinephrine (noradrenaline) are homologous with the cells of the peripheral sympathetic ganglia.

Most of the abdominal visceral organs (stomach, small intestine, liver, large intestine, urinary bladder and sexual organs) are innervated by postganglionic neurons arising from one of three collateral sympathetic ganglia, including the celiac, the superior mesenteric, and the inferior mesenteric, all the which are in the abdomen.

Overall excitation of the sympathetic nervous system enables the body to cope with stress. Sympathetic activity increases heart rate, blood pressure, blood flow to muscles, and blood glucose levels, while inhibiting gastrointestinal activity. Each of these effects increases the body's capacity to respond to stress.

Parasympathetic Nervous System

The parasympathetic nervous system is divided into two divisions: cranial and sacral (*The sacral region (sacrum) is at the bottom of the spine and lies between the fifth segment of the lumbar spine (L5) and the coccyx (tailbone). The sacrum is a triangular-shaped bone and consists of five segments (S1-S5) that are fused together.*)

Parasympathetic preganglionic neurons are located both in the visceral nuclei of the cranial nerves (III, VII, IX and X) and in the lateral horn of the sacral spinal cord. Postganglionic neurons are close to the visceral structures that they innervate. The postganglionic neurons are very short, many of them are embedded in the walls of the organ that they supply.

The fibres of the vagus nerve provide the major parasympathetic pathway. They connect with most of the thoraco-abdominal visceral organs, including heart, trachea, bronchi, small intestine and liver. Visceral structures in the head (salivary glands, tear glands and blood vessels, among others) receive their parasympathetic innervation for fibres in the other cranial nerves (III, VII and IX). The sacral division provides parasympathetic innervation to the rectum, kidney, bladder and sexual organs.

Parasympathetic activity is concerned with the recovery and restoration of body resources. Major effects of parasympathetic activity are decreased heart rate and blood pressure and increased gastrointestinal activity are associated with body rest and restoration.

Autonomic Function of Medulla

The major neural centres for the control of the cardiovascular and respiratory systems are in the medulla. These vital centres control the major cardiovascular and respiratory reflexes. They receive inputs from both baroreceptor cells are sensitive to direct stimulation by CO_2 and H^+ levels in the blood. The cardiovascular and respiratory reflexes which these centres control are critical to the individual's survival. In addition to these, medulla also has neural centres that control reflexes like coughing, sneezing, swallowing and vomiting. These reflexes require coordinated activity of the pharynx, upper respiratory tract and upper digestive tract.

Autonomic Function of Limbic Cortex

The limbic system, containing the highest centres of visceral integration is formed by the interconnection of several cortical and subcortical areas of the telencephalon.

A close anatomical and functional relationship exists with the hypothalamus; indeed some authorities include the hypothalamus as part of the limbic system.

The limbic system is the highest level of control of autonomic nervous activity and pituitary gland secretion. It is the site of integration of three kinds of information. They are (1) Visceral activity; (2) Olfactory inputs and (3) The activity of the association areas of the cerebral cortex-both motor and sensory. It is concerned with levels of motivation and the production of complex behavioural patterns that require coordination of both visceral and somatic motor activities for their successful execution.

Anatomically the limbic cortex forms a ring at the base of the cerebral cortex which surrounds the upper end of the brain stem. It includes the olfactory cortical areas and the hippocampus.

The limbic cortex forms a ring at the base of the cerebral cortex which surrounds the upper end of the brain stem. It includes the olfactory cortical areas and the hippocampus.

The limbic cortex is formed from a 'primitive' kind of cortical tissue, the allocortex which contains only three layers of cortical neurons. In contrast, the sensory, motor and association areas of the cerebral cortex are formed of neocortex, which contains six layers of cortical neurons.

Few direct connections exist between the limbic system and the remainder of the cerebral cortex; this may explain the difficulty of consciously controlling one's emotions.

The major subcortical structures associated with the limbic system include the amygdala and septums in the telencephalon and the anterior thalamic nucleus and hypothalamus in the diencephalon. Limbic system also connects with the olfactory bulb. Inputs from the sensory, motor and association areas of the cortex must pass through the anterior thalamus to reach the limbic system. The only exception is the connections between the limbic system and frontal cortex. Other major inputs to the limbic system are olfactory and viscerosensory (from the hypothalamus and visceral nuclei of the brain stem).

Outputs from the limbic system are directed primarily at the visceral centres in the hypothalamus, the pituitary gland via the hypothalamus and the autonomic nervous system. The limbic system can affect somatic motor activity through its interconnections with the basal ganglia, anterior thalamus and reticular formation.

A variety of complex behavioural patterns associated with feeding, reproduction, aggression and flight is evoked when electrical stimuli are applied to different areas of the limbic system, including pleasure, rage, distaste and fear-emotions that are associated with these complex behaviours. The activity of the limbic system is closely correlated with that of the hypothalamus. There is evidence that various areas of the limbic system regulate the secretion of the releasing hormones in the hypothalamus.

The behavioural patterns controlled by the limbic system are concerned with the preservation of either the individual or the species.

Stimulation of amygdala produces behaviour associated with feeding, e.g., chewing, swallowing and licking. Lesions of the amygdala are associated with docility, increased feeding to the point of obesity and hypersexuality. During stimulation of the septum, an aggressive animal becomes docile. Lesions of the septums produce a furious and aggressive subject. Stimulation of many regions of the septum elicit sexual and maternal behavioural patterns.

Factors Affecting Impulse Conduction Velocity in Nerves

1- Factors attributable to generation of action potential

I. Temperature

Decrease temperature ⟶ Marked increase in duration of action potential ⟶ Delayed conduction ⟶ Slow down conduction velocity

II. Level of resting membrane potential

When resting membrane potential is less negative ⟶ Slow down both generation of action potential and electrotonic conduction

III. Level of threshold potential (firing level)

2- Factors attributable to electrotonic conduction

I. Axon diameter

a . In myelinated nerve fibers, conduction velocity is directly proportional to axon diameter.

II. Myelination

Conduction velocity in myelinated fibers (m/sec.) = 6 X axonal diameter (μm)

Greater diameter of nerve fiber

- Increases speed
- Increases magnitude of spike potential
- Decreases threshold
- Decreases duration of spike and refractory period

Speed of conduction (m/sec)

1. In myelinated fibers is proportional to 6 times of the fiber diameter

Speed of conduction a 6 times of the fiber diameter

2 . In unmyelinated fibers is proportional to square root of diameter

Classification of Nerve Fibers

1- Erlanger and Gasser's classification

a) A type nerve fibers (large and medium sized myelinated fibers of spinal nerves)

i. a nerve fiber ii. b nerve fiber iii. g nerve fiber iv. d nerve fiber

b) B type nerve fibers c) C type nerve fibers

2- Numerical classification

a) Based on origin of nerve fibers

b) Some time used for sensory neurons

3- Physio-clinical classification

I. Based on sensitivity to hypoxia, pressure and anesthetic agents a) Based on sensitivity to hypoxia: Preganglionic B fibers are most susceptible to it

b) Based on sensitivity to local anesthetic agents: Block transmission of pain sensation in group C fibers before they affect touch fiber in group A

Appearance of multiple peaks in action potential is known as 'compound action potential'.

In general

Type of nerve fiber Contribution to compound action potential

Group A fibers Maximum

Group C fibers Minimum

Type of Summation

1- Spatial summation

- The increase in depolarization occurs because of the additive effect of synaptic currents originating at more than one synapse and it is termed as 'spatial summation'.

2- Temporal summation

- When a second postsynaptic potential is elicited within a short time, it will ride piggyback upon first. This effect is known as 'temporal summation'.
- Modification of neuronal functions as a result of experience is known as plasticity.
- Synaptic efficiency: It is the effectiveness of presynaptic impulse in producing a postsynaptic potential change.

Mechanoreceptors

Respond to displacement of tissue.

Four histologically distinct mechanoreceptors have been identified in skin

1. Merkel's disk
2. Ruffini's endings
3. Meissner's corpuscles
4. Pacinian corpuscles

Mechanoreceptors (Adaptability, Receptive Action field)

Merkel's disk-Slow Small Respond to skin indentation & velocity of skin displacement

Ruffini's endings-Slow Large Proprioceptive property

Meissner's-Rapid Small Present at hair less corpuscles skin and more sensitive to low frequency vibrations

Pacinian-Rapid Large Present at hairy skin and best corpuscles respond to high frequency vibrations

Neurotransmitter

Neurotransmitters are often referred to as the body's chemical messengers. Neurotransmitters are the chemical substances which are responsible for transmission of an impulse through a synapse. They are a type of chemical messenger which transmits signals across a chemical synapse from one neuron (nerve cell) to another 'target' neuron, to a muscle cell, or to a gland cell. The first neurotransmitter to be discovered was a small molecule called acetylcholine. It plays a major role in the peripheral nervous system, where it is released by motor neurons and neurons of the autonomic nervous system. It also plays an important role in the central nervous system in maintaining cognitive function. Damage to the cholinergic neurons of the CNS is associated with Alzheimer disease.

Most neurotransmitters are either small amine molecules, amino acids, or neuropeptides. There are about a dozen known small-molecule neurotransmitters and more than 100 different neuropeptides. These chemicals and their interactions are involved in countless functions of the nervous system as well as controlling bodily functions.

Neurotransmitters can be divided into two groups.

Excitatory Neurotransmitters and Inhibitory Neurotransmitters

1. Excitatory neurotransmitters can cause an action potential (if the target cell is another neuron), contraction (if the target cell is a muscle) or secretion (if the target cell is a gland). The most common excitatory neurotransmitter within the CNS is glutamate. Other excitatory neurotransmitters are acetylcholine, aspartic acid etc.
2. Inhibitory neurotransmitters reduce or block the activity of the postsynaptic cell. They produce a hyperpolarization of the postsynaptic membrane called the inhibitory postsynaptic potential. The most common inhibitory neurotransmitters within the CNS are glycine or GABA (γ-aminobutyric acid). Other inhibitory neurotransmitters include dopamine.

Neuromodulators are a bit different, as they are not restricted to the synaptic cleft between two neurons, and so can affect large numbers of neurons at once. Neuromodulators therefore regulate populations of neurons, while also operating over a slower time course than excitatory and inhibitory transmitters. Many neuromodulators, such as **dopamine**, are monoamines. There are several dopamine pathways in the brain, and this neurotransmitter is involved in many functions, including motor control, reward and reinforcement, and motivation.

Wakefulness, Sleep Cycle

The sleep cycle of most mammals consists of slow-wave sleep or quiet sleep, followed by REM sleep (Rapid Eye Movement sleep, also called active sleep), and then wakefulness. The sleep–wake cycle in healthy humans is a 24-hour cycle composed of approximately one-third sleep and two-thirds wake.

Sleep is characterized by a stereotypic posture, minimal movement, reduced responsivity to stimuli, reversibility, and species-specific diurnal timing and duration. Sleep is the state when an animal is unaware of his environment. This does not mean that the animal is unconscious, but means that the subject is only less conscious of its environment. The sleep state can be differentiated from death, coma, and hibernation by the characteristics of arousability and rapid reversibility. The difference between sleep and unconscious state lies in the fact that sleep is a normal recurring state during which the individual can be aroused, whereas in the unconscious state he cannot be aroused.

There are two states of sleep; light sleep or slow wave sleep and deep sleep or fast wave sleep. Light sleep is characterised by some electrical activity in the cerebral cortex and by the presence of some muscle tone. The deep sleep; also called as dreaming sleep, is a state characterised by loss of muscle tone, rapid eye movement and fast electrical waves. The brain wave pattern during REM sleep among animals is similar to humans. Scientists still don't know if animals dream during REM sleep, as humans do.

The sleep-wake cycle is regulated by two opposing processes, the circadian rhythm and the homeostatic drive for sleep. The circadian rhythm is set by the suprachiasmatic nucleus of the hypothalamus, which regulates the sleep-wake cycle. The suprachiasmatic nucleus projects to the pineal gland to release melatonin, which promotes sleep.

There are certain physiological factors that are involved in sleep. During sleep there is a slowing up of the heart rate, decrease in arterial blood pressure and the basal metabolic rate.The muscles also relax and become atonic. There may also be a decrease in body temperature. Sleep–wake cycles have profound influence on the activity of the brain stem respiratory network. Respiratory sensitivities to arterial levels of PO^2 and PCO^2 are reduced during sleep, and the apneic threshold is raised. Breathing during sleep is often disordered and frequently interrupted by periods of apnea. Sleep is also associated with increases in upper airway resistance.

However, during fast wave sleep while dreaming, there may be elevation of blood pressure and heart rate may also go up. Besides these, a number of other changes take place, such as increased blood flow to the cerebral cortex, elevation of brain temperature, increased gastric juice secretion, enhanced secretion of the adrenal cortex, and changes in the urine production. There is high central nervous activity during fast sleep.

Animals can be classified on the basis of their activity cycles into monophasic *or* **polyphasic.** Monophasic animals tend to have a long rest period each day, usually at night following the activities of the day. Most domestic animals tend to be monophasic such as sheep, pig. Polyphasic animals show several alternating periods of rest and activity in a 24-hour period. Most mammalian youngs have a polyphasic sleep pattern wherein they awaken every few hours, nurse and then return to sleep.Activity cycles are subject to modifications by environmental changes; many domestic animals adjust to man's activity cycles.

Wakefulness, Sleep Cycle in Ruminants

Several studies indicate that adult ruminants do not sleep during their inactive periods but young ruminants do sleep. The inactive periods in ruminants are mostly spent **cud-**chewing and the eyes are seldom closed for more than 30 minutes per day. However, sheep and goats have shown typical sign of sleep when the EEG was studied.Horses can sleep even while they are standing. Adult ruminants rest in sternal recumbency so that rumen function is possible, while very young ruminants will lie in lateral recumbency.When healthy cattle lie in sternal recumbency, most of the fore weight is borne by the sternum.

Sleep is necessary for health and animals deprived of sleep will eventually become ill. Animals which do not get proper rest periods become irritable.

There are several states in animals which resemble sleep such as hibernation, hypnosis, chemical anaesthesia, electrosleep and electro anaesthesia.

The mechanisms controlling sleep are not completely understood but two major theories are current to explain the initiation of sleep.

Neuronal Fatigue theory states that sleep occurs due to the neuronal fatigue in the reticular activating system. *Sleep centres* theory postulates several areas in the brain which when stimulated can cause sleep. Several of them are located in the basal forebrain, thalamus and caudal reticular formation. Stimulation of sleep centres induces sleep. Lesions in the sleep centres of the basal forebrain or the caudal reticular formation cause insomnia or sleeplessness . Insomnia is the most common sleep disorder in human beings and can be due to psychiatric problems, systemic illness , alcoholic illness or drug addiction.

Slow wave sleep is believed to depend on a system of serotonin (5 hydroxytryptamine) containing neurons located in the median raphe nuclei. Second neurochemical system is formed by norepinephrine containing neurons in the dorsal pons which is concerned with the control of REM (rapid eye movement, paradoxical or dreaming) sleep.

Higher Function of Nervous System –learning, Memory

Communication is one higher function of the nervous system which is highly developed in human beings in the sense that human beings can communicate through language. But communication is no less important for domestic animals although not developed to the extent found in human beings. Communication which involves learning and memory is very much important even for the survival of animals.

Learning and memory are closely related. Learning is impossible without memory and memory has no meaning without learning. Learning refers to a neural mechanism by which the individual changes behavior on the basis of the past experience. Memory refers to the acquisition, storage and retrieval of sensory information, while learning is the change in behavior based on the sensory information stored in the brain.

Associative Learning

In associative learning, the subject learns about the relationship between two stimuli or **between a stimulus and a behaviour**. Two forms of associative learning have been distinguished based on the experimental procedures used to establish the learning:

Classical Conditioning or Pavlovian Conditioning

A conditioned reflex is a reflex response to the stimulus that is acquired by repeatedly pairing the stimulus with another stimulus that normally does produce the response. Ivan Pavlov was a Russian psychologist best known for his work in classical conditioning. In 1904, this work earned him the Nobel Prize in physiology or medicine. It depends for its appearance on the formation of new functional connections in CNS.

Reinforcement, i.e. a process of following a conditioned stimulus with the basic unconditional stimulus is must for retaining a conditioned reflex, otherwise it will get extinct.

Operant conditioning- is a trial and error conditioning.Operant conditioning is of two types. Reward conditioning. In it a naturally occurring response is strengthened by positive reinforcement (reward). Adversive conditioning. In it a naturally occurring (innate) response is weakened by a negative reinforcement (punishment)

Only a small fraction of the important sensory information causes an immediate motor response. Much of the remainder is stored for future control of motor activities and for use in the thinking process. Most of this storage occur in the cerebral cortex, but not all, for even the basal regions of the brain and perhaps even the spinal cord can store small amounts of information. The main parts of the brain involved with memory are the amygdala, the hippocampus, the cerebellum, and the prefrontal cortex . The amygdala is involved in fear and fear memories. The hippocampus is associated with declarative and episodic memory as well as recognition memory.

The storage of information is the process we call memory and this is a function of the synapses. This is, each time a particular sensory signal passes through a sequence of synapses, the respective synapses become more capable of transmitting the same signal the next time, which process is called facilitation. After the sensory signal has passed through a synapse a large number of times, the synapses become so facilitated that signals from the 'control center' of the brain can also cause transmission of impulses throughout the same sequence of synapses even though the sensory input has not been excited. This gives the person a perception of experiencing the original sensations though in effect it is only a memory of the sensation.

In animals the memory function is less developed as compared to man and this is manifest in the poor development of the cerebral cortex. However, experiments do indicate that they also have some semblance of memory function of human beings.

Classification of Memory

Classification of Memory (on the basis of duration of memory)

1. Short term memory (working memory) lasts for seconds to hours. Example of short-term memory includes memory of a new telephone number after a looking into the directory. Most of the time such a telephone number is forgotten after a few minutes.
    i. Phonological memory (left cerebral hemisphere)
    ii. Visuospatial memory (right cerebral hemisphere)

2. Intermediate memory- or secondary memory: Lasts for days-to-weeks, but is eventually lost.
3. Long term memory-or tertiary memory, which once stored, can be recalled years later or for a lifetime.

Memory can also be classified on how the information is stored or recalled in two forms: Implicit memory and Explicit memory. Implicit memory is information about how to perform something. Implicity memory is rigid and tightly connected to original stimulus conditions under which the learning occurred. Explicit memory refers to factual knowledge of people, places, things and what these facts mean. Explicit memory is highly flexible and involves the association of multiple bits and pieces of information.

Mechanism for simple forms of learning results from changes in the effectiveness of synaptic transmission which involves habituation and sensitization.

The process by which transient short-term memory is converted into a stable long-term memory is called consolidation. Consolidation of long term implicit memory for simple forms of learning involves gene expression, new protein synthesis and growth of synaptic connections.

Familiarization with Common Equipments Used in Neurophysiology (Oscilloscope, Electroencephalography, Machine Stimulators etc)

An **oscilloscope** is a laboratory instrument commonly used to display and analyze the waveform of electronic signals. In effect, the device draws a graph of the instantaneous signal voltage as a function of time. Oscilloscopes display the change of an electrical signal over time, with voltage and time as the Y- and X-axes, respectively, on a calibrated scale. The waveform can then be analyzed for properties such as amplitude, frequency, rise time, time interval, distortion, and others. Special-purpose oscilloscopes may be used to display the waveform of the heartbeat as an electrocardiogram.

Electroencephalography: An EEG, or electroencephalogram, is a test that records the electrical signals of the brain.An EEG is very useful test in human medicine for the diagnosis of epilepsy and sleep disorders.It is typically noninvasive, with the electrodes placed along the scalp.

The stereotactic apparatus uses a set of three coordinates (x, y and z) in an orthogonal frame of reference (cartesian coordinates), or, alternatively, a cylindrical coordinates system, also with three coordinates: angle, depth and antero-posterior (or axial) location. The mechanical device has head-holding clamps and bars which puts the head in a fixed position in reference to the coordinate system (the so-called zero or origin). In small laboratory animals, these are usually bone landmarks which are known to bear a constant spatial relation to soft tissue. Stereotactic surgery is a minimally invasive form of surgical intervention which makes use of a three-dimensional coordinate system to locate small targets inside the body and to perform on them some action such as ablation, biopsy, lesion, injection, stimulation, implantation, radiosurgery (SRS), etc.

Multiparametric Magnetic Resonance Imaging (MRI) has achieved tremendous advances in applications to amyotrophic lateral sclerosis (ALS) to increase the understanding of the associated pathophysiology. fMRI is used to measure local amount of oxygenated blood. The technique makes it possible to determine the activity of various parts of the brain. MRI provides high quality images with excellent detail and resolution of the brain and spinal cord compared to other imaging tools, such as computed tomography. Common examples of MRI use in animals include paralyzed dogs with disc herniation, brain tumors, stroke, and many other conditions such as rupture cranial cruciate ligament.

MRI techniques for animals are exactly the same as those for humans. The imaging technique is exactly the same whether a "human MRI" machine or a "veterinary MRI" machine is used. The only difference between people and animals receiving an MRI is that animals will not lie still when asked. In general, it takes approximately 45 minutes to perform a MRI scan. Thus, animals must be under anesthesia for the scan. Magnetic resonance imaging (MRI) is the newest form of imaging in general use today. In this imaging modality, a powerful magnet, up to 60,000 times as strong as the magnetic field of the earth, is used to transiently align the hydrogen atoms in the body with the magnetic field.

Positron emission tomographic scanning (PET scanning) is used to measure local glucose metabolism, which is proportionate to neural activity.

Neurological Problems in Domestic Animals

Veterinary neurologists treat nervous-system problems of all shapes and sizes, from dogs with back pain and dogs and cats with seizures. Neurological problems in animals can be caused by a reaction to medication, hereditary disorders, infection or trauma. Tumors, herniated disks and traumatic injuries are often treated with surgery, but many neurological conditions also respond to medications – antibiotics, immunosuppressive drugs, anti-seizure medication, and chemotherapy.

Listeriosis is defined as an acute bacterial meningoencephalitis of ruminants characterized by circling and cranial nerve deficits. Polioencephalomalacia (Polio) is defined as a neurologic disease of young (usually) ruminants characterized by blindness due in part to thiamine deficiency. Tetanus is a neurologic disease characterized as a progressive muscular rigidity due to a Clostridium tetani neurotoxin.

Cysts are common in sheep and goat brain and have to be removed surgically. Cerebral Coenurosis (Gid) is a neural disease found in sheep and goat and is caused by larval stage of taenia multiceps known as coenurus cerebralis.

Summary

- Nervous system acts as a control network within the body.
- The nerve cells are excitable, i.e. capable of generation of electrical impulses at their membranes.
- A neuron is the basic unit of nervous tissue. It is specialized for the function of reception, integration and transmission of information in the body.

- The electrical impulses generated in the nervous tissue are used to transmit signals along the membranes.
- The neurons are linked together in a highly intricate manner and through these connections the body is made aware of changes in the environment or of those inside the animal body and appropriate responses to such changes are produced.
- The nervous system is broadly classified into two divisions: the central nervous system and the peripheral nervous system. Central nervous system (CNS), which occupies the central axis of the body, includes the brain and spinal cord. Peripheral nervous system is the part of the nervous system which lies outside the CNS.
- Functionally, the nervous system can be divided into two parts: Somatic nervous system and Autonomic nervous system.
- The autonomic nervous system (ANS) collects the information about the changes that take place in the internal environment (i.e. internal viscera), interprets these changes, guides the action and gets the plan executed with the help of smooth muscles of viscera, cardiac muscles and secretory epithelium of glandular tissues (which are effector organs of ANS).
- The ANS has two main divisions: sympathetic and parasympathetic, each having a central and a peripheral component.

7

Sense Organs and Receptor Physiology

Sense Organs and Receptors Physiology of Special Senses

Detection of sensations allow the body to be aware of changes (or **stimuli**) that occur in the environment or inside the body. These senses permit the central nervous system to produce reactions for the stimuli and maintain body homeostasis. Somatic senses ("soma" means body) detect touch, pain , pressure, temperature, and tension on the skin and in internal organs. Special senses detect the sensations of taste, smell, hearing, equilibrium, and sight, only in special sense organs in the head region. All senses are detected by sensory receptors, and after integration and processing being done in the central nervous system, motor nerves produce a response.

Types of Receptors

Sensory receptors present throughout the body provide sensory input to the central nervous system. The sensory receptors present in the body include as follows

- Chemoreceptors
- Thermoreceptors
- Nociceptors
- Photoreceptors
- Mechanoreceptors
- Baroreceptors

Chemoreceptors detect chemical concentrations. b) in somatic senses, chemoreceptors can detect ionic, glucose, oxygen, and carbon dioxide concentrations in the blood and tissue fluids. c) in special senses Chemoreceptors are responsible for the senses of taste (in oral cavity) and smell (in nasal cavity).

The taste (gustatory) stimuli are detected by specialized chemoreceptors called taste receptors or taste cells. The taste receptors are clustered in the taste buds located on the tongue, palate, pharynx, epiglottis and upper-third of oesophagus.

1. Nociceptors

Pain receptors,also called nociceptors,are the most common and widely distributed sensory receptors inside and on the surface of the body. Nociceptors can be found in the skin and many visceral organs detecting tissue damages. Nociceptors detect pain or tissue damage due to excessive mechanical, electrical, thermal, or chemical forces.

They are found almost everywhere. They range from simple, free nerve endings that respond to intense stimuli of all types, to more specialized structures that detect mechanical forces, temperature, and so on. Pain receptors are not found in the brain. Their purpose is to protect the body from damage by alerting the CNS to potentially harmful stimuli. Pain can be superficial or deep. Pain can be acute or chronic.

2. Thermoreceptors

a) detect temperature changes.

b) in somatic senses, certain thermoreceptors detect cold temperatures in the skin and some visceral organs, while other thermoreceptors detect high temperatures only.

3. Mechanoreceptors

a) detect mechanical forces.

b) in somatic senses, proprioceptors detect muscle tension, pressoreceptors detect blood pressure, and stretch receptors detect lung inflation, stomach distention, and urinary bladder expansion.

c) in special senses, mechanoreceptors in the inner ear detect the senses of hearing (in cochlea)and equilibrium (in semicircular canals).

4. Baroreceptors

a) Baroreceptors are specialized stretch receptors located within thin areas of blood vessels and heart chambers that respond to the degree of stretch caused by the presence of blood. They send impulses to the cardiovascular center to regulate blood pressure. Vascular baroreceptors are found primarily in sinuses (small cavities) within the aorta and carotid arteries. The aortic sinuses are found in the walls of the ascending aorta just superior to the aortic valve, whereas the carotid sinuses are located in the base of the internal carotid arteries. There are also low-pressure baroreceptors located in the walls of the venae cavae and right atrium.

b) When blood pressure increases, the baroreceptors are stretched more tightly and initiate action potentials at a higher rate. At lower blood pressures, the degree of stretch is lower and the rate of firing is slower. When the cardiovascular center in the medulla oblongata receives this input, it triggers a reflex that maintains homeostasis.

5. Photoreceptors

The photoreceptors are found in the rod and cone cells present in the retina of the eye. Their distinguishing feature is the presence of large amounts of tightly packed membrane that contains the photopigment rhodopsin or a related molecule. Photoreceptors are special cells in the eye's retina that are responsible for converting light into signals that are sent to the brain. Photoreceptors give us our color vision and night vision. Photoreceptors

a) detect light intensity.

b) in special senses, photoreceptors in the eye detect the tones (by rods photoreceptors) and colors (by cones photoreceptors) of visual images

Eye: Functional Morphology, Nourishment and Protection Neural Pathway

Vision is a fundamental sensory phenomenon that affords a distinct survival advantage to most animals. Ophthalmology is the study of the eye. Sense of vision is a complex function of the two eyes and their neural connections. Domestic animals have the capacity to respond to light. They are able to do so with the help of specialized organ, the eye. Human beings have a greater visual activity but most domestic mammals have a much larger visual field and greater ability to see in dim light.

Many mammals are born blind but they start seeing shortly after birth. Mammals such as cows and horses are born with perfectly functional eyes and ears because they may need to run away from a predator within minutes of being born. Cats and dogs are born with their eyes and ears sealed completely shut which start opening by themselves by 2 weeks of age.

Most domestic animals are dichromatic, meaning they possess 2 photopigment populations. So, contrary to popular belief, domestic animals do not see in black and white. They have color vision. Primates and humans possess unique dichromatic color vision which enables them to differentiate between colors such as violet, green, and yellow-green, which are the short wave, medium wave, and long wave respectively.

The eye is composed of a spherical eyeball situated in the orbit. The movement of the eyeball is controlled by a set of six extrinsic muscles, which are named according to the region where they are inserted.Domestic animals tend to have eyes placed more laterally. This allows them to have a wider range of vision but less depth perception. For this reason it is best not to approach a horse directly from the front as it will startle it.Flat faced dogs have many problems related to the eye. The eyes do not fit well in the eye orbit. Bulldog breed of dogs therefore commonly have problem of glaucoma, characterized by increased fluid pressure in the eye and can cause blindness if not treated.

Camels have three eyelids. Two of these eyelids have eyelashes which help protect their eyes from sand. The third is a very thin lid which works as sort of "windshield wiper" to clean off their eyes. Called a nictitating membrane, the transparent lid helps keep out sand and dust; it can even improve vision, like a contact lens. Many animals, including dogs, cats, sharks, and some birds and amphibians, also have third eyelids

The eyeball is composed of three layers. The outermost layer is made of dense fibrous connective tissue and serves as a protective and opaque layer. This is known as the *sclerotic coat.* In the front part, the sclera is modified into a transparent glassy part, the cornea which is covered by a thin, transparent and vascular conjunctiva. The middle layer is called the choroid coat. It is composed of highly vascular connective tissue with some pigment cells. In the front, the choroid separated from the sclerotic coat forming an iris.

The innermost layer of the eye is called the retina which is a thin, light sensitive nervous layer containing sensory epithelium. Retina is a thin, delicate, transparent membrane. It is the most highly developed tissue of the eye. The optic nerve fibres originate from the retina. The images are formed on this layer and so it is comparable to the film plate of a camera.Microscopically retina consists of ten layers most important of which is layer of rod and cones. Photoreceptors are the end organs of vision.

Behind the iris is a transparent biconvex lens which is attached to the ciliary body. The eye has fluid filled in the two chambers. The anterior chamber, between the cornea and the lens is filled with aqueous humour. The aqueous humour is a clear, watery fluid filling the anterior chamber (0.25 mL) and posterior chamber (0.06 mL) of the eyeball. In addition to its role in maintaining a proper intraocular pressure, it also plays an important metabolic role by providing substrates and removing metabolites from the avascular cornea and lens. Aqueous humour is derived from plasma within the capillary network of ciliary processes.

The posterior chamber behind the lens is filled with transparent jelly like fluid called vitreous humour.The major factor responsible for transparency of the ocular media is their avascularity.

Tears consist of a complex and usually clear fluid that is diffused between the eye and the eyelid. Tears are constantly secreted at a relatively regular rate from the lacrimal glands located in the superior upper lip.

Lacrimal glands of most domestic animals are less active than in men. The secretions of these glands are useful for lubrication of the globe and for the removal of desquamated cellular tissue. The secretions of the *Harders gland* and those of ***nictitans gland*** compliments that of the lacrimal gland in its function.

Lacrimal fluid also called tear fluid contains water, mucin, lipids, lysozyme, lactoferrin, lacritin, immunoglobulins, glucose, urea, sodium and potassium. Lacrimal fluid helps in fighting against bacterial infection. The intraocular pressure keeps the external coats of the eye rigid and closely positioned to each other. Tonometry is the procedure eye care professionals perform to determine the intraocular pressure (IOP), the fluid pressure inside the eye. It is an important test in the evaluation of patients at risk from glaucoma. Most tonometers are calibrated to measure pressure in millimeters of mercury (mmHg).

Eyes are filled with different fluids that keep them healthy. New fluid is constantly being made and old fluid drained out. But if this drainage system gets plugged, the fluids build up. That causes the pressure inside your eyes to rise. Sometimes the pressure is caused by an eye injury or trauma. Over time, high pressure inside your eye can damage your optic nerve, which sends images from your eyes to your brain. Left untreated, it can cause glaucoma. Eye pressure is different from person to person. Normally, it lies somewhere between 12-22 mmHg ("millimeters of Mercury"). Most people diagnosed with glaucoma have an eye pressure above 20 mmHg.

Receptors-optics

The vertebrate eye is the most sophisticated receptor known. The retina, the sensory portion of the eye is embryologically part of the brain, and is consequently sufficiently complex to permit extensive analysis of photic information, before relaying it to higher centres of the brain. The actual photoreceptors that detect the image and generate visual nerve impulses are in a single layer of cells in the Retina. Accessory structures of the eye contribute to the focusing of images on the retina, control of brightness and blocking of the extraneous light.

Two kinds of photoreceptor cells are found in the retina : rods, which respond to dim light (scotoptic vision) and cones, which mediate color vision in brighter light (photic vision). Photoreceptors

1- Rods are sensitive to dim light. Rods are having pigment known as rhodopsin also known as visual purple or 11-cis retinene scotopsin.

2- Cones are sensitive to bright light. There number is highest in central region of retina, particularly in the fovea.The fovea is in a zone of retina known as area centralis. Cones are densest in central area and sparse in peripheral area whereas rods are densest in peripheral area and sparse in central area. There are three kinds of cones in primates. The peak absorbance wavelength of the 'blue', 'green' and 'red' sensitive cones lie at about 435, 535 and 580 nm, respectively.

Young-Helmholtz Trichrome Theory

Color perceived by any individual is the function of 3 different visual pigments, each pigments being associated with different cones i.e. animal with color vision have inherited at least 2 and in higher mammals 3 different types of cones.Young-Helmholtz theory of color vision postulates the existence of 3 kinds of cones, each containing a different photopigment and that are maximally sensitive to one of the 3 primary color. The time resolving ability of the eye is determined by measuring the critical fusion frequency (CFF).

Most domestic animals can see colors to some extent, but because most have a **lot of rods** and not as many cones, colors probably appear washed out to them. Retina of domestic animals has mostly rods (their number is highest in central region). Birds have mostly cones. Since only one pigment is involved in scotopic vision for most animals, no colors are perceived. Dim light vision is known as scotopic vision; whereas bright light vision is known as photopic vision.

Domestic animals have very sensitive night (scotopic) vision. Several physiological and anatomical mechanisms account for this improved visual performance in the dark. The first is the amount of light entering the eye. Animals (especially cats, cattle and horses) have very large corneas and pupils. Therefore more light can pass through their cornea and pupil and reach the retina. It has been calculated that the amount of light that falls on a feline retina is x 6 the amount of light that reaches a human retina. About 10% of environmental light actually reaches the photoreceptors; this percentage is increased by tapetum lucidum. The eyes of many animals can see in the dark due to the presence of tapetum lucidum. Tapetum is absent in pigs. As Table below demonstrates, cats have a much higher concentration of rods than humans throughout the retina, thus contributing significantly to their night vision, while detracting from their visual acuity.

The light rays striking the retina generate potentials in the rods and cones. Thus the eye converts energy in the visible spectrum into action potentials in the optic nerve. Optic nerve and its connections convey the impulses generated in the retina to the occipital region of the cerebral cortex where they produce sensation of vision. Optic nerve fibres are axons of the retinal ganglion cells and carry the total output of the retina.

Rhodopsin is the photosensitive visual pigment present in the discs of the rod outer segments. It consists of a protein opsin (called scotopsin) and a carotenoid called retinal (the aldehyde of vitamin A).The visual pigments consist of retinal, an aldehyde (oxidation product) of retinol, bound as the chromophore to a protein molecule called opsin.

During a photochemical reaction of the eye, rhodopsin, the pigment of mammalian rod cells, when exposed in vitro to light, breaks down into all trans retinal and opsin. The absorption of a single photon by a pigment complex, can initiate the reaction which results in the transformation of retinal to all trans configuration. The trans configuration will not fit opsin. It is the freeing of the retinal moiety which in some obscure way leads to an excitation in a retinal neuron that eventually registers in the brain as the sensation of light. In cats the amino acids 'taurine' is necessary for photoreceptor cell function and viability.

Vitamin A (all-trans-retinol) is a precursor of rhodopsin, the photopigment found in rods within the retina of our eye that helps us to see at night. Without vitamin A, "night blindness" occurs. Vitamin A, is a well known fat soluble vitamin found in many supplements and foods.

Cataract is a common lens abnormality in elderly human beings which can be corrected by surgical removal of the entire lens.

Ocular Muscles and Movements

Ocular muscles are capable of a wide range of movements that allow the eyes to track and examine objects with great precision. The extraocular eye muscles attach to the sclera of the eye .

There are 2 types of muscles of iris

1. Circular muscle - Having parasympathetic innervations
2. Radial muscle - Having sympathetic innervations

Accommodation is the process by which the refractive power of the eye may be increased.Accommodation in most domestic animals is performed by alteration of the shape of the lens. Equine having 'ramp retina' which could focus on the grazed objects and far objects simultaneously. In birds cornea may play a role in accommodation.

Cornea : Is strongest optical portion of the eye because of the air- to-tissue surface. Intraocular pressure in animals is 10-25 mmHg. Tremor of iris muscle is known as hippus.

Photochemistry, Eye Defects and Eye Examinations (As An Aid to Clinical Evaluation)

Color-blindness is the inability to distinguish the differences between certain colors. This condition results from an absence of color-sensitive pigment in the cone cells of the retina, the nerve layer at the back of the eye. Most color vision problems are inherited and are present at birth.

Different animals have different kinds of color vision. Some have very poor color vision and others have very good color vision. Dogs, cats, mice, rats and rabbits have very poor color vision. Bulls, along with all other cattle, are color-blind to red. Why do bulls charge when they see red. The bull is likely irritated not by the muleta's color, but by the cape's movement as the matador whips it around. In support of this is the fact that a bull charges the matador's other cape — the larger capote — with equal fury. Some animals do have good color vision. Monkeys, ground squirrels, birds, insects, and many fish can see a fairly good range of color.

The typical test for color-blindness is based on a person's ability to see numbers inside a circle.

Ear: Physiology of Hearing and Common Hearing Impairment

The receptors for hearing and equilibrium are located in the ear. Auditory function plays a significant role in domesticated animals as they interact with fellow animals, other animals, and humans, and in non-domesticated animals as they interact with other animals, prey species, and predator species. Diminished or absent audition can present danger or even be lethal, whether it be a deaf dog struck by an undetected motor vehicle, or a deaf wild animal succumbing to an undetected predator. Some animals can move their ears like radar antennas to seek out sound. Hearing is a function of the cerebral cortex. Hearing requires an intact auditory pathway from the ears to primary auditory areas. Primary auditory areas include the Brodmann's area located in the middle of superior temporal gyrus on the upper margin and on its deep or insular aspect.

The mechanism of hearing is closely associated with the mechanism of equilibrium; therefore, the inner ear acts as an organ of hearing and equilibrium.

The external ear, the middle ear and the cochlea of the inner ear are concerned with hearing. The external ear funnels sound waves to the external auditory meatus and subsequently to receptors for hearing in the inner ear.

External ear

Middle ear

Cochlea of Inner Ear

The **external ear** acts as a funnel to collect sound wave vibrations and direct them to the eardrum. The middle ear amplifies and transmits the vibrations from the eardrum to the inner ear. The inner ear contains the actual sensory receptors that convert the mechanical vibrations to nerve impulses, along with receptors for the equilibrium sense.

The external auditory canal is a soft, membrane-lined tube that begins at the base of the pinna and carries sound waves to the tympanic membrane (eardrum). In most domestic animal species, it is somewhat L-shaped with an

outer, vertical portion and an inner, horizontal portion. It ends blindly at the tympanic membrane. The tympanic membrane is susceptible to perforation, most commonly secondary to conditions such as otitis media, neoplasms, or traumatic injury.

Tympanic membrane, also called eardrum, thin layer of tissue in the ear covered by skin on the outside and mucosa on the internal surface, that receives sound vibrations from the outer air and transmits them to the auditory ossicles, which are tiny bones in the tympanic (middle-ear) cavity. When sound waves reach the tympanic membrane they cause it to vibrate.

Middle ear is It is filled with air and contains three small bones called ossicles and the opening of the Eustachian tube, which connects it with the pharynx (throat).The ossicles (malleus, incus, and stapes) within the middle ear are responsible for sound transduction from low-impedance air to high-impedance perilymph in the inner ear.

When sound waves hit the tympanic membrane, they stimulate the three auditory ossicles, which form a chain suspended in the tympanic cavity. These bones articulate with each other as a lever system, amplifying sound waves that ultimately produce vibrations in the inner ear and allow animals to hear.

Three small bones called ossicles link the tympanic membrane with the cochlea of the inner ear, where the receptors for hearing are located. The outermost bone, the malleus (hammer), is attached to the tympanic membrane. The malleus forms a complete synovial joint with the middle bone, the incus, which in turn forms a joint with the medial-most bone, the stapes. The other end of the stapes is attached to the membrane that covers the oval window of the cochlea.

The Eustachian tube connects the middle ear cavity with the pharynx. Its purpose is to equalize the air pressure on the two sides of the tympanic membrane. The slitlike opening of the tube in the pharynx is stretched open whenever the animal swallows or yawns. This allows air to enter or leave as necessary to equalize the pressure in the middle ear cavity with that of the outside air. The inner ear is made up of structures that contribute to both hearing and equilibrium. The hearing portion of the inner ear is contained in a snail shell-shaped spiral cavity in the temporal bone called the cochlea. Within the hollowed-out bony cavity of the cochlea is a soft, multilayered, fluid-filled portion that contains the receptor organ of hearing—the organ of Corti. The organ of corti has tiny, hairlike projections which are receptor cells of hearing. The nerve impulses so generated travel to the brain to be deciphered as sound.

If under extreme acoustic stress, the stereocilia gets destroyed due to excessive movement, hearing loss occurs.

Vestibule Apparatus

The vestibular system is the sensory system that provides the leading contribution to the sense of balance and spatial orientation for the purpose of coordinating movement with balance. The vestibular system is part of the inner ear. The vestibular system consists of two structures of the bony labyrinth of the inner ear, the vestibule and the semicircular canals, and the structures of the membranous labyrinth contained within them. Movement of the head bends the vestibular apparatus, which generates nerve impulses that give the brain information about the position of the head.

The brain relies on the vestibular system, the eyes, and the proprioceptors around the body for information about how and where the body is moving so that it can keep the animal upright and maintain balance. The brain relies on the vestibular system, the eyes, and the proprioceptors around the body for information about how and where the body is moving so that it can keep the animal upright and maintain balance. In each utricle and saccule is a patch of sensory epithelium called the macula. It consists of hair cells and supporting cells covered by a gelatinous matrix that contains tiny crystals of calcium carbonate called otoliths.

Physiology of Olfaction and Taste

The sense of smell plays an important role in our interaction with the environment and therefore it can have a direct influence on animal and human behavior. The sense of smell or olfaction is well developed in animals like dog and rabbit to give warning of the environmental dangers. In humans, apes and monkeys (primates), the sense of smell is comparatively less developed, but still it is important for pleasure and for enjoying the taste of food. Domestic animals and Human beings can detect and distinguish thousands of different compounds by smell, often with considerable sensitivity and specificity. Most odorants are relatively small organic compounds with sufficient volatility that they can be carried as vapors into the nose. The smell produced by an **odorant** depends on the compound's interaction with a specific binding surface, most likely a protein receptor. Average dog's nose is tens of thousands of times as sensitive to odors as compared to human beings. Dogs possess up to 300 million olfactory receptors in their noses, compared to about six million in human beings.Some dog breeds are famous for their sense of smell such as German Shepherd, Blood Hound and Pointer etc. The ability of the dog to detect scents varies between breeds, with long-nosed dogs able to distinguish scents better than the short-faced ones.

Some human beings (and other animals) suffer from specific anosmias; that is, they are incapable of smelling specific compounds even though their olfactory systems are otherwise normal. Such anosmias are often inherited. These observations suggest that mutations in individual receptor genes lead to the loss of the ability to detect a small subset of compounds.

Olfaction involves a pathway of biochemical and electrophysiological processes, which allows the conversion of molecular information into sensations. The initial sensory process starts at the olfactory epithelium and then the signal is brought through the axons from the thousands of cells expressing the odor receptor converging in the olfactory bulb.

Odorants are detected in a specific region of the nose, called the main olfactory epithelium, that lies at the top of the nasal cavity. The olfactory membrane lies in the superior part of each nostril. Their receptor cells for the smell sensations are the olfactory cells. Which are actually bipolar nerve cells derived originally from the central nervous system itself. There are about several million of these cells in the olfactory epithelium interspersed among sustentacular cells. The mucosal end of the olfactory cell forms a knob called the olfactory vesicle from which a large numbers of olfactory hairs of cilia, 0.3 micron in diameter and 50 to 150 microns in length, project into the mucus that coats the inner surface of the nasal cavity. Approximately 1 million sensory neurons line the surface of this region. These are there to stimulate the olfactory cells. Spaced among the olfactory cells in the olfactory membrane are many small *glands of Bowmen* that secrete mucus into the surface of the olfactory membrane.

Stimulus Necessary for Smell

The following are the physical characteristics of the substances that cause olfactory stimulation.

1. First the substance must be volatile so that it can be sniffed into the nostrils.
2. Second it must be at least slightly water soluble so that it can pass through the mucus of the olfactory cells.
3. Third it must be lipid soluble, presumably because the olfactory hairs and outer tips of the olfactory cells are composed principally of lipid materials.

Around 20 years after the start of their pioneering studies on the function of the nose and brain in odor perception, R. Axel and L. Buck have received the 2004 Nobel Prize for Medicine or Physiology. Olfactory receptor gene clusters are located in proximity to key locus of susceptibility for autoimmune diseases such as the major histocompatibility complex. Linda Buck and Richard Axel (2004 Nobel Prize awardees) have discovered that mammals usually have 1,000 genes for odor receptors. Genes associated with olfactory receptors are distributed on all but two chromosomes, with the majority being on chromosome 11 and most others spread along chromosomes 1, 6, and 9.

Anosmia is a total loss of sense of smell as has been reported in some cases of corona infection. Hyposmia refers to a diminished olfactory sensitivity.

Sense of Taste

The sense of taste, also called the gustatory sense, is a chemical sense. Its receptors are located in the mouth in structures called taste buds. The taste buds are located on the tongue, palate, pharynx, epiglottis and upper-third of oesophagus. When taste buds detect chemical substances dissolved in the saliva, the taste receptors generate nerve impulses that travel to the brain and are interpreted as tastes. The importance of taste lies in the fact that it allows the animal to select his food in accord with his desires and perhaps also in accord with the need of the tissues for specific nutritive substances. The sense of taste affords an animal the ability to evaluate what it eats and drinks. At the most basic level, this evaluation is to promote ingestion of nutritious substances and prevent consumption of potential poisons or toxins.

Tongue, the main site of taste detection, contains numerous taste buds on its dorsal surface. The mucous membrane of the dorsal surface of tongue exhibits numerous papillae, which increase the surface area of the mucosa available for taste receptors. The sense of taste is mediated by taste receptor cells which are bundled in clusters called taste buds. Taste receptor cells sample oral concentrations of a large number of small molecules and report a sensation of taste to centers in the brainstem. Each taste bud contains 50 to 100 taste receptor cells. The taste receptor cells within a bud are arranged such that their tips form a small taste pore, and through this pore extend microvilli from the taste cells. The microvilli of the taste cells bear taste receptors.

The Taste Bud and Its Functions

The taste buds are concerned with the sensation of taste. Each taste bud is barrel shaped and measures about 50–70 mm in diameter. It consists of cluster of cells with a small opening (taste pore) on the surface.The taste bud is composed of modified epithelial cells called taste cells. The outer tip of the taste cells are arranged around a minute taste pore. From the tip of each cell, several microvilli or taste hairs about 2 to 3 microns in length and 0.2 micron in width, protrude outward through the taste pore to approach the cavity of the mouth.

These microvilli are believed to provide the receptors surface for taste. Interwoven among the taste cells is a branching terminal network of several taste nerve fibres that are stimulated by the taste cells. These fibres invaginate deeply into the folds of the taste cell membranes, so that there is an extremely intimate contact between the same taste fibre. The taste buds are located on the papillae of the tongue. The sense of smell is quite important in the taste perception.

The sense of taste is equivalent to excitation of taste receptors, and receptors for a large number of specific chemicals have been identified to contribute to the reception of taste. The sensation of taste includes five established basic tastes: sweetness, sourness, saltiness, bitterness, and umami.

Sweet - usually indicates energy rich nutrients. There are many non-carbohydrate molecules that trigger a sweet response, leading to the development of many artificial sweeteners, including saccharin, sucralose, and aspartame. Some of these artificial sweeteners are taken by diabetic people as a substitute for natural sugars.

Umami - the taste of amino acids (e.g. meat broth or aged cheese)

Salty - allows modulating diet for electrolyte balance

Sour - typically the taste of acids

Bitter - allows sensing of diverse natural toxins.The bitter taste, when it occurs in high intensity, usually causes the animal to reject the food. This is undoubtedly an important purposive function of the bitter taste sensation because many of the deadly toxins found in poisonous plants are alkaloids and these all cause an intensely bitter taste.

There are some clear differences among animals in what they can taste. Cats, for example, do not respond to sweets due to a deletion in the gene that encodes one of the sweet receptors.

Threshold for Taste

The different ruminant species differ in their threshold for taste. Goats are reputed to have a higher threshold for bitter taste.

Summary

- The nerve cells are excitable, i.e. capable of generation of electrical impulses at their membranes.
- Sense of vision is a complex function of the two eyes and their central connections.
- The mechanism of hearing is closely associated with the mechanism of equilibrium; therefore, the inner ear acts as an organ of hearing and equilibrium.
- The sense of smell or olfaction is well developed in animals like dogs to give warning of the environmental dangers.

8

Monogastric and Polygastric Digestive System

Digestion is the process by which food is converted into substances that can be absorbed and assimilated by a living organism. In most animals it is accomplished in the digestive tract by the mechanical and enzymatic breakdown of foods into simpler chemical compounds. Digestion usually consists of two elements: a mechanical/ physical stage, e.g. mastication, churning, emulsification, in which no chemical bonds are broken and no enzymes are required; and a chemical stage requiring enzymes in which complex food molecules are broken down by hydrolysis into a state in which they can be absorbed. In most heterotrophic organisms digestion is 'extracellular', the enzymes being released outside the cell and the digested products absorbed. In the majority of heterotrophs digestion takes place in a specialized cavity or internal tube, the alimentary canal, which is usually muscular, with food being squeezed through the digestive system by a process of peristalsis.

The digestive tract may be described as a tube extending from the lips to the anus. The mammalian gastrointestinal tract spans from the mouth to the anus, with an average length of approximately 5 m in humans.The digestive process begins with the prehension, or taking up of food; continues with its mastication (chewing), insalivation (mixing with the salivary secretions), deglutition (swallowing), and the digestion, absorption, and assimilation of those food elements that are of nutritive value; and terminates with defecation, or the excretion of the remaining ingested matter not capable of being absorbed or utilized as nourishment.

The primary functions of gastrointestinal tract are the maintenance of water homeostasis, the digestion, and absorption of macro- and micronutrients and electrolytes, trafficking of the fraction of macromolecular antigens that survive digestion, and the exclusion of pathogens.The specific purpose of digestion is to convert food substances into simple and soluble materials fit for absorption and assimilation. The gastrointestinal tract is a continuous tube i.e. alimentary canal and the glands associated with it that stretches from mouth to anus.

The powers of sight and smell are useful to all animals in finding their food. The mouth and teeth of ruminants are well adapted for the prehension and grinding of plant parts and there are well developed salivary glands in the mouth. The large amount of saliva secreted aids in mastication of the feed. The digestive systems of animals are divided into three main categories: ruminants (cranial fermenter) and monogastrics and Hind gut (caudal fermenter). The hind gut fermenters have a simple stomach, but a very large and complex large intestine.The notable hind gut fermenter is horse.The large intestine of hind gut fermentors is analogous to the rumen in ruminants.

- Large, anaerobic fermentation vat.
- Microbes digest structural carbohydrates (cellulose, hemicellulose) and soluble carbohydrates that escape digestion in small intestine to VFA's.
- VFA's absorbed from large intestine and utilized by the animal.
- Microbial protein produced in large intestine is wasted (only very limited absorption from large intestine).

The digestive system of ruminants differ from that of non-ruminants. The food supplies energy to the body and supplies nutrients for its growth and maintenance. The type of digestive system influences the dietary foodstuffs the animal can effectively utilize.

Monogastrics, also known as nonruminants, are animals with relatively small, simple, one-compartment stomachs containing limited microorganisms. Monogastric animals include the pig, chicken,dog, cat and horse. The monogastric stomach is a C-shaped organ located just behind the diaphragm in the left cranial abdomen.

Body needs energy for the functioning of various processes for the nutrition and repair of damaged tissue. This energy comes from the food nutrients. The food nutrients undergo a series of chemical reactions in the body to release the necessary energy.

The higher animals are dependent on plants and other animals for their nutrients. They can be classified into two groups.

Carnivores : Those animals which obtain most of their food by eating other animals are carnivores. In these species digestion is mainly enzymatic in nature and microbial digestion is minimal.

Herbivores : These animals obtain most of their food nutrients from herbage and other plant parts. In the herbivores, microbial digestion is of great significance and allows utilization of plant materials that are not broken down by the enzymes present in the digestive secretions.

Most of the domesticated animals except cat & dog fall in the category of herbivores. The domesticated herbivores can be divided into three groups:

1. Ruminants : Those possessing a rumen (cow, buffalo, sheep, goat, camel etc.) in which there is extensive microbial fermentation of the herbage diet in a specialized region of the digestive tract, prior to its digestion by the alimentary enzymes.
2. Psedoruminants eg members of the camelidae family eg camel, Ilama, alpaca, vicuna etc. In pseudo ruminants animal third compartment of the compound stomach is absent.
3. Non-Ruminant : The second group is those with simple stomachs (Horse, Pig) in which fermentation takes place in the posterior part of the digestive tract.

Morphological Characteristic of Monogastric and Polygastric Digestive System

Most foodstuffs contain a mixture of nutrients viz proteins, fats, carbohydrates, minerals, vitamins and water. As few of these can be absorbed directly by the animals, they must be prepared or notified to make them available. This is accomplished by the process of digestion in which foodstuffs are converted to diffusible or assimilatable substances with the help of enzymes secreted in the digestive tract or especially in herbivores, by the actions of microorganisms living in symbolic association with the animal. Thus the digestive system is concerned with the ingestion, digestion and assimilation of food nutrients. The food nutrients undergo a series of chemical reactions in the body to release the necessary energy. The sum total of these reactions is termed as metabolism.

Digestive System : The digestive system includes the digestive tract and its associated glands. The tract itself is a tubular structure for the ingestion and digestion of food. The tract includes the mouth, pharynx, esophagus, stomach, small intestines (duodenum, jejunum, ileum) large intestines (caecum, colon, rectum) and anus. The macroscopic compartments, separated from each other by sphincters, are the buccal cavity, esophagus, stomach, small intestine, and large intestine. The accessory structures are located outside the limits of the tract proper and empty into it through ducts. They are salivary glands, liver and pancreas.

The continuous multilayer stratified squamous epithelium in contact with the lumen of the buccal cavity and esophagus is adapted to handle the high volume of quickly passing food.

Regulations of Food Intake : Animal eats food to provide energy required for the various body functions. In higher vertebrates food must be actively sought, ingested and digested before it can be of use to the animal. Appetite is the drive causing an animal to eat. Several theories have been propounded to explain the regulation of food intake in domestic animals.

Central control of food intake is affected by the hypothalamus. Stimulation of various centres in the hypothalamus can cause an animal to eat several times of its requirement or in some cases may stop an hungry animal from eating. The ventromedial nucleus is called the satiety centre and lateral hypothalamus as hunger center. Damage to the ventromedial hypothalamus (satiety center) causes overeating and obesity while lesions in the lateral hypothalamus (hunger center) causes under eating followed in some cases by death. Goats eat excessively following similar lesions and fill their rumen to the extent that breathing becomes difficult.

The intake of food in most domestic is adjusted to the energy expenditure. If the animal is used for heavy draft, the food intake is increased to adjust the excess energy expenditure. Among the peripheral mechanisms which regulate food intake include blood glucose level. The VFA (volatile fatty acids) production in the rumen and gastric filling also regulate food intake in these animals. In the horse, the VFA concentration in the colon is an important regulator of food intake.The sensory qualities of a food will provide inputs to the brain which will be integrated with inputs from gut, liver and other sensitive areas to determine whether, and at what rate, an animal eats. The control of food intake is thus multifactorial. The feed intake in ruminants is controlled by factors which are not necessarily the same as in non ruminants. Ruminants have the capacity to eat a heavy bulk of food which is rich in crude fibre. Physiology factors such as gastrointestinal fill are important in these animals in the regulation of food intake. Food intake by the lactating cow and buffalo depends upon several animal, food, as well as management factors. The animals factors include the body weight, milk yield, stage of lactation and other metabolic factors. The food factors include the forage type its preparation, concentrate forage ratio and protein content of the food. The management factors include frequency of feeding and access time. Palatability of the food also determines the amount of food taken in. Roughages high in lignin have poor palatability and there is less feed intake than from fodders low in lignin. Small particle size causes higher feed intake as compared to larger particle size. Thus feed preparation such as chafing, palleting etc. are important regulators of food intake in ruminants.

The ruminants are known to possess taste receptors the threshold of which vary between different species. The goat has a higher threshold for the bitter taste as compared to cattle. The taste responses can be modified by feeding taste modifiers such as gymnemic acid, inosinic acid or monosodium glutamate.

Capacity of Digestive System

The herbivorous animals are equipped with a more capacious digestive system as compared to non herbivores . The ox, for example, in proportion to high weight relative to man has about nine times the digestive tract capacity. Such an arrangement by the herbivores is necessary for processing the relatively enormous quantities of food of low usable energy & high bulk (such as the roughages) necessarily consumed to obtain the quantity and energy and nutrients necessary for normal maintenance and production. Most of the bulk of the digestive tract in ruminants is due to the large rumen which constitutes about 90% of total stomach capacity and weight about 40% of total digestive tract in adult buffalo.

Prehension

Prehension is the process of seizing or grasping or otherwise getting food into the mouth. Different species use different techniques to prehend food - for example, horses and goats rely considerably on their lips, whereas cattle, dogs and cats don't use their lips to any extent, but rather, gather many foods with their tongues.

Mastication, or chewing, is the first step in the breakdown of complex foodstuffs and serves several functions, including ;breaking large pieces into small pieces, resulting in a massive increase in surface area, which is where digestive enzymes work;softening of food and transformation into a size conducive to swallowing:lubrication of food by impregnating it with saliva

Chewing is, to a large extent, a reflex. The presence of food in the mouth causes a reflex inhibition of the muscles of the lower jaw. Those muscles relax and the lower jaw drops, causing a stretch reflex which causes muscle contraction and closure of the mouth. During mastication, the tongue and, to a lesser extent, the lips and cheeks acts to keep food between the grinding surfaces of the teeth. Tongue forces mix the food with salivary fluid secreted from the parotid and salivary glands.

Deficits in the ability to effectively masticate are a very common cause of digestive disease in animals. Many of these problems are associated with poor teeth.

Sense of Taste

Taste is a function of the taste buds in the mouth and its importance lies in the fact that it allows the animal to select his food in accord with his desires and perhaps also in accord with the need of the tissues for specific nutritive substances.

There are at least four primary sensations of taste, sour, salty, sweet and bitter.

The bitter taste, when it occurs in high intensity, usually causes the animal to reject the food. This is undoubtedly an important purposive function of the bitter taste sensation because many of the deadly toxins found in poisonous plants are alkaloids and these all cause an intensely bitter taste.

Threshold for Taste

The different ruminant species differ in their threshold for taste. Goats are reputed to have a higher threshold for bitter taste.

The Taste Bud and Its Functions

The taste bud is composed of modified epithelial cells called taste cells. The outer tip of the taste cells are arranged around a minute taste pore. From the tip of each cell, several microvilli or taste hairs about 2 to 3 microns in length and 0.2 micron in width, protrude outward through the taste pore to approach the cavity of the mouth. These microvilli are believed to provide the receptors surface for taste.

Interwoven among the taste cells is a branching terminal network of several taste nerve fibres that are stimulated by the taste cells. These fibres invaginate deeply into the folds of the taste cell membranes, so that there is an extremely intimate contact between the same taste fibre. The taste buds are located on the papillae of the tongue. The sense of smell is quite important in the taste perception.

The final part in pregastric digestion is *swallowing*, also known as *deglutition*. During swallowing, boluses of food are propelled through the esophagus by strong peristaltic contractions. In dogs and humans, it takes 4-5 seconds for the bolus to traverse the esophagus.

Mastication or chewing : Perhaps the most important mechanical preparation of food is mastication or chewing, which breaks up large particles, and mixes saliva with the food to serve as a lubricant to allow easy swallowing. Animals differ in their ability to masticate their food, depending upon the physical structure of their mouth & teeth and also on the kind of food they eat. Ruminants usually swallow small seed grains with little chewing. However, forages are ground thoroughly during the rumination, when the boluses are regurgitated and remasticated rather than at the time the forage is consumed. Poultry have no teeth and they swallow their food whole. Any grinding that occurs is in the bird's gizzard. The carnivorous animals usually don't masticate or chew their food. The thorough mastication is essential for the microbial action of the rumen microorganisms.

Eructation is the mechanism whereby the ruminant animal belches or gets rid of the large quantities of gas produced in the forestomach as a result of microbial fermentation. Normally a cow weighing 500 kg with 70 kg of rumen contents produces about 2 litres of gas per minute. The quantity and rate of gas production in the rumen vary greatly with the quality of feed.

Methane and carbon dioxide are produced as end products of fermentation and are largely eliminated by eructation.The rumen gas consists of carbon dioxide, methane, nitrogen, oxygen, hydrogen and hydrogen sulphide. The methane is a type of greenhouse gas which has recently become a centre of attraction. Low methanogenic feeds have been advocated to be fed to ruminants in order to decrease the greenhouse gases in our environment.

Esophagus : Once the food has been swallowed by the animal, the food mass is known as *bolus* and moves by peristaltic waves of the esophagus and gravity to the stomach.

Peristalsis consists of alternate contractions and relaxations of the smooth muscle of the oesophagus and is carried out entirely in a reflex manner by the autonomic nervous system, which sends visceral efferent impulses to the smooth muscle in the walls of the digestive tract.

No digestive enzymes are secreted by the esophagus and, therefore, no digestion takes place there. No absorption takes place in the lumen of the buccal cavity and esophagus.

Nonruminants are better adapted to processing and utilizing concentrated feeds such as grains.

A ruminant is any hooved animal that digests its food in two steps-a) By eating the raw material and regurgitating a semi digested form known as cud. Ruminants are animals that have a complex stomach consisting of four chambers namely the rumen, reticulum, omasum, and abomasum. The largest compartment is the rumen. Because the rumen can store large quantities of roughages, ruminants have a greater ability to process and utilize large quantities of bulky roughages. Examples of ruminants are cattle, buffalo,camel,sheep and goats. The size or volume of the stomach varies depending on how full or empty it is. Fermentative digestion which precedes gastric and intestinal digestion is buffered by salivary secretions.

The gastric mucosa is made up of simple columnar epithelium containing surface mucous cells that produce a layer of mucus. This helps protect the stomach from the acidity of the gastric secretions. If the surface mucous cells are not producing adequate mucus, this can lead to the development of gastric ulcers in monogastric animals as well as human beings. Mucus is compsed of mucin glycoproteins that form viscoelastic gels resulting in an adherent unstirred layer coating the GI wall.

The glandular portion of the stomach can be divided into three basic regions, called the cardia, fundus and pylorus. The muscle contractions of the monogastric stomach wall contribute to the mechanical breakdown of food particles that will be further digested in the small intestine.Hormones such as secretin, cholecystokinin (CCK) and gastric inhibitory peptides released by the small intestine, play a role in delaying gastric emptying by inhibiting pyloric antral contractions and further constricting the pyloric sphincter.

Rumen gases, particularly methane, are increasingly in the news because of their contribution to greenhouse gas and climate change.

The ruminant stomach is composed of four parts; the rumen, reticulum, omasum and abomasum. These compartments give the cow and other ruminants a decided advantage in digesting and utilizing those parts of the plants and other compounds which are practically useless to animals with simple stomach. Substances such as cellulose, a major constituent of plant tissues and urea, a non protein nitrogen compound, are of limited use of non ruminants. However ruminants through fermenting and synthesizing action of microorganisms in their complex stomach, can efficiently utilize these substances for productive purposes. The dairy cow converts this feed into milk and meat, two highly nutritious and palatable food for humans. This ability to make use of feed which otherwise would go waste because it is not directly consumable for humans is one of the most compelling justifications for the existence of cattle and buffaloes, in a world which must make use of all possible food resources.

Different Parts of Compound Stomach

1. ***Rumen*** : The rumen or paunch is divided into areas by muscular bands called pillars. There are a dorsal, a ventral and 2 posterior sacs. Action of the muscular pillars forces the feed in the rumen to move in a rotary fashion so that it thoroughly mixes with the ruminal fluid. Many finger-like projections, the papillae, line the rumen wall, resulting in a greatly increased surface area for absorption of nutrients from the rumen.

At regular intervals the portions of the ruminal and reticular contents are returned to the mouth for remastication and reinsalivation. In the rumen the ingesta are subjected to energetic mixing, kneading and churning by *rumen and reticular movements*.

There are two waves of contraction 1. The primary waves and 2. Secondary waves. In contraction, the movements of rumen and reticulum are closely associated. First the reticulum undergoes a sharp contraction followed by the rumen. This helps in passing the liquid material from reticulum and rumen.

During contractions, the rumen produces sounds which are heard readily by auscultation.Reticulum also produces sounds which can be heard ventrally over the seventh rib on the left side. The major contractions of the rumen and reticulum are under vagal control.

2. Reticulum : The reticulum is only partially separated from the rumen by a low partition. Ruminal and reticular contents intermix freely and the two compartments frequently are referred to as the reticulo-rumen. The thick walls of the reticulum resembles a honeycomb, a name which has been used in the past for this part of the ruminant stomach. An opening on the right side of the reticulum leads into the omasum, an organ into which food passes after action by microorganisms in the rumen and reticulum. A groove in the reticulum between the esophagus and the omasum, is called oesophageal groove. In the nursing calf, the sides of the groove extend upward by reflex action and form a conduit through which milk passes directly from the esophagus to the omasum before the rumen and reticulum are developed and functioning. Even if ruminal action were normal, it is more efficient for milk to bypass fermentation in the rumen and be digested directly in the abomasum and intestines. Fermenting action by ruminal microorganisms is wasteful of energy and reduces the protein quality of an easily digested, high quality food such as milk.

3. Omasum : After fermenting action in the rumen and reticulum, feed passes through the reticulo-omasal orifice into the omasum. This organ consists of many layers of muscular leaves, which resulted in its being called the many plies. The reticulo-omasal orifice is a "valve" which retains feed particles within the rumen until they are reduced to 1 to 2 mm in diameter. In the particles leaving the rumen have most of the fermentable carbohydrates solubilized. Much of the water and electrolytes are absorbed in the omasum.

4. Abomasum : The abomasum is the true stomach of the cow. It is the only part of the ruminant stomach which contains tissue for secretion of gastric juices. The walls of the abomasum are lined with many folds, greatly increasing the surface area within the organ. This organ makes up 80% or more of the total stomach volume of a newborn calf. The other compartments grow at a much faster rate once the calf starts eating the dry feeds and less than 10% of the stomach capacity in the adult cow is in the abomasum. In the abomasum the pH is decreased from 6 to 2.5. Abomasal secretions contain proteolytic enzymes.

Rumination

Ruminants differ from other animals in having a greatly enlarged forestomach consisting of three additional stomach compartments and in relation to their method of eating food. In contrast to other animals, the ruminants quickly crop (tears) and swallow large amounts of herbage with relatively little chewing. Ruminants graze and swallow their food as soon as it is well lubricated. Cattle usually graze for 4 to 9 hours a day and sheep and goats for 9 to 11 hours a day. Cattle, buffalo, sheep, goat and horses have palatability preferences for certain plants.The four compartments are rumen, reticulum, omasum and abomasum. Of these the rumen and reticulum together have more than 50 % of the total digestive tract capacity of mature cattle. This large capacity is essential to allow feed retention so that microorganisms can break down cellulose and other complex carbohydrates which mammalian stomach enzymes cannot hydrolyse.

After having taken in sufficient fodder, the animal will stop eating, lie down and then slowly start regurgitating one bolus or 'cud' after another. Each bolus, this time, is thoroughly and slowly chewed and again swallowed. This process is called rumination or 'chewing the cud'. Rumination consists of four processes, regurgitation, remastication, reinsalivation and redeglutition. Rumination is a reflex that is initiated by mechanical stimulation of receptors in the mucosa of the reticulum, rumino-reticular fold and rumen in the area of the cardia. The coarseness of the ration influences the time spent in rumination. Thus rumination time is longer on a roughage based ration than on a concentrate based ration.

Rumen Movements

The rumen moves regularly and contracts about once every minute. By putting your fist on the left flank (in the hollow behind the ribs) you will be able to detect the contractions. Regular contractions are a sign of good health. An orderly pattern of ruminal motility is initiated early in life and except for temporary periods of disruption, persists for the lifetime of the animal. These movements serve to mix the ingesta, aid in eructation of gas, and propel fluid and fermented foodstuffs into the omasum. If motility is suppressed for a significant length of time, ruminal impaction may result.

Two types of contractions are identified:

Primary contractions originate in the reticulum and pass caudally around the rumen. This process involves a wave of contraction followed by a wave of relaxation, so as parts of the rumen are contracting, other sacs are dilating.

Secondary contractions occur in only parts of the rumen and are usually associated with eructation.

The forestomachs possess a rich enteric nervous system, but coordinated contractions require central input. Motility centers in the brainstem control both the rate and strength of contraction via vagal afferents. Cutting the vagus nerve in a ruminat abolishes coordinated reticulo ruminal motility. There are also vagal afferents from the rumen to the motility centers which allow stretch receptors and chemoreceptors in the rumen to modulate contractility. Animals on a high roughage diet have a higher frequency of contractions than those on a diet rich in concentrates.

Regurgitation is initiated with a reticular contraction distinct from the primary contraction. This contraction, in conjunction with relaxation of the distal esophageal sphincter, allows a bolus of ingesta to enter the esophagus. The bolus is carried into the mouth by reverse peristalsis. The fluid in the bolus is squeezed out with the tongue and reswallowed, and the bolus itself is remasticated, then reswallowed. Rumination occurs predominantly when the animal is resting and not eating.

Rumen fermentation produces an enormous quantity of gas. Ruminants remove this gas through the process of eructation or belching. Eructation is associated with almost every secondary ruminal contraction Anything that interferes with eructation is life threatening to the ruminant because the expanding rumen rapidly interferes with breathing. Animals suffering ruminal tympany (bloat) die from asphyxiation. Fever has been associated with decreased rumen motility. Pain may be associated with rumen hypomotility or atony.

Several physiological and physical factors contribute to the buffalo's ability to utilize poor quality roughage and crop residues. Among these factors are the large rumen volume, high rate of salivation, slower rate of passage of digesta through the reticulorumen, slow rumen motility, and higher cellular activity.

Rumen Microorganisms

The ruminants have got unique ability to utilize lignocellulosic feed with the help of very well developed rumen microbial community in the fore stomach of livestock . Rumen is a fermentation chamber filled with microorganisms. These include rumen bacteria, protozoa and fungi. Among the different microbial communities, the bacteria are most abundant (10^{10} -10^{11}/ml) followed by protozoa (10^5 -10^6 /ml). The fungi are less in numbers (10^3 -10^4 /ml). The digestion of nutrients in the rumen is accomplished with the help of rumen microorganisms. Bacteria , protozoa, and fungi have been shown to be the microorganisms involved in plant cell wall digestion in the rumen. In spite of complicated interrelationships among the microorganisms (e.g., bacteria, protozoa, and fungi) in the rumen ecosystem, bacteria are believed to play a major role because of their numerical predominance and metabolic diversity.

The rumen bacteria constitute around 40-60% of the microbial biomass produced in the rumen and primarily responsible for fibre degradation.However, protozoa have been shown to digest from 25 to 30% of total fiber. Fungal activity is responsible for most of the cell wall degradation. Enzymatic activities of fungi, combined with the particular penetrating growth of the rhizoidal system, leads to weakening and particle size reduction of plant cell walls.

Bacterial concentration may be as high as 2.1×10^{10} bacteria/ ml of the rumen liquor in zebu cattle and approximately 2.5×10^{10}/ml of rumen liquor in buffaloes. Bacteria in the rumen are cellulolytic, amylolytic and methane producing.

Bacterial and protozoal number varies greatly with the type and quantity of diet, age and breed of the animals. The protozoal number in the rumen may be as high as 1×10^6 per gm of rumen contents. The protozoa are single cell organisms which feed on the bacteria and ingested feed.

Microorganisms are introduced by feeding but protozoa are found in the rumen only after weaning. This question of origin of rumen microorganism is more complex than it appears. The argument against this theory is that although microorganisms are certainly present in grasses and hay, these are different from those found in the rumen. However, it is also not clear how aerobic microorganisms of feed get converted to anaerobic microorganisms of the rumen. Rumen microorganisms are highly susceptible to changes in rumen pH.

Rumen protozoa are large (20-200 microns) unicellular organisms. Protozoa engulf feed particles and digest carbohydrates, proteins and fats. Recently it has been advocated that protozoa are parasites in the rumen and selective destruction of protozoa can lead to increased efficiency of utilization of food by the ruminants. Several methods of selective defaunation of the rumen are being currently experimented with.

The rumen bacteria and protozoa are anaerobic i.e. they will die or will not survive in the presence of air or oxygen. That is why rumen contains a large amount of CO_2 which is favourable for the survival of these bacteria. This CO_2 is produced as a result of fermentation of food by the bacteria themselves. The requirement of CO_2 by the anaerobic bacteria is very large and rumen provides a completely anaerobic environment.

A variety of bacteria and protozoa occur in the rumen, the composition of the population being largely determined by an equilibrium established in relation to the diet. The fate of the rumen microorganisms is that they eventually will pass into the abomasum and intestines where they are digested by secretions of the digestive tract and provide nutrients for the host animals.

These microorganisms break down the complex carbohydrates, such as cellulose and hemicellulose, by fermenting them to short chain fatty acids through action of their enzymes. The fatty acids then are absorbed directly from the rumen and reticulum into the bloodstream of ruminants for use as energy sources and for milk fat synthesis.

Anaerobic rumen fungi have been reported in a wide range of herbivores fed on high fibre diets. Six genera of fungi in the rumen have been described, namely, the monocentric Neocallimastix, Caecomyces and Piromyces and the polycentric Anaeromyces, Orpinomyces and Cyllamyces. The extensive colonization and degradation of fibrous plant tissues by the fungi suggest that they have a role in fibre digestion. All rumen fungi studied so far are fibrinolytic. They produce a range of hydrolytic enzymes, which include the cellulases, hemicellulases, pectinases and phenolic acid esterases, to enable them to invade and degrade the lignocellulosic plant tissues. Although rumen fungi may not seem to be essential to general rumen function since they may be absent in animals fed on low fibre diets, they, nevertheless, could contribute to the digestion of high fibre poor-quality forages.

Development of genetically modified microbes and their establishment in the rumen of domestic ruminants will be an interesting area in future with immense implications in ensuring food security in the world.

Digestion of Carbohydrates in the Rumen

The diet of ruminants consist in large parts of crosslinked polymerised carbohydrates - such as cellulose, hemicellulose and lignin.These polymerized carbohydrates occur in all plant cell walls .The lignin strengthens the plant structure but microbes in the rumen degrade lignin slowly. The quantity of lignin limits the utilization of many plants by the ruminant stomach.Unlignified plant cell wall materials are generally digested through microbial fermentation into volatile fatty acids. The crosslinked polymerised carbohydrates are broken down in the rumen to simple carbohydrates which are ultimately fermented to volatile fatty acids. This breakdown process occurs due to presence of enzyme cellulase secreted by rumen microorganisms. This is the reason why very little sugar and glycogen is present in animal's blood and tissues although carbohydrates form the largest part of the ruminants diet.

Lignin reduces digestibility of carbohydrates in the rumen by hydrogen bonding at critical sites which limit cellulase action. Alkali treatment of straws improves palatability, nutritive value and growth rate due to its ability to dissociate the lignin from the cell wall.

Glucose is the major breakdown product of starch and cellulose whilst hemicelluloses mainly yield pentoses. The pentoses are converted to hexoses before further catabolism.

The great majority of the carbohydrate metabolism thus proceeds via hexose which is then fermented to yield pyruvate, lactate and subsequently CO_2, volatile fatty acids, methane and of course ATP. A simple scheme for these reactions is shown below:

Thus it is clear from the foregoing discussions that carbohydrates are converted in the rumen into acetic, propionic and butyric acids.

As little glucose is absorbed as such in the case of ruminants, the blood glucose in ruminants is low. This blood glucose comes from the conversion of volatile fatty acids to glucose in the liver. This process is known as gluconeogenesis. Thus gluconeogenesis can be defined as the process of formation of glucose from materials other than sugars. Propionate is the principal glycogenic fatty acid in the ruminants. The estimates of the contribution of VFA to nutrition of ruminants range from 36 to 80% of the energy digested and absorbed from the gut. The figures illustrate the dominant role of the rumen as a site of digestion.

The rumen fermentation and digestion of plant cell wall material by microbes in the rumen decided the feed resources that are commonly used as diets for ruminants which include fibrous residues from cereal production, particularly from rice, wheat, maize etc and fermentable carbohydrate rich by products from agro-industries such a molasses from sugar extraction and bran's from processing of cereals and pastures.

Gas Production

Ruminal digestion of feed by the microorganisms, under anaerobic conditions, results in the production of acetate, propionate and butyrate(volatile fatty acids) which are used by the animal as energy source, and the production of ruminal gases such as $CO_2$and CH_4. The ruminal gas comprises carbon dioxide (65%), Methane (25-27%), nitrogen (7%) and trace amounts of oxygen, hydrogen and hydrogen sulphide. This gas is get rid of from the rumen by the process of eructation. Production of excessive amount of gas under pathological conditions may result in production of bloat, which may even be fatal.

Methane, which has a high energy equivalent, represents a direct loss of energy to the animals. Ruminal methanogenesis represents an energy loss to the animal besides contribution to greenhouse gases emissions.Methane emissions represent the second major contributors to global warming. Several techniques have been tried to reduce rumen methanogenesis with varying degree of success, which include immunization against ruminal methanogenesis, defaunation, uses of chemicals additives,ionophore antibiotics, plant extracts or feeding of methane reducing special plant species.

Lipid Metabolism in The Rumen

Lipid consumption by herbivorous animals is low because most forages contain only a limited amount of lipids.

The herbage lipids contain a high percentage of unsaturated fatty acids. The lipids are present in the form of galactosyl diglycerides.

In the rumen, the fat is hydrolysed to produce free fatty acids and glycerol. Rumen microbes also modify the unsaturated fatty acids by either saturating the or causing changing in the location of double bonds or altering the normal cis bond to a trans double bond. These changes in fatty acids are reflected in changes in the composition of fatty acids present in tissue or milk fat.

Some de novo synthesis of fatty acids also takes place resulting in the production of odd length and branched chain fatty acids. The rumen microbes are intolerant to high dietary levels of fat. When added fat is used, it is fed normally at no more than 5 to 7% of the total diet. Higher levels are apt to result in abnormal rumen fermentation unless the fat is protected from the rumen microorganisms by coating fat droplets with casein which is then treated with formaldehyde (protected fat feeding).

Protein Metabolism in The Rumen

The ruminants are able to use poor quality protein for the synthesis of body proteins. This is made possible because of the fact that the dietary proteins are taken up by the rumen microbes which break them down to constituent amino acids and these amino acids are used for the synthesis of high biological value protein by the rumen microbes. Proteins are degraded in the rumen by the action of proteases of microbial origin. Not all the microbial population possess exopeptidases, estimates range from 10 to 40% having such activity. Although the proteolytic enzymes are extracellular, there is little proteolytic activity in the rumen fluid.

The peptides released by protease activity are further catabolized to yield amino acids and ammonia. The ammonia concentration in the rumen is normally in the order of 10^{-2} while that of the free amino acids is much lower ($2.6\text{-}6.5 \times 10^{-5}$ M).

The high biological value proteins formed by the rumen microbes are again broken down in the abomasum or true stomach and used by the body. By the same reasoning the ruminants can use nonprotein nitrogen compounds such as urea and biuret which cannot be utilized by nonruminants. Thus ruminants differ from nonruminants in their protein metabolism in that they do not need high biological value protein in their diets.

Some of the ammonia present in the rumen is absorbed by blood and converted to urea in the liver. In ruminants, this urea instead of being completely excreted by the kidney, is secreted in the saliva. The salivary urea when it enters the rumen, again produces ammonia. Thus, there is recycling of urea in the ruminants which is absent in most nonruminants. Urea recycling has been found important in the horse too. Simultaneously with these breakdown reactions there is synthesis of microbial protein from the NPN compounds including ammonia, in the rumen.

About 200 g of microbial protein is produced per kg of organic matter digested in the rumen. The recycling of urea described above is more efficient on a low nitrogen intake.

Not all rumen bacteria possess urease activity. The total activity of urease in the rumen can be affected by the diet. Protozoa on the other hand possess little, if any, urease activity.

Urea $\rightarrow$ urease $\rightarrow$ NH_3

Some amino acids can also be synthesized in the rumen provided adequate quantities of precursors are made available in the diet. Thus the synthesis of methionine and cysteine by rumen microorganisms requires sulphur and its intake may limit protein synthesis when large amounts of non protein nitrogen are used. The synthesis of the nucleic acid involved in protein synthesis requires phosphorus and it is therefore also essential to ensure an adequate supply in the diet.

Vitamin Synthesis in the Rumen

Ruminants do not require a dietary source of B-complex vitamins as required by nonruminants. This is because of the fact that most of the complex vitamins can be synthesized by the rumen microorganisms. These vitamins are then utilized by the animal. However, in animals on cobalt deficient diet , symptoms characteristic of B_{12} deficiency can be produced. This is due to the fact that cobalt is a necessary precursor for the synthesis of vitamin B_{12} (cyanocobalamin) by the rumen bacteria. The water soluble vitamins (B-complex) are not stored in the body.

Metabolism in the Ruminant Animals

The ruminant animal is able to absorb nutrients required for its metabolism from the digestive tract. These nutrients are protein, fat and carbohydrates. The various energy & protein sources from the digestive tract are as below.

1. A large portion of the digestible energy is absorbed from the rumen in the form of VFA (Volatile Fatty Acids).
2. Another important source of energy is absorption of bacterial cell wall constituents digested in the lower gastrointestinal tract.
3. The third important source of energy to the animal comes from the long chain fatty acids of the ration of these animals.

Use of NPN by Ruminants

Urea and other NPN compounds (non protein nitrogen compounds such as biuret) can meet a part of the dietary protein requirement of the ruminants. NPN feeding to ruminants is more economical than natural protein However, the factors affecting the efficient utilization of urea nitrogen are varied and complex. For example carbohydrates not only supply energy for the growth and multiplication of rumen microorganisms but may also provide Carbon template for synthesis of microbial proteins.

Efficiency of Utilization of VFA in Ruminants

Theoretically on complete oxidation acetyl CoA, propionyl CoA and butyryl CoA give rise to 12, 20 and 29 moles of ATP per mole respectively. Two moles of ATP are required per mole of VFA activated.

In immature ruminants, the rumen is not developed and their digestive tracts function more like those of monogastric animals.

Defecation

Defecation is the final act of digestion, by which organisms eliminate solid, semisolid, or liquid waste material from the digestive tract via the anus. Waves of muscular contraction (known as peristalsis) in the walls of the colon move fecal matter through the digestive tract towards the rectum. Feces are the solid or semisolid remains of food that could not be digested in the small intestine. Feces contain a relatively small amount of metabolic waste products such as bacterially altered bilirubin, and the dead epithelial cells from the lining of the gut. The forces required to expel the feces are generated through muscular contractions and a build-up of gases inside the gut, prompting the sphincter to relieve the pressure and to release the feces.

Defecation is a temporary reflex that interrupts anal continence as the muscles comprising the anal sphincters are normally kept tightly shut. Defecation reflex is initiated when the fecal matter reaches the rectum. In some animals the external anal sphincter can help in delaying the defecation reflex eg dog to a limited extent.

The frequency of defecation varies among animals but can occur 5 to 10 times daily in horses and 10 to 20 times daily in cattle.

Constipation is the infrequent or difficult evacuation of feces, which are typically dry and hard. Constipation is a common clinical problem in small animals. Peristaltic waves are responsible for the aboral movement of fecal material in the colon. Giant migrating waves that occur intermittently throughout the day move this matter farther and more rapidly. These waves constitute the "gastrocolic reflex" and are common after ingestion of a meal. A reduction or loss of these waves may contribute to constipation.

Mild constipation can often be treated by dietary adjustment consisting of avoidance of dietary indiscretion, ready access to water and high-fiber diets, and use of suppository laxatives.

Vomition

Vomiting is the reflexive, forceful expulsion of part or all of the contents of the stomach and proximal small intestines through the mouth. It involves a series of involuntary spasmic movements requiring visceral, diaphragmatic, and abdominal muscular contractions. The reflex act of vomiting is initiated by the vomiting (or emetic) center, located in the reticular formation of the medulla. The vomiting center is responsive to input from 4 major sources: 1) afferent receptors from a variety of peripheral structures (the GI tract, pancreas, heart, liver, urogenital tract, and peritoneum) carried by the vagus and sympathetic nerves; 2) the chemoreceptor trigger zone (CRTZ) of the area postrema of the medulla; 3) the cerebral cortex and limbic system; and 4) the vestibular apparatus.

Vomition or Emesis is a protective mechanism that provides animals with the ability to remove harmful or toxic substances from the stomach or upper intestine.Some species, such as dogs and cats vomit easily. The vomiting reflex is controlled by the vomiting center in the medulla.

Horses rarely vomit because their cardiac sphincter is very strong. Ruminants have evolved to consume and subsist on roughage - grasses and shrubs built predominantly of cellulose.The rumen is a fermentation vat par excellence, providing an anaerobic environment, constant temperature and pH, and good mixing. Well-masticated substrates are delivered through the esophagus on a regular schedule, and fermentation products are either absorbed in the rumen itself or flow out for further digestion and absorption downstream.

Regulation of Secretory Function of Saliva

Food is mixed with saliva during the process of mastication which besides lubrication also contains some digestion enzymes. Three pairs of salivary glands pour their secretion of saliva along short ducts into the mouth. The water soluble components of food are dissolved in the saliva in the mouth and then able to activate the taste buds, which initiate further secretory activity. Salvia also seems to contain an antimicrobial substance that reduces the incidence of mouth infections and tooth decay.

Salivary Secretion

Food is mixed with saliva during the process of mastication which besides lubrication also contains some digestive enzymes. There are three main pairs of salivary glands in the body, the parotid, the submandibular and sublingual glands. Many small buccal glands in the mucous membrane lining the mouth also secrete saliva.

The parotid glands, largest of the salivary glands are located in the tissue below and in front of the ears. A duct delivers secretion from each parotid gland into the mouth through an opening in the inner surface of each cheek opposite the second molar of the upper jaw.

The parotid glands become swollen and infected during mumps in human beings.

Increased secretion of saliva occurs during ptyalism. Decreased secretion occurs during fever, dehydration and salivary gland disease. Specific inflammation of the salivary glands in domestic animals are unusual.

The submandibular and sublingual glands lie below the jaw and under the tonguc, respectively. Their ducts open into the floor of the mouth below the tongue.

Secretory unit of the salivary gland is an acinus. Each acinus is lined by glandular epithelium secretion of which enters the lumen which later on continues as intercalated duct . A serous acinus contains cells, the nucleus of which is more towards the base and they have zymogen granules. These granules are precursors of salivary enzyme ptyalin which is also known as salivary amylase.There are two types of acini in the salivary glands namely serous and mucous type. The acini, myoepithelial cells and the blood vessels of salivary glands are well supplied by sympathetic and parasympathetic nerve fibers. Saliva consists of two main components.

1. A serous (thin, watery) secretion containing the digestive enzymes called salivary amylase (also called ptyalin). Amylase is an enzyme that catalyses the hydrolysis of starch (Latin amylum) into sugars.Salivary amylase, initiates carbohydrates digestion by catalyzing the hydrolysis of polysaccharides into disaccharides. Foods that contain large amounts of starch but little sugar, such as rice and potatoes, may acquire a slightly sweet taste as they are chewed because amylase degrades some of their starch into sugar.

Under normal conditions, salivary amylase cannot produce complete degradation of starch molecules due to the rapid oral transit. Ptyalin continues functioning in the stomach, although briefly, since the gastric juice, which has a very low pH (about 1.5), completely inactivates it. This is why the role of ptyalin in starch digestion is limited.

However, the main site for carbohydrate digestion is the small intestine. Amylase from the pancreas completes the breakdown of starch polysaccharides into disaccharides that are then hydrolyzed into glucose, fructose, and galactose. These monosaccharide units are then absorbed into the intestinal cell and eventually enter the bloodstream either by passive diffusion (fructose) or through a sodium and energy-dependent active transport mechanism (glucose and galactose).

2. A Mucous secretion which lubricates the mouth. Mucous acini have cells which contain mucinogen granules which are precursors of mucin. The parotid glands secrete the serous component, the sublingual and buccal glands, the mucous, and the submandibular gland release both components. Some antibacterial substances are also found in the saliva.

Functions of the Saliva

The saliva has several functions.

1. It continuously lubricates the tissues of the mouth and throat, thereby facilitate chewing. By moistening the food it helps the tongue to convert it to semisolid mass (bolus) that can be easily swallowed.
2. By dissolving the food molecules, it helps in the perception of its taste.
3. Saliva washes away food particles and bacteria and also contains antibacterial substances, thus reducing the chances of dental decay.
4. Its enzymes, salivary amylase, initiates carbohydrates digestion.
5. The saliva protects the oral mucosa from drying.
6. Saliva also neutralizes the organic acids produced by bacteria normally present in the mouth.
7. The saliva also helps in thermoregulation in species like dogs & cats. In addition, the saliva of ruminants perform the following function.
8. The high buffering capacity of the ruminant saliva helps to stabilize the pH of the rumen.
9. Recycling & conservation of nitrogen: Return of nitrogen as urea through saliva to the rumen is an important adaptation of ruminants to inadequacies of the diet, especially diets low in protein.

Saliva is continuously added to the rumen and maintains the contents in a fluid state, facilitating access of microorganisms to the plant materials.

Saliva of Ruminants & Nonruminants

Ruminants produce a much greater quantity of saliva than simple stomach animals. The large volume is important for lubricating the large quantities of high fibre diets & for maintenance of the fluid conditions in the rumen. The saliva has a higher pH. Ruminant saliva is a bicarbonate-phosphate buffer secreted in large quantities. In ruminants, saliva serves unique functions. It is required for the maintenance of the contents of the rumen. The great buffering capacity is necessary to neutralize the large amounts of short-chain fatty acids which are the major end products of rumen fermentation. The urea in saliva can be utilized by rumen bacteria for protein synthesis. Protein synthesized in the rumen is then used to meet dietary protein requirements. In this way, urea nitrogen can be recycled through the amino acid pool of the body and in ruminants need not be considered an end stage in protein catabolism. The ability to neutralize urea has also been demonstrated in the horse and may be of particular benefit during periods of the protein deficiency. Urea present in the saliva is produced by the liver from ammonia absorbed from the rumen and subsequently extracted from the blood by the salivary glands.

The buffering effect is maintained by the continuous nature of parotid salivary secretions partly brought about by the wider distribution of the reflex salivary pathway in the ruminant.

The volume of saliva secreted by ruminants is dependent on diet. The salivary secretion rate is about 1 litre a day in case of humans. The value is as high as 100-200 litres a day in case of cattle and 8-12 litres a day in case of sheep.

Structure of Salivary glands : The secretory cells of the salivary glands are organized into small lobules which are composed of pyramidal secretory cells surrounding a central lumen. These secretory units are referred to as acini. The secretory acini may be composed of mucous cells, serous cells or seromucous cells. Serous cells produce a watery secretion which is high in enzyme content. Mucous cells produce a viscous fluid which is high in mucopolysaccharides. Seromucous cells produce a material which is somewhat similar to a mixture of the secretions of the serous and mucous cells.

Regulation of secretory functions of saliva: The secretion of the saliva is under neural control. However the parotid gland in ruminants seems to function without neural stimulation. The sight, smell or merely the thought of food can initiate the reflex secretion of saliva.

Composition of Saliva :The saliva is a buffered bicarbonate solution with a pH around 8 and contains high concentration of sodium and phosphate ions. Mixed saliva obtained from the mouth is a colourless slightly opalescent fluid. The main constituent of saliva is water. In addition small amounts of carbohydrates, enzymes, proteins, sialic acid inorganic ions, hormones and blood group substances are also present. The saliva of ruminants also contain significant amounts of urea.

The saliva contains enzymes principal of which is amylase. However, ruminants produce little or no salivary amylase. Amylase is also said to be absent in the saliva of dogs, cats and horses. The other important enzyme in saliva is lysozyme which may be important for antibacterial activity.

The salivary pH in the nonruminants is on the alkaline side (Approx. pH 8.5).

Numerous other enzymes are present in the saliva, for example, lipase, maltase, phosphatase and peroxidase but it is probable that these originate from the oral bacteria and unlikely that they play an important role in the digestive process. A lipase active against milk fat glyceride containing short chain fatty acids is secreted by the buccal glands in a number of species, particularly the calf. The major cations in the saliva include Na+ and K+ while Ca++ and Mg++ are of lesser importance. The major anions include the Cl-, HPO - and HCO- . These anions are responsible for the buffering capacity of saliva.

In addition the saliva contains mucoproteins. The mucoproteins are composed of N-acetylneuraminic acid and N-acetylgalactosamine as the carbohydrate portion bound to protein mucin. The composition of the saliva in different species of domestic animals is shown below (Table).

Forces Governing Absorption, Control Intestinal Transport of Electrolyte and Water

A large portion of the alimentary canal is primarily concerned with absorption of digested food and water. Absorption of food is a slow process compared with digestion. For the organism to maximize the efficiency of absorbing food, a large surface area needs to be available. A large surface area is made available by the folding of the intestinal surface into villi and microvilli.

A large portion of major nutrients is broken down to their basic building blocks before being absorbed.

The animal needs to degrade its food into basic organic molecules like glucose, amino acids and fatty acids because of the two reasons.

1. The food is not in the form required by the body.
2. Large molecules such as starches and proteins are not readily absorbed across biological membranes.

Absorption of VFA

The major proportion of the VFA are absorbed from the rumen by diffusion alone. However, some VFA move to the omasum and abomasum in the fluid transported along the tract and are absorbed from these organs.

Absorption of Water & Electrolytes

Most of the water and electrolytes particularly HCO^- are absorbed from the omasum.

Absorption of Glucose

In ruminants, the soluble sugar and starches of the ration are mainly fermented and not absorbed as such. However, some glucose may be absorbed in the lower tract which may come from grains resistant to ruminal fermentation and some reserved polysaccharides of bacteria passing to the lower gut. It has been estimated that only 5-10 gm of dietary glucose may become available for absorption each day in sheep.

Absorption of Long Chain Fatty Acids

Long chain fatty acids liberated from the dietary lipids by hydrolysing in the rumen are largely saturated in the rumen, but are otherwise unchanged. These compounds are efficiently absorbed in the small intestine.

Storage of Energy in The Body

Some amount of chemical energy is stored in the body of most living organisms, for use during scarcity. The most common forms of stored chemical energy in the body is lipids and polysaccharides. The storage of large amounts of polysaccharides is characteristic of plants, in which, with the exception of seeds, lipid storage is scanty. Among higher animals, including farm animals, lipids account for the bulk of energy storage, whereas polysaccharides storage occurs only in the form of relatively small amounts of glycogen.

The large stores of chemical energy in the form of lipids or polysaccharides do not have any effect on osmotic pressure, as lipids are not soluble in water and large molecular weight polysaccharides are only sparingly soluble.

Although glycogen occurs in most tissues, including the cells of adipose tissue, the glycogen of liver and of skeletal muscle has attracted most attention. The glycogen of tissues is metabolically active and is undergoing constant turnover, unlike lipids which are relatively less active. Liver is one of the most prominent source of glycogen storage as is evident from the fact that between 2 and 8% of the wet weight of the liver is glycogen depending on the species. The liver of an animal fasted for 24 hours is virtually depleted of glycogen. Refeeding with glycogenic materials e.g. glucose results in prompt reaccumulation of liver glycogen.

Enzymatic Digestion in Monogastric and Fermentative Digestion in Rumen

Digestive enzymes are responsible for the chemical digestion of food in the stomach. Mechanical digestion in the mouth and in the stomach serves the purpose of increasing the amount of food surface area that can be exposed to the digestive enzymes.

Ruminants have to consume large quantities of highly fibrous and less nutritive diet and to digest this food properly, they require a more complex digestion process than non ruminants. To increase the surface area of such food for action by the digestive enzymes or rumen enzymes, they need to ruminate or chew the cud. This involves several processes like re-insalivation, re-matication and re-swallowing. The rumination cycle is more when the animal eats fiber rich diet as compared to when a low fiber diet is consumed.

The ruminal mucosa contains numerous papillae, which help to increase the surface area for absorption.

In the rumen of ruminants, cellulase enzymes bound to the surfaces of cellulolytic bacteria break down complex carbohydrates through hydrolysis, releasing specific monosaccharides (simple sugars) such as glucose and less complex polysaccharides.

In both ruminants and non ruminants, the starch and soluble sugars are digested by the enzyme amylase.

Lipid digestion is not very important in the ruminants as lipids constitute a very small portion of the diet of ruminants. Lipase secreted by the rumen microorganisms hydrolyse triglycerides into fatty acids and glycerol. The glycerol goes through the process of fermentation, producing VFAs and fatty acids go through the process of hydrogenation which are absorbed in the small intestine. The fatty acids so absorbed are used by the body for energy or for storage as adipose tissue.

Peptidases from rumen bacteria break down proteins to form small peptide chains. Some of the peptides are used by rumen bacteria to synthesize microbial protein and which is further digested to form peptides or amino acids. The amino acids in ruminants are deaminates to produce ammonium which can again be used to resynthesize amino acids or to produce VFAs.Amino acids can also be synthesized from non-protein nitrogen compounds such as urea by the rumen microbes, which is not possible in non ruminants. In facts, NPN compounds are added to ruminant diets as compound feed to make it cheaper.

Proteins in ruminants as wells non ruminants are broken down by proteolytic enzymes and absorbed in the small intestine. Bypass proteins pass through the rumen unaltered and are degraded enzymatically in the small intestine. The amino acids so produced are absorbed across the intestinal mucosa into the blood-stream and transported to the liver. Absorbed amino acids are metabolized to make proteins in the liver.

In the liver, urea is produced as a waste product from the metabolism of amino acids which is excreted by the kidneys in the non ruminants but gets reutilized in the ruminants as it gets secreted in the saliva and into the rumen to be reutilized by the rumen microbes to synthesize the proteins again. Thus ruminants are more efficient in N metabolism and utilization as compared to non ruminants.

In the ruminants, the glucose is not absorbed in the small intestine as all the carbohydrates get converted into VFAs in the rumen. So the glucose requirement of ruminants is through gluconeogenesis in the liver from non carbohydrate sources. Propionate, a waste product of microbial metabolism, is absorbed from the rumen into the blood and reaches the liver where it is converted into glucose through gluconeogenesis.

As we know that carbohydrates are metabolized to acetic, propionic and butyric acids in the rumen, butyric acid is converted to beta hyroxybutyrate in the liver. Beta hydroxybutyrate is a ketone which can be metabolized but not used to make glucose.

Acetic acid or acetate is the most abundant VFA which is absorbed and reaches the liver but cannot be used to make glucose.

Acetate and Butyric Acids so Absorbed from the Rumen are Used in the Mammary Glands to Synthesize Fatty Acids

Stomach

Digestion in the simple stomach : The stomach function in the storage and digestion of food taken in by the mouth. Food in the stomach is digested and mixed with gastric secretion, as a result of which it becomes more fluid and is called **chyme**.

The gastric secretions are produced from gastric glands present in the lining of the stomach. The gastric secretions contain digestive enzymes and the acid. Thus the function of the stomach is to continue the digestion of food, change its consistency and to store it for release a little at a time to the small intestine, where the greater part of digestion occurs. The stomach has mainly a preparatory function rather than a vital one, and, if certain precautions are taken, the complete removal of the stomach is compatible with life.

Control of the Secretion of Gastric Glands

The best example of dual control of secretion by the nervous system and by hormones is seen in the stomach. Secretion in the stomach has been studied in man by direct observation of the gastric juice produced in a few individuals who have a gastric fistula (an opening from the stomach to the exterior, usually produced by some accident). It has been studied in much more detail in experimental animals, starting with the classic work of Pavlovian dogs.

Nervous Phase of Gastric Secretion

When the animals with an exteriorised oesophageal tube are fed, no food or stimulus reaches the stomach. In such a situation one quarter of the normal amount of gastric juice is secreted, through reflex stimulation. The pathway is similar to that involved in salivary secretion, except that parasympathetic impulses are carried to the gastric glands via the vagus nerve. If the branches of vagi to the stomach are cut, this phase of gastric secretion does not occur.

Hormonal Phase of Gastric Secretion

If food is placed directly in the stomach, the gastric juice starts to flow. This secretion is not abolished by cutting the nerves to the stomach and is, therefore, not reflex in nature. It is mediated by hormone **gastrin**. Food in the stomach causes the release of gastrin from certain cells in the gastric mucosa. Gastrin passes into the bloodstream, circulates around the body back to stomach, and stimulates the gastric glands to secrete **pepsinogen** and acid.

Composition of the Gastric Juice

The Gastric juice is mainly composed of enzyme & acid.

(a) ***Gastric hydrochloric acid*** : The most important constituents of gastric juice is hydrochloric acid which provides the optimal low pH for pepsin activity. This acid is secreted by the oxyntic cells of the stomach. Recent evidence indicates that prostaglandins possess potent gastric anti ulcer properties independent of their known inhibitory effects on acid secretion.

(b) Protein digestion in the stomach : Several enzymes are responsible for the proteolytic activity of gastric juice. These include pepsinogens, pepsins & renin.

The chief cells secrete pepsinogens, which is inactive zymogen. The secretions of zymogens are stimulated by the cholinergic impulses and by the hormones gastrin and secretin. Pepsinogen is converted to proteolytically active pepsin when it mixes with acid secreted by the oxyntic cells.

(c) ***Pancreatic amylase*** is an alpha amylase and splits glycosidic bond to hydrolyse starch and glycogen to the disaccharide maltose. Amylase requires chloride for activation and calcium appears to be an integral portion of the enzyme.

(d) ***Renin***: The gastric juice of new born calves contains a milk clotting enzyme, called renin. The enzyme **chymosin** is found in the stomach lining of animals because it aids in the digestion of their mother's milk. Rennet made from animal chymosin is usually called "rennet"

(e) ***Lipase***: Gastric juice also contains a lipase.

In addition to hydrochloric acid and enzymes, the gastric juice contains mucus. This substance provides lubrication and protects the epithelial cells of the stomach from the hydrochloric acid.

Fat digestion in the stomach: Muscle contractions of the stomach produce the shear forces sufficient for emulsification. Potential emulsifiers that can function in the acidic mileu of the stomach include peptic digesta of dietary proteins, complex polysaccharides and membrane derived phospholipids. Enzymatic hydrolysis of triglycerides also begins in the stomach, and since triglyceride are stored for 2-4 hours, 30% of the total dietary triglyceride may be digested. However, quantitative hydrolysis and absorption, especially of the long chain fatty acids, require less acidic conditions, appropriate lipases detergents (bile salts) and specialized absorptive cells. This environment is provided by the lumen and mucosa of the upper small intestine.

Intestine

Small Intestine

Intestinal digestion is a terminal phase in the preparation of materials for absorption from the intestinal tract. The digestible proteins, carbohydrates and lipids are completely hydrolysed to absorbable materials, prepared for absorption through the intestinal mucosa.

Secretin : Secretin is released from the upper small intestine mucosa.

The small intestine is the main absorption site and contains a series of microscopic finger-like projections, the villi, which greatly increase the surface area available for the absorption of nutrients. Each villus contain an arteriole and venule, together with a drainage tube of the lymphatic system, a lacteal. The venules ultimately drain into the portal system and the lacteals into the thoracic lymphatic duct. Four secretions enter the small intestine; duodenal juice, bile, pancreatic juice and succus entericus.

Duodenal juice: The duodenal (Brunner's) glands produce an alkaline secretion which enters the duodenum through ducts situated between the villi. This secretion acts as a lubricant and also protects the duodenal wall from the hydrochloric acid entering from the stomach.

Succus entericus: It is produced in the crypts of Lieberkuhn, the tubular depressions between the villi. by the entry of H+ ions into the duodenum and this in turn stimulate the centro acinar and ductal cells of the pancreas to secrete the electrolyte containing fluid. The HCO^- secreted by the pancreas neutralizes the HCl secreted by the stomach.

Cholecystokinin: Cholecystokinin is released from the duodenal mucosal cells in response to products of protein digestion and this hormone causes some secretion of the pancreatic enzymes and contraction of the gallbladder.

Vasoactive Intestinal peptide *(VIP)*: It is liberated from intestine and shares a structural and functional homology with secretin. Each of these peptides inhibits gastric secretions, stimulates pancreatic secretion, increased adenylate cyclase activity in plasma membranes of the exocrine pancreas and raises cellular cyclic AMP content in the pancreas.

Motility of small intestine: Rhythmic contractions of the muscular coat of the intestinal wall provide for movement of materials through the small intestine and the mixing of these materials with digestive juices of the intestinal contents.

Large Intestine

The large intestine comprises the caecum, colon, rectum and is the final region of the tract through which digesta pass before they are voided as the faeces.

The caecum is a simple tubular structure with a blind end and is of considerable size in the non-ruminant herbivores to allow for the extensive microbial fermentation which takes place in these species.

The colon is a major site for water, electrolyte and VFA absorption from the ileal and cecal contents which pass into it and in the ruminant and the pig, is both extensive and much coiled to provide the necessary surface area. Large intestine is lined with mucus-secretory cells which assist the passage of the progressively more dehydrated digesta.

In the nonruminants the bacterial action occurs to a certain extent in the large intestine and is of major significance in the case of the horse and rabbit. The main site of absorption of digested nutrients is the small intestine, so that by the time food material has reached the entrance to the colon most of the hydrolysed nutrients will have been absorbed.

The large intestine of horses and other hindgut fermenters is a fermentation system analogous to the rumen.The caecum in horse is a blind sack approximately 1.2m long that can hold around 28-36 litres of feed and fluid. The caecum is a inoculation vat, similar to the rumen in a cow. The microbes break down feed that was not digested in the small intestine, particularly fibrous feeds like hay or pasture. The caecum in horse is odd in design because its entrance and exit are both at the top of the organ. This means that the feed enters at the top, mixes throughout, and is then expelled up at the top. In horses caecum, volatile fatty acids are produced in large quantities, absorbed through the cecal and colonic epithelium, and distributed for use throughout the body. However, large quantity of microbial protein generated in the equine large gut is wasted because there is no opportunity there for significant absorption of amino acids.

Pancreas

The pancreas is both an **exocrine** and **endocrine gland**.

Structure : The pancreas is a U shaped organ lying along the duodenum and is composed primarily of pancreatic acini which secrete the pancreatic enzymes. Scattered throughout the pancreas are small islets of cells that are structurally quite different from those of the acini.

Light microscopic images of the pancreas of the camel, using immunostaining of insulin-producing cells (IN), glucagon-producing cells (GL), somatostatin producing cells (ST), and pancreatic polypeptide producing cells (PP). Beta cells were distributed throughout the islet in the center and the periphery. Alpha cells were mostly observed as clumps in the periphery area. Clumps of small number of Δ-cells and a few PP-cells were found throughout the islet.

Pancreatic juice : The pancreatic juice is composed of two portions.

1. ***Viscid enzyme rich Proteinaceous portion***: This portion is largely enzymatic. These enzymes are synthesized by the acinar cells which are arranged in clusters around the terminal pancreatic ductules.
2. ***Watery portion rich in fluid and electrolytes:*** The epithelial cells lining, the terminal and interlobular ductuli which carry the pancreatic juice toward the intestine form the fluid and electrolyte portion of the pancreatic juice.

The pancreatic juice contains bicarbonate as its main anion and this is the major factor responsible for reducing the acidity of the stomach contents when they enter the duodenum. The chloride is another principal anion.

The pancreatic juice of ruminants contains less amylase and lipase as compared to the non-ruminants.

Pancreatic juice contains enzymes for digesting all the three major nutrients in the food, viz. proteins, carbohydrates & fats.The proteolytic enzymes are trypsin, chymotrypsin , carboxypeptidase, ribonuclease and deoxyribonuclease.Trypsin and chymotrypsin split whole or partially digested proteins, while carboxypeptidase splits a particular peptide linkage of small peptides.

The nucleases split the two types of nucleic acids; the ribonucleic acid (RNA) and deoxyribonucleic acid (DNA).

The pancreatic amylase digests the carbohydrates by hydrolysing starches, glycogen and most other carbohydrates except cellulose, to form disaccharides.

Pancreatic lipase digests the fat by hydrolysing triglycerides into glycerol and fatty acids. Pancreatic lipase is secreted in an active form but its activity is enhanced by bile salts. Bile salts enhance the efficacy of lipolysis by increasing the surface area of oil water interfaces at which water soluble lipase is effective.

The proteolytic enzymes synthesized in the pancreatic cells are in the inactive forms ,trypsinogen,chymotrypsinogen and procarboxypeptidase, which are all inactive in nature. These become activated only after they are secreted into the intestinal tract. Trypsinogen is activated by an enzyme called enterokinase, which is released from the intestinal mucosa whenever chyme comes in contact with the mucosa. Also, trypsinogen can be activated to a slight extent by the trypsin that has already been formed. Chymotrypsinogen is activated by trypsin to form chymotrypsin and procarboxypeptidase is presumably activated in some similar manner.

Trypsin inhibitor : It is important that the proteolytic enzymes of the pancreatic juice do not become activated until they have been secreted into the intestine, for the trypsin and other enzymes would digest the pancreas itself. Fortunately, the same cells that secrete the proteolytic enzymes into the acini of the pancreas secrete simultaneously another substance called trypsin inhibitor. This substance is stored in the cytoplasm of the glandular cells surrounding the enzymes granules, and it prevents activation of trypsin both inside the secretory cells and in the acini and ducts of the pancreas. Since it is trypsin that activates the other pancreatic proteolytic enzymes, trypsin inhibitor also prevents the subsequent activation of all these.

The Volume of Pancreatic Juice Secreted by the ox is 2 to 2.48 Litres per day and 0.32- 0.42 Litres for Sheep per day.

Regulation: Neurohumoral regulation of pancreatic juice secretion is largely under the control of the vagus and two hormones secretin & CCK (Cholecystokinin). The vagus stimulation or parasympathetic drugs causes both enzyme and fluid secretion by the pancreas.

Hormones Secreted by the Pancreas

The islets of Langerhans in the pancreas are responsible for secretion of four hormones namely Insulin, glucagon, somatostatin and pancreatic polypeptide. All the four hormones are associated with glucose metabolism in the body.

Insulin

Blood glucose concentration is normally maintained within a narrow range despite marked variations in the availability of glucose absorbed from the gut. Two hormones have a central role in the regulation of blood glucose concentration, insulin and glucagon.Insulin is involved in the regulation of glucose metabolism in the body. Basal plasma insulin of 10 to 50μU/ml for sheep, and about 40 μU/ml for goats have been reported. Insulin is a protein secreted rapidly from the β-cells of the islets of Langerhans in the pancreas in response to a small rise in blood glucose; its secretion is inhibited by a fall in blood glucose .

Insulin consists of two peptide chains, A and B, connected by two disulphide bridges.

The actions of insulin affect carbohydrate, lipid, and protein metabolism. Insulin facilitates the use of glucose through glycolysis which involves the oxidation of glucose to pyruvate and lactate through glucokinase, phosphofructokinase and pyruvate kinase enzymes. Secretin and pancreozymin are involved in bringing about the rise in plasma insulin in cattle within 1 hr after feeding and that glucose and, possibly, short-chain fatty acids produced in the rumen are involved in maintaining elevated plasma insulin for about 6 hr after feeding.

Alloxan and streptozotocin have each been used to induce chronic diabetic states in laboratory animals by their toxic effects on the beta cells of the islets of Langerhans.

Insulin deficiency produces diabetes mellitus which can further cause diabetic ketoacidosis. Diabetes mellitus is caused by autoimmune destruction of beta cells of pancreas. Diabetes mellitus (DM) is a chronic metabolic disorder in which the body's ability to produce or respond to the hormone insulin is impaired, resulting in abnormal metabolism of carbohydrates and elevated levels of glucose in the blood and urine. In diabetes, glucose is overproduced by the liver and underutilized by other organs.DM is one of the common and prominent metabolic diseases that have been diagnosed in canine and feline family after human beings. The classic symptoms of diabetes in dogs are excessive thirst, increased urination, and weight loss despite normal or increased food consumption. Acute blindness resulting from cataract can also be a sign. The diagnosis is easy to confirm with simple tests for glucose (sugar) in the blood and urine. A striking feature of diabetes is the shift in fuel usage from carbohydrates to fats; glucose, more abundant than ever, is spurned. In high concentrations, ketone bodies overwhelm the kidney's capacity to maintain acid-base balance. The untreated diabetic can go into a coma because of a lowered blood pH level and dehydration.

Glucagon

Glucagon is secreted by the alpha cells of the pancreas and has direct stimulatory effect on beta cells to secrete insulin. Glucagon is a polypeptide hormone consisting of a single chain of 29 amino acids. Glucagon is released from the alpha cells of pancreas by the process of exocytosis.

Somatostatin

Somatostatin is a 14 amino acid polypeptide that inhibits growth hormone secretion by the pars distalis.The actions of somatostatin can be classified as inhibitory.

Pancreatic Polypeptide

Pancreatic polypeptide is a hormone which inhibits pancreatic secretion of digestive enzymes.

Bile secretion

The **liver** plays a central role in the biochemical coordination of various physiological processes. The liver and the biliary system serve both as a secretory organ for the assistance of intestinal digestion and as an excretory organ for the elimination of by products of tissue metabolism from the body. The liver is the largest gland in the body & its size reflects the multiplicity of its functions.

The liver is composed of a great number of small lobules, separated by interlobular connective tissue. The liver cells are polygonal in structure and often have two or more nuclei. These cells are called hepatocytes, which act as multipurpose epithelial cells. The liver consists of multiple lobes in animals, the number and arrangement varies considerably among domestic animal species and 70%-80% of the liver mass is composed of hepatocytes

Functions

- Secretion of bile.
- Important blood forming organ of the fetus.
- Storage of glycogen, which it synthesizes from the carbohydrates absorbed from portal blood.
- It can temporarily store fats & small amounts of protein.

- It converts end products of protein catabolism to urea and which are discharged into the blood stream and then removed by the kidneys. In ruminants the urea is recycled to the gastrointestinal tract via the salivary glands.
- It removes waste products resulting from the breakdown of red blood cells from the blood. These wastes are the end products of the haemoglobin catabolism and are discharged in the bile as bile pigments.
- The liver is also capable of extracting harmful substances from the blood and detoxifying them.
- Liver is a storehouse for vitamin A & iron.
- It is involved in metabolic reactions including catabolism of glucose, glycogen, fatty acids, amino acids, synthesis of triglycerides, ATP, glycogen, urea.

Filters the portal blood through the activity of phagocytic reticuloendothelial cells (Van Kupffer cells) found in the sinusoids. Bacteria entering the blood through the intestines are removed by these cells.

Bile pigment metabolism produces bilirubin, which is then conjugated with glucuronic acid and excreted into the intestine. Reduction in the intestine produces urobilinogen. Reabsorption of bile by the intestine results in the return of bilirubin and/or urobilinogen.

Jaundice

Excessive accumulation of bile pigments results in Jaundice. In Jaundice, free or conjugated bilirubin accumulates in the blood, the skin and mucus membrane turns yellow . The total bilirubin is greater than 2mg/dl. The term icterus (or jaundice) denotes a yellow discoloration of mucous membranes of the gums, nostrils, genitals, and other areas due to a high concentration of bilirubin, a normal bile pigment formed as a result of a breakdown of hemoglobin present in red blood cells (RBCs). Higher concentrations of bilirubin are toxic and may cause discoloration of the skin (i.e., jaundice), liver and kidney injury, and may also affect brain tissue. All breeds of dogs can be affected. An inflamed liver or obstructed bile duct can lead to jaundice.

Bile consists of certain salts such as sodium glycocholate and sodium tauroglycocholate, which reduce surface tension and are important in emulsifying fats. This process makes them more readily digested by the lipase from the pancreas which will only function normally in the presence of these salts. The bile also contains breakdown products from blood haemoglobin which are bilirubin and biliverdin,which colour the faeces. A quantity of HCO^{-3} is released with the bile fluids giving them a pH of 7 and helping to make the duodenum alkaline. Bile also stimulates the peristaltic movement of the gut.

Hunger, Appetite Control

Appetite is controlled by feelings of hunger and satiety, and is regulated centrally through the hypothalamus of the forebrain, as well as the midbrain and brainstem. The hypothalamus is the main regulatory effector organ of appetite, and controls the volume of food consumed. It communicates with other central nervous system (CNS) areas of the brain stem, as well as the reward-related limbic pathways of the midbrain.

It acts as a sensor via numerous hormones, and as a biological clock that stimulates hunger. Hunger occurs when the body's store of nutrients is depleted. Glucose regulates short-term control over appetite. The hypothalamus interprets and integrates the input of neural and humoral (circulating) factors that result in the body's coordinated feeding and energy expenditure responses.

The hypothalamus induces the secretion of adiponectin (a hormone that regulates insulin secretion and fatty acid oxidation), as well as leptin and ghrelin (the "stop" and "go" hunger hormones, respectively). Leptin comes from white adipose tissue cells and decreases appetite. Basically, these hormones act as signals for satiety, thereby regulating food intake. Leptin and another biomarker, serotonin, function in separate systems to control appetite. Adiponectin and leptin are the fat-regulating hormones.

The leptin is a 16 kD protein consisting of 146 amino acids which is synthesized primarily by adipose tissue and is secreted into the bloodstream after cleavage of the 21 amino acid signal peptide. Leptin was first identified as the gene product found deficient in the obese ob/ob mouse. The hypothalamus appears to be the primary site of action, since leptin receptors are located within hypothalamic areas associated with control of appetite, reproduction and growth.

Developmental Aspects of Digestion

The alimentary canal is a continuous tube by the fifth week of development. Digestive glands bud from the mucosa of the alimentary tube.

The developing fetus receives all nutrients through the placenta

In newborns, feeding must be frequent, peristalsis is inefficient, and vomiting is common.

- Teething begins around age six months
- Metabolism decreases with old age

Middle age digestive problems

Ulcers

Gallbladder problems

Activity of digestive tract in old age

Fewer digestive juices

Peristalsis slows

Diverticulosis and cancer are more common

Luminous, Membranous and Microbial Digestion in Rumen and Intestine

The primary functions of GI tract include digestion and absorption of nutrients, secretions, and immune response. GI tract is divided into four layers: the mucosa (epithelium, lamina propria, and muscularis mucosae), the submucosa, the muscularis propria (inner circular muscle layer, intermuscular space, and outer longitudinal muscle layer), and the serosa.

Permeability Characteristics of Intestine

Intestinal permeability is a term describing the control of material passing from inside the gastrointestinal tract through the cells lining the gut wall, into the rest of the body. Intestinal mucosa facilitates the uptake of dietary nutrients, electrolytes, water and various other beneficial substances from the intestinal lumen. The barrier formed by the intestinal epithelium separates the external environment (the contents of the intestinal lumen) from the body. The intestinal epithelium is composed of a single layer of cells and helps in absorption of nutrients and filtration of harmful substances such as foreign antigens, toxins and microorganisms.

Selective permeability is mediated via two major routes:

Transepithelial or transcellular permeability. This consists of specific transport of solutes across the epithelial cells. It is predominantly regulated by the activities of specialised transporters that translocate specific electrolytes, amino acids, sugars, short chain fatty acids and other molecules into or out of the cell

Paracellular permeability. It depends on transport through the spaces that exist between epithelial cells. It is regulated by cellular junctions that are localized in the laminal membranes of the cells. This is the main route of passive flow of water and solutes across the intestinal epithelium. Regulation depends on the intercellular tight junctions which have the most influence on paracellular transport. Disruption of the tight junction barrier can be a trigger for the development of intestinal diseases.

Forces Governing Absorption

Final stages of digestion and most of the nutrient absorption occur in the small intestine, where the food is dissolved into the juices from the pancreas, liver, and intestine. All of the digested nutrients are absorbed through the intestinal walls.

Primary form of amino acid absorption in the ruminant is as peptides, not as free amino acids. Production of ammonia in, and the absorption of ammonia from, the rumen and on NPN utilization are also important in ruminants. By pass protein is the protein that passes through the intestine as unaltered.

Fats and fat-soluble vitamins are also digested in and absorbed from the small intestine.

Control Intestinal Transport of Electrolyte and Water

Intestine plays an important role in transport of electrolyte and water through the intestinal lumen.Failure to efficiently absorbing water and electrolyte, it will lead to dehydration and electrolyte imbalance.

The cells relevant to intestinal water and electrolyte transport can be roughly divided into two major groups: those involved in electrolyte transport and those having predominantly a regulatory role, i.e. integrating the functional responses of the first group. The gut is capable of absorbing greater than 98 % of the fluid load it is presented with making it a highly efficient organ for absorption of water and electrolytes. The absorption of water and electrolytes is mainly carried out by epithelial cells of the intestine. Epithelial cells represent the largest population of cells of the intestinal mucosa , of which there are four major types: (1) columnar, polarized epithelial cells, capable of vectorial transport of nutrients and electrolytes; (2) mucosal endocrine cells; (3) mucus producing and secreting goblet cells ; and (4) defense-producing Paneth cells located at the base of intestinal crypts.

The striated ducts consist of columnar epithelial cells that possess deep infoldings of their basal membrane. These deep infoldings produce their striated appearance from which the striated ducts derive their name.Striated ductal cells are responsible for water and electrolyte transport. The presence of Na+, K+-ATPases in the basolateral regions of the striated ductal cells are responsible for this transport. Carbonic anhydrase (CA) -I and -II are localized in striated ductal cells and these enzymes are also involved in water and electrolyte transport. Angiotensin II exerts important effects on water and electrolyte transport by indirect and direct mechanisms. Circulating aldosterone can also regulate ductal cell function. Aldosterone is a mineralocorticoid hormone that is responsible for the absorption of NaCl and the secretion of K+. Angiotensin II modulates water and electrolyte transport indirectly, via the stimulation of aldosterone secretion, and directly, by stimulating NaCl reabsorption.

Blood capillaries and lymphatics have a major role in intestinal water and electrolyte transport. Coordinated patterns of intestinal motility ensure that mixing and propulsive activity of luminal contents proceed appropriately.

Electrolyte transport in the intestine is also under neural control.

Diarrhea , which results when the absorptive capacity of the gut is exceeded, infrequently occurs under physiological circumstances.

Modification of Toxic Substances in Rumen

Biotransformation is a key body defense mechanism whereby chemical reactions transform toxic compounds in the body. Plants that are poisonous to some animals can be harmless to others. In general, ruminants are more tolerant of poisons in plants than are nonruminants; but some plants are more toxic to ruminants. Even among ruminants, there are striking differences in tolerance of plant toxicants.

In ruminants, gastrointestinal microbes can detoxify plant compounds,and this capacity has been enhanced in a few cases by deliberate modification of rumen microbial populations. In ruminants, tolerance of poisonous plants may be modified by microbial fermentation of ingesta in the reticulorumen (which can diminish toxicity of some plant compounds and increase toxicity of others). Rumen act as a bio transformer for some toxic substances, whereby some toxic compounds gets converted to less toxic compounds, a process called inactivation or detoxification.Ruminants are relatively tolerant of tannins due to the ruminal mechanisms of dilution, protein binding and microbial degradation. Rumen fermentation is known to reduce fescue seed toxicity. Ruminants can also tolerate Gossypol present in cotton seed cake fed commonly in India) although gossypol is known to be toxic to several physiological systems in animals, with cardiac, reproductive , pulmonary and hepatic lesions being observed. The ability of cattle and buffalo to tolerate gossypol toxin is due to the binding of free gossypol by soluble ruminal proteins and microbial degradation in the rumen.

Ruminants tolerate many poisonous plants far better than nonruminants. It has been suggested that rumen microbial detoxification of poisonous plants might have been as important as rumen microbial degradation of cellulose for the evolutionary development and ecological expansion of ruminants as herbivores. Microbial populations change gradually with prolonged, increasing exposure to toxic substances, and such gradual adaptations allow ruminants to increase their tolerance of some poisonous plants. Absorption of toxic substances from the gastrointestinal tract into blood and lymph may be modified by feeding binding agents such as clay, resins, and indigestible fibers, or by pharmaceuticals that interfere with absorption of toxicants.

Activated charcoal has been used effectively to adsorb some kinds of poisons and prevent their absorption Substances absorbed from the gut into blood usually pass to the liver which, therefore, has "first pass" in metabolism of nutrients and biotransformations of non nutrient substances.

Digestion in Birds

In nature, birds are faced with variable food sources that may differ in composition (protein vs. carbohydrates) and quality (highly digestible material vs. indigestible fiber).Birds have several peculiarities as regards their diet and digestive processes. The molecule capsaicin, which is responsible for the fiery taste of chillies and peppers, is repellent to many mammals, but birds feed on these fruits with impunity. The gastrointestinal tract of poultry can respond to varying diet composition and quality by changing morphology and/or activities of digestive enzymes.

Chicken and other birds have some structural peculiarities of the digestive tract. The esophagus empties directly into the crop where the food is stored and soaked. The digestive system of birds include the following parts. From the crop the food passes through the proventriculus, an enlarged glandular portion where digestive juices are copiously secreted and mixed with the food as it passes to the gizzard. This is a very muscular organ which normally contains stones or grit that aid in grinding hard seeds and grains before they move into the small intestine. The grinding of food and seeds and grains in gizzard is similar to mastication in domestic animals and it allows the mixing of the feed with the saliva for its lubrication and initiation of enzymatic digestion before swallowing.

Birds including chicken have two ceca, but they do not have much nutritional significance.

Mouth: Birds have no teeth and their jaws are covered by a beak. Food is taken in with the beak. Birds do not really masticate, and mechanical disruption of food is accomplished by the beak and gizzard. Chickens are omnivores. A small bit of saliva and digestive enzymes are added as the food moves from the mouth into the esophagus.

Esophagus (Gullet): Transports food from the mouth to the stomach.

Crop: A pouch in the esophagus used to store food temporarily before moving it on to the stomach. Probably because of the high metabolic rate of the fowl, a more or less continuous supply of food is required by the digestive system. This is provided for by the crop that acts as a reservoir for the storage of food prior to its digestion and consequently permits the fowl to eat its food as periodic meals.

Stomach (Proventriculus/Gizzard): Principally the organ where food is broken into smaller units. It has two parts: the proventriculus for storage and the gizzard. The **gizzard** is a muscular part of the stomach that uses grit to grind grains and fiber into smaller particles.The gizzard almost always contains quantities of hard objects such as gravel or other grit that aids in the disintegration of food, which is the primary function of the gizzard.

Small Intestine: Birds have a small intestine that seems very similar to the small intestine of mammals. Aids in digestion and nutrient absorption. Composed of the duodenum, jejunum and ileum.Of the three parts of the mammalian small intestine, the duodenum, jejunum and ileum, only the duodenum can be easily distinguished in the fowl. Much of the digestion of the food and all of the absorption of the nutrients takes place in the small intestine and hence its structure is quite important.

The duodenum receives digestive enzymes and bicarbonate (to counter the hydrochloric acid from the proventriculus) from the pancreas and bile from the liver (via the gallbladder). The digestive juices produced by the pancreas are involved primarily in protein digestion. Bile is a detergent that is important in the digestion of lipids and the absorption of fat-soluble vitamins (A, D, E, and K).The proximal small intestine receives digestive enzymes from the pancreas, and the absorptive epithelial cells are decorated with essentially the same enzymes and transporters as in mammals.

Liver: The largest glandular organ in the body. Aids in the metabolism of carbohydrates, fats and proteins.

Ceca: Bacterial action in the ceca helps break down undigested food passing through the intestine. The ceca turns into the large intestine, which connects with the cloaca.

Large Intestine: The large intestine consists of a short colon and, typically, a pair of ceca. Short villi extend into the lumen of the colon, unlike what is seen in mammals. The cloaca is an expanded, tubular structure that serves as the common opening of the digestive, reproductive and urinary systems, which opens to the outside of the bird as the vent. Functions primarily to absorb water, dry out indigestible foods and eliminate waste products.

Cloaca: Where the digestive, urinary and reproductive systems meet.

Urinary System: Consists of two kidneys and two ureters. The kidneys are located in the pelvic bones. They filter waste from the blood and pass it through the ureter to the outside via the cloaca.

Vent: The external opening of the cloaca that passes waste to the outside.

Antiperistalsis that originates in the cloaca is a prominent pattern of motility in the avian colon and has been suggested to assist not only in filling the ceca, but to flush urine from the cloaca into the large gut for absorption of water. In some birds, the ceca appear dispensable and can be removed without apparent harm.

Vitamins and Minerals

Before the turn of present century, it was considered that carbohydrates, fats, proteins and minerals were sufficient for fulfilling the nutritional needs of animals. Later it was recognised that several other factors also need to be provided in the diet in small quantities, the absence of which resulted in diseases like beriberi, scurvy, pellagra and rickets. Funk in 1912 proposed the term vitamine for such factors, vita for being essential and amine because these factors were thought to be amines in chemical structure. Later it was discovered that not all such factors were amines, hence the last 'e' from the word vitamine was dropped.

Vitamins, a group of complex organic compounds that are present in minute amounts in natural foodstuffs, are essential for normal metabolism, and a lack of these compounds in the diet causes deficiency diseases.

The quantities of vitamins needed by the body are small, in the range of milligrams or micrograms. Thus vitamins came to be regarded as essential dietary factors which are required by an organism in small quantities and whose absence results in deficiency diseases. Many of these vitamins act as coenzymes in important metabolic reactions of the body. Most of the history of vitamins is linked to efforts to find cures for human diseases such as night blindness, xerophthalmia, scurvy, beriberi, rickets and pellagra.

The vitamins have been broadly classified on the basis of their solubility. Fat soluble vitamins - A, D, E and K. Water soluble vitamins- B complex and C. This classification has proved useful from the functional point of view also for an extended period of time and is now an established classification scheme. The water soluble vitamins cannot be stored in the body over extended periods of time during periods of opulence and used during periods of scarcity and therefore need to be supplemented on regular intervals or almost daily.

Most vitamins cannot be synthesized by the body hence the need for dietary supplement. However, ruminants have an advantage in that the rumen microorganisms can manufacture most of the B-complex vitamins which are utilized and required by the animal. Vitamin C is required only by human beings and guinea pig, hence is not of importance as a dietary ingredient for domestic animals. Most other animals are able to synthesize adequate amounts of vitamin C required by them. The site of synthesis of vitamin C is not well established but it seems that the liver and adrenal glands are actively involved. There appears to be no microbial synthesis of vitamin C in the intestine

At this stage it should be clarified about the dietary and physiological requirements. All vitamins are physiologically required by the domestic animals but only a few are required to be an essential dietary ingredient. Bioavailability is defined as the proportion of a consumed nutrient that is available for normal physiological functions and storage. Several factors affect the bioavailability of a vitamin or precursor in the diet for human beings and animals. Bioavailability of carotenoids in raw vegetables is estimated to be 5–10% for humans and rats, while it may be as high as 50% when dissolved in oils. Parasitic infection may reduce the bioavailability of vitamins or pro vitamins.

Fat Soluble Vitamins

Vitamin A

Vitamin A is essential for life in all vertebrate animals. Vitamin A is one of the fat soluble vitamins (along with vitamins D, E and K). All animals require vitamin A for proper nutrition.

Vitamin A is necessary for many functions in ruminants including: vision, bone growth, immunity and maintenance of epithelial tissue. Vitamin A is required for normal cellular differentiation, development, and immune function. Because of their strongly lipophilic nature, carotenes are found in the lipid core of the cell membrane.

Vitamin A is essential for proper vision and is utilized in the retina in the chemical reactions necessary for sight. Vitamin A deficiency results in night blindness and formation of ulcers on the cornea. Retinoic acid interacts with the nearly ubiquitously expressed nuclear retinoid receptors (RAR and RXR) to regulate gene expression.

Vitamin A affects bone development through its effect on bone metabolism. Essentially, vitamin A deficiency results in unchecked bone growth that in turn manifests as malformed bones and joints. Vitamin A directly affects immunity through both production of antibodies and through maintaining an adequate barrier to infection with healthy epithelial cells. Vitamin A deficiency reduces the primary antibody response in the event of infection.

Vitamin A is actually a family of compounds that are structurally similar to and have the essential functions and biological activity of retinol. Retinol is a long-chain, unsaturated alcohol containing five double bonds and a β-ionone ring. Retinol and most other naturally occurring retinoids are lipid-soluble compounds. The most physiologically active forms of Vitamin A are retinoic acid and retinal (also known as retinaldehyde).

Additionally, vitamin A's role in the maintenance of mucous membranes and epithelial linings directly affects other production parameters. Deficiency often results in keratinization (a form of thickening and hardening of tissues) and thus a loss of tissue function and increased susceptibility to infection. Keratinization of the digestive and respiratory tracts results in diarrhea and pneumonia. These are typical secondary symptoms of vitamin A deficiency. Keratinization of the reproductive tract results in poor sperm production in males and early abortion in females.

The body cannot make enough vitamin A, thus it must be provided by the diet. Major sources of preformed vitamin A include liver, fish, eggs, and fortified foods such as milk, cereals, and margarine. Vitamin A requirement can be met from dietary preformed vitamin A or provitamin A carotenoids, the most important of which is β-carotene. Plants cannot manufacture vitamin A. Plants are able to make β-carotene, which is a precursor to vitamin A. The animal converts β-carotene into vitamin A within its body. Omnivores and herbivores are more efficient at converting β-carotene to vitamin A than carnivores. Plants contain β-carotene to varying degrees. A relatively good indicator of carotene content is the degree of greenness of the plant. Fresh forages and early cut, leafy, green hays have high carotene content. Cereal grains (excluding yellow corn) have poor carotene content. The metabolism of β-carotene, including its intestinal absorption, accumulation in tissues, and conversion to vitamin A, varies widely across animal species and determines the role that β-carotene plays in meeting vitamin A requirement.

Sheep and goats are efficient convertors of β-carotene to vitamin A. Sheep and goats have colorless fat, indicating that they do not accumulate β-carotene in their adipose tissue. Horses have yellow fat so they seem to accumulate β-carotene in adipose tissue.

Vitamin A is stored in the liver and can be built up during times of abundance to help animals cope during scarce periods. It is believed that healthy adult livestock can store sufficient vitamin A to last 6 months if necessary. The storage capacity of young animals is much less than this. Borderline deficiency is much more common than severe deficiency, as with most nutrient deficiencies. The need for vitamin A is greatest during calving (kidding or lambing), breeding and other times of stress.

Vitamin A deficiency results in xerophthalmia, metaplasia, epithelial differentiation, anorexia, and compromised function of both innate and adaptive immunity. Ruminants deficient in vitamin A are more susceptible to eye infections. They are also more susceptible to respiratory diseases and exhibit poor heat tolerance. A lack of vitamin A results in decreased reproductive efficiency in both males and females.

Vitamin D

Vitamin D is a fat-soluble vitamin also known as sunshine vitamin, that helps maintain the balance of calcium in the body, important for normal growth and mineralization of bones and teeth. Extensive and ongoing research on Vitamin D has also brought to light new roles of this vitamin in modulation of cell growth, neuromuscular and immune functions.

The observed beneficial effect of sunlight on rickets is due to the cutaneous photoproduction of cholecalciferol (Vitamin D_3) from its provitamin, 7-dehydrocholecalciferal

Structure: The vitamin D is group of compounds that are sterols. In 1927 Dr. E. H. Reerink and Dr. A. van Wijk, two young scientists in the Phillips' Physics Laboratory in Eindhoven, the Netherlands, used the newly developed high pressure ultraviolet lamp to obtain reaction products from ergosterol by careful wavelength monitoring. They achieved the first industrial scale photochemical transformation of ergosterol into an anti-rachitic substance which was a synthetic method of producing pure Vitamin D.

Mode of Action

The epidermis and dermis layers of the skin contain 7-dehydrocholesterol also known as provitamin D_3 which on exposure to UltraViolet radiation between 290 – 315 nm (UVB range) is converted to Vitamin D_3. In the kidney 25(OH)D_3 is converted into 1,25(OH)2D3 i.e. 1,25 dihydroxyvitamin D_3 or calcitriol which is the active form of Vitamin D_3 required by the body. The *in vivo* synthesis of the major biologically active metabolites of vitamin D occurs in two steps. The first hydroxylation of ergocalciferol takes place in the liver (to 25-hydroxyvitamin D) and the second in the kidneys (to 1,25-dihydroxyvitamin D). Vitamin D metabolites promote the active absorption of calcium and phosphorus by the small intestine, thus elevating serum calcium and phosphate levels sufficiently to permit bone mineralization. Vitamin D metabolites also mobilize calcium and phosphate from bone and probably increase the reabsorption of calcium and perhaps also of phosphate by the renal tubules.

The main role of Vitamin D3 in mammals, birds, and reptiles is to control bone metabolism by regulating calcium absorption.Vitamin D helps in the absorption of Ca^{++} from the intestine with the help of calcium binding protein. The active metabolite of vitamin D for this purpose is 1, 25- dihydroxy Vitamin D_3.

Vitamin D helps in the absorption of phosphorus by the intestinal epithelium. Vitamin D3 regulates calcium metabolism through its interaction with its major target tissues, the bone and the intestine. Various factors, including serum phosphorus (Pi) and parathyroid hormone (PTH), regulate the renal production of D3.

Deficiency of vitamin D causes osteoporosis. Osteoporosis is a quantitative reduction in the amount of bony material per unit volume of bone as an organ. This reduction causes increased bone fragility.

Rickets *:* The most common deficiency symptom of vitamin D deficiency is rickets. This disease is characterised by a decreased concentration of calcium and phosphorus in the organic matrix of cartilage and bone. Rickets is a particularly devastating disease characterized by softened bones (leading to deformity) as well as muscle spasms and seizures. Rickets was first identified as a rare disorder in the 1600s. However, in the late 1700s, it became rampant in Europe as people began to stay indoors and live in large, polluted cities, with reduced exposure to sunlight. In the 1890s, scientists began to search for specific foods that could prevent rickets.Later, it was shown that cod liver oil could prevent rickets. It was discovered that exposure to sunlight was also completely effective in curing and preventing rickets. Companies such as Hoffmann-La Roche and BASF produce large quantities of the primary form of vitamin D, also known as vitamin D3 or cholecalciferol.

Osteomalacia *:* Osteomalacia is equivalent to rickets in the adult. This disease is characterised by a decreased concentration of calcium and phosphorus in the bone matrix only.

Vitamin D3 is an essential nutrient in feed for animals. Vitamin D3 supplementation is linked to better egg productivity from poultry resulting in fewer breakages and more eggs per hen.

Vitamin E

Vitamin E is an antioxidant vitamin present in the form of several closely related active compounds. The structure of the most active form is called alpha-Tocopherol.

Vitamin E is very widely distributed in foods. Green fodders are good sources of alpha tocopherol, young grass being a better source than mature herbage. Losses during hay making may be as high as 90% but losses during ensilage and artificial drying are small.

Functions : Vitamin E is attributed to have two metabolic roles, firstly it acts as a non specific biological antioxidant and secondly it has a more specific action associated with selenium, in which it protects vital phospholipids from peroxidative damage.

Deficiency symptoms include sterility and muscle dystrophy in young ruminants. The popular names of these diseases include white muscle disease and Stiff Lamb disease.

Fatal syncope is a vitamin E deficiency symptom in pig and calves in which the heart muscle is affected and sudden death may occur.

Vitamin K

Vitamin K was originally discovered in 1935 to be an essential factor in the prevention of hemorrhagic symptoms produced in chicks. Vitamin K is necessary for the formation of prothrombin and factors VII, IX and X required for blood clotting. Liver cells synthesize prothrombin.Vitamin K is a group of fat soluble vitamins that are needed for the modification of certain proteins, mostly required for blood coagulation but also involved in metabolism pathways in bone and other tissue. Three types of vitamin K, namely K1- Phylloquinone, K2 – Menaquinone and K3-Menadione are recognised. Vitamin K3 is easily synthesized and available commercially.

Vitamin K is absorbed from the intestine into the blood. Some foods, specially green plants, contain this vitamin in the phylloquinone form. It is also synthesized by bacteria present in the digestive tract . Since these bacteria are not present in the newborn animals, they require a dietary supplement of vitamin K.

Because vitamin K is fat soluble, its absorption requires bile salts. If therefore, the bile ducts become obstructed and bile cannot enter the intestine, a vitamin K deficiency develops. The liver cannot then produce prothrombin at its normal rate and blood prothrombin concentration soon falls below normal. A prothrombin deficiency gives rise to a bleeding tendency. As a pre-operative safeguard, therefore, patients with obstructive jaundice are generally given some kind of vitamin K preparation.

Deficiency of vitamin K results in haemorrhages because of the failure of the blood to clot.

It is generally considered that bacterial synthesis of vitamin K in the digestive tract supplies sufficient vitamin K for the animals' need.

A hemorrhagic disease in cattle called Sweet Clover disease is associated with vitamin K deficiency. This is because spoiled clover (Melilotus officinalis) contains a compound, dicoumarol, which lowers the prothrombin content of the blood. This disease can be overcome by administering vitamin K to the animals. For this reason, dicoumarol is sometimes referred to as an antivitamin.

Water Soluble Vitamins

Vitamin C

Vitamin C is a water soluble vitamin called ascorbic acid ($C_6H_8O_6$). Vitamin C is very important in human nutrition but do not have the dietary requirement in ruminants. Vitamin C present in fresh vegetables and green fruits such as guava, oranges, limes, turnip, peppers etc. Vitamin C is destroyed by cooking. Blood concentration of vitamin C in domestic animals varies from 2-6 mg/litre. However, the milk or cow/buffalo is generally deficient in Vitamin C.

Domestic livestock including ruminants have the ability to biosynthesize L-ascorbic acid through glucuronic acid pathway in liver (in mammals) using either D-glucose or D-galactose although young ruminants may not produce adequate endogenous ascorbic acid until four months of age. It has been suggested that calves less than four months of age may have a marginal vitamin C deficiency and that this deficiency may affect disease resistance early in life . Cattle are essentially dependent on this endogenous synthesis as dietary vitamin C is almost totally destroyed by rumen microorganisms. Ascorbic acid need not be added to dairy cattle rations. However, several studies have conclusively documented the decrease of vitamin C level in the blood during stress and diseases in cattle and other ruminants. Decrease in the vitamin C level during stress and diseases may be the end result of decreased endogenous synthesis or increased demand or a combination of both.

Human beings lack the ability to synthesize vitamin C as they lack the enzyme gulonolactone oxidase that converts L-gulonolactone to ascorbic acid.

Vitamin C is a powerful reducing agent required in the hydroxylation of proline and lysine for the biosynthesis of collagen. Thus vitamin supports wound healing and formation of blood vessels, bone and teeth. Vitamin C is regarded to have critical functions in the brain including its role as a cofactor of dopamine-hydroxylase, and is thereby involved in catecholamine biosynthesis.

The antioxidant role of vitamin C appears to be a common link in its role in the function and integrity of various cell types in the body, in detoxification functions and in the normal functioning of the adrenal glands, lungs, brain, eye and immune system.

Dermatosis in calves has been associated with vitamin C deficiency. Demand of vitamin C increases during various infections . Classic symptoms of vitamin C deficiency, or scurvy, are marked deterioration of mucosal integrity and health and subsequent loss of disease resistance. Because ruminants possess the metabolic pathway to synthesize ascorbic acid, they are only likely to experience outright deficiency symptoms in the neonatal period, before synthesis reaches full capacity. Young ruminants are susceptible to vitamin C deficiency during the first few weeks of life, particularly when subjected to stress, disease exposure or limited colostrum intake. Vitamin C is not an essential dietary nutrient for adult ruminants, however benefits have been shown for supplemental vitamin C for animals under stress or disease conditions, such as mastitis. Vitamin C addition has been advocated to be added to cryopotecting media for semen or embryos because of antioxidant activity.

Vitamin C deficiency in human beings can cause scurvy and muscle and joint pain.

B-Complex

Many years ago, Osborne and Mendel showed that rats fed on a highly purified diet, failed to grow and developed other abnormalities, but when given an extract of yeast, growth was resumed. They named the factor in yeast extract as vitamin B. However, it was later shown that the yeast extract could be fractionated into many different compounds, so now it is called the B complex. Since B vitamins are synthesized by microflora in the rumen, as well as being relatively abundant in ordinary feeds, they have been of less concern in the nutrition of ruminants.

The vitamins of the B complex are thiamine (B1), Riboflavin(B2), Niacin, Pyridoxine (B6), Pantothenic acid, Biotin, Folic acid, Choline, and vitamin B_{12}. These vitamins are water soluble and cannot be stored in the body i.e. they need to be provided in the diet daily or regularly in the simple stomached animals. A single high dose may not be as effective as large number of small daily doses taken,in alleviating the deficiency symptoms. In herbivores, other than ruminants such as horse and rabbit, the microbial synthesis of B-complex vitamins occurs in the colon or caecum. Thus they do not need to be dietary essential for these species too. However, for pigs, poultry and other simple stomached animals including humans, dietary sources are essential. Animals with a functional rumen were once thought to synthesize B-vitamins and therefore to have no need for supplementation. However, deficiencies do occur under special conditions and supplementation has proven beneficial in the case of thiamin, niacin, vitamin B_{12}, choline and biotin.

The rumen does not become functional with respect to vitamin synthesis for some time after birth. For the first few days of life, the young ruminant resembles a non ruminant in that it requires dietary sources of the B vitamins. Beginning as early as eight days, and certainly by two months of age, the ruminal flora has developed to the point that it contributes significant amounts of B vitamins. Production of these vitamins at the proximal end of the gastrointestinal tract makes them available to the host as they pass down the digestive tract.

These vitamins like hormones and trace minerals, are trace compounds i.e. present in the body in extremely small quantities. However, their effects are tremendous on the body metabolism. All the members of the B-complex vitamins are organic compounds but are unrelated to each other in structure. In many of the reactions involved in intermediate metabolism vitamins of the B complex play an important role.

Thiamine (B_1)

Thiamine consists of one molecule of pyrimidine joined with one of thiazole.Thiamine is phosphorylated in the liver to form co-enzyme, co-carboxylase or thiamine pyrophosphate (TPP). Thiamine pyrophosphate is involved in the decarboxylation of alpha keto acid eg. decarboxylation of pyruvic acid to acetaldehyde.

The pig is somewhat unique in that it stores appreciable thiamine in its tissues. This accounts for the fact that pork is an excellent source of dietary thiamine. A thiamine binding protein is present in the blood plasma of pregnant rats and has been implicated to play a role in the transfer of thiamine across the placenta.

In mature ruminants the microflora of the rumen synthesizes sufficient riboflavin and other water soluble vitamins to eliminate a dietary need under most conditions. Young pre ruminant animals (lambs and calves) have dietary requirement early in life, however, and deficiency signs can be induced with synthetic milk diets. Diets low in riboflavin produce lesions in the corners of mouth and on the lips, anorexia, loss of hair and diarrhoea in calves and lambs. The type of diet fed to immature ruminants appears to be a controlling factor in the development of the rumen microbial population that synthesizes riboflavin.Riboflavin is heat stable but destroyed by light.

Deficiency : Thiamine deficiency is known to produce Beri Beri in human beings. This disease is characterised by the numbness of the extremities, weakness and stiffness of the thighs, oedema of the feet and legs, unsteady gait and paralytic symptoms and pain along the spine.

In chickens, a disease known as polyneuritis occurs in the absence or deficiency of thiamine.

Thiamine is heat labile i.e. destroyed by heat. Thiamine toxicity has not been reported since excess thiamine is always excreted rapidly in the urine.

Riboflavin (B_2)

Riboflavin is a yellow fluorescent pigment consisting of ribose and alloxazine.

Functions : Riboflavin functions as a coenzyme (FAD and FMN)

which occurs in a large number of enzyme systems.

Deficiency Symptoms: The most common effect, as with most of the water soluble vitamin deficiencies is reduced growth rate in young animals. In rats, conjunctivitis, corneal opacity and vascularization of the cornea are common signs of deficiency.

Niacin, sometimes called nicotinic acid, is the vitamin component in two important coenzymes called NAD (nicotinamide adenine dinucleotide) and NADP (nicotinamide adenine dinucleotide phosphate). The coenzymes NAD and NADP are concerned with carbohydrate, fat, and protein metabolism systems for all animals. Niacin was isolated in 1937 and demonstrated to be effective in curing black tongue in dogs and pellagra in man. The word pellagra means rough skin, which relates to dermatitis. In the 1940s, it was discovered that the amino acid tryptophan could be converted in the body to niacin in most animals. It is not known how much tryptophan is converted to niacin in the ruminant animal by rumen microorganisms, but they are known to synthesize some niacin. In recent findings, research has shown a beneficial effect from niacin supplementation for ruminants under certain situations.

In 1948, Rickes and his colleagues in the United States and Smith in England isolated vitamin B_{12} and identified it as the anti pernicious anemia factor. Since the mineral cobalt is an integral part of the vitamin B12 molecule, a deficiency of cobalt would naturally lead to a deficiency of vitamin B_{12}. A deficiency of cobalt and vitamin B_{12} will result in anemia. Simple monogastric animals were found to require the vitamin, whereas ruminants and other species with large microbial populations (e.g. horses) require dietary cobalt rather than vitamin B_{12}. Cobalamin plays an essential role in the synthesis of nucleic acids. Cyanocobalamin is the common term used to refer to the most active and stable supplemental form of vitamin B_{12}.

Bio-synthesized vitamins are more available to animals (rabbit, rat and others) that habitually practice coprophagy and thus recycle products of the lower gut. This behavior provides significant amounts of B vitamins to the host animal. Intestinal synthesis of B vitamins in non-ruminants occurs in the lower intestinal tract for example horses.

Minerals

Vitamins, minerals and trace elements are dynamic nutrients which are usually required to be added in feed rations as they have a positive effect on maintenance, growth, health and milk production. Minerals are inorganic compounds which are important both as constituents of body tissues as well as catalysts to metabolic reactions. Major elements, constitutes a large part of the body organism. Minor or Trace elements whose function is only biochemical i.e. catalytic rather than structural.

Microminerals can be divided into two groups.

Macro elements, such as

1. Calcium (Ca),
2. Phosphorus (P),
3. Sodium (Na),
4. Chlorine (Cl)
5. Magnesium (Mg),
6. Potassium (K),
7. Sulphur (S)

Trace elements such as

1. iron (Fe),
2. copper (Cu),
3. zinc (Zn),
4. manganese (Mn),
5. cobalt (Co),
6. selenium (Se),
7. iodine (I) and
8. molybdenum (Mo).

Beside these ones, other trace elements exist in nature, such as fluorine, nickel, boron, chromium, cadmium, arsenic, mercury etc but these are not essential for the body , and can even be toxic.

The bioavailability of a mineral or trace element is defined as the fraction of the ingested nutrient that is absorbed and subsequently utilized for normal physiological functions. Physiological requirements for different inorganic nutrients vary widely, depending upon age, sex, stage of growth, pregnancy, and lactation. Dietary requirements are calculated from physiological requirements and efficiency of absorption from the diet.

Often, synergistic effects are seen between macro and trace elements and vitamins. For example vitamin D and calcium. Furthermore, calcium absorption is increased when there is magnesium and phosphorus available as well. Another example is vitamin B_{12}

and cobalt. Cobalt deficiency can cause vitamin B12 deficiency and hence anorexia, low rumen functionality, susceptibility to microbial infestations etc. Vitamin E and selenium also act synergistically. Vitamin E can boost immunity of livestock. Also, in a synergistic role with selenium, it influences the concentration of polyunsaturated fatty acids which are then converted to saturated in order to be absorbed into the rumen The use of trace elements in animal nutrition has moved to increasing the bioavailability for better absorption and meeting animal demands and avoiding overdose while feeding less absorbable forms.

Macro Elements

Major elements, constitutes a large part of the body organism.

1. calcium (Ca)
2. phosphorus (P)
3. sodium (Na)
4. chlorine (Cl)
5. magnesium (Mg)
6. potassium (K)
7. sulphur (S)

Calcium and Phosphorus elements are quantitatively the most important minerals. Calcium is required for a wide variety of functions including bone and teeth formation, muscle contraction, nerve conduction, neurotransmitter release, blood coagulation, activation of specific enzymes, endocrine secretion, cell differentiation, cell motility and cell division. The major crystalline form of Ca and P in bone is hydroxyapatite Ca^{10} (PO4) $(OH)^2$. Obviously the exchangeable Ca and P form a very small part of the total body content.

Hepatic transglutaminase displays an absolute requirement for Ca^{+2} . Most intracellular activities including functions of the neuromuscular system and endocrine system are primed by the first increase of permeability of Ca^{+2} ions into the cell. Thus this step is the key to the secretion of several hormones like catecholamines from the adrenal medulla, insulin from beta cells of the islets of Langerhans in Pancreas, steroids of the adrenal cortex stimulated by ACTH and secretion of neuro hypophysial hormones and renin secretion from the kidney. Thus Ca+2 ion is the key to the functioning of several hormones in the cell where it is bound by calcium binding protein called calmodulin.

A number of proteins and other factors have been proposed as participants in the transfer of calcium from the intestinal lumen to the lamina propria.

Contrary to the normal belief, bone is not a static tissue, but has a very rapid turnover of minerals, which decreases with ageing. The true digestibility of calcium is very high in young (milk fed) animals, but decreases in adults. Calcium digestibility increases when dietary calcium is low. Bone is the body reserve of Ca and P.

As mentioned earlier, Ca is important in four steps of the blood clotting process. Complement activation also requires Ca^{2+} ions.The conversion of 'phosphorylase b' to 'phosphorylase a' by phosphorylase b kinase is stimulated by Ca^{+2} ions. Thus calcium modulation couples glycogenolysis and contraction of skeletal muscle.

Ca is critical for so many essential functions of the body. Ca concentration in the blood is regulated accurately by the elegant interplay of several hormones which include thyrocalcitonin and parathormone.

Parathormone is a polypeptide hormone secreted by the parathyroid gland. Its secretion is triggered by low amounts of ionized calcium in the plasma. Parathormone induces a drop in the renal Tm of phosphates (Tm = maximal tubular rate of reabsorption), inducing a phosphate diuresis and hypophosphatemia, a stimulation of the formation of the active metabolite of vitamin D (1,25 - dihyroxycholecalciferol) in the kidney and an increase in bone calcium turnover, with a predominance of osteolysis.

Calcitonin is also a polypeptide hormone, secreted mainly by the thyroid gland in the parafollicular cells. Its secretion is triggered by high amounts of ionized calcium in the plasma. It induces a decrease in the renal Tm of phosphates, and stops calcium metabolism without modifying accretion. The resulting effect is a decrease of Ca and P in the blood and an increase in bone mass.

Vitamin D is also concerned with the stimulation of intestinal absorption of Ca and P and stimulation of bone mineral turnover. A deficiency of either Ca and P or Vit. D can cause rickets in young animals, a disease in which the bone becomes deformed or osteomalacia in adults. An excess of Ca in the diet during late pregnancy causes the appearance of milk fever in cows at subsequent calvings.

Potassium is essentially an intracellular element, in contrast to the extracellular localization of sodium. This is significant metabolically since a considerable expenditure of energy is required to maintain constant concentration gradient across the cell wall. The sodium transcellular gradient seems to be the major factor in the transport of a variety of substances against their concentration gradient.

Chloride ion is mainly extracellular. During Na deficiency, the plasma osmotic pressure decreases; the osmo receptors feed back to the hypothalamus; which decreases the secretion of antidiuretic hormone from the neurohypophysis. This leads to a reequilibration of the osmotic pressure and decrease in extracellular volume and blood pressure. The low blood pressure induces thirst through brain baro receptors and stimulates the secretion of renin by the juxtaglomerular cells of the kidney : kidney renin catalyses the cleavage of circulating angiotensinogen (secreted by the liver) to form pro angiotensin, subsequently transformed to angiotensin. Angiotensin increases the blood pressure and stimulates the glomerular cells at the periphery of the adrenal cortex, to secrete aldosterone. Aldosterone stimulates Na^+ K^+ exchange in the nephron and thus promotes Na^+ conservation and K^+ excretion, which increases both osmotic pressure and extracellular volume.

Thus Na deficiency in the adult results in salt hunger, thirst, polyuria, decrease in extracellular volume, blood pressure, plasma sodium and plasma osmolality, loss of weight due to decrease in extracellular volume and, in chronic cases to the lack of appetite.

An increase in temperature induces ADH and aldosterone secretion with water and sodium retention and an increased volume of extracellular fluid. This could be an adaptive mechanism anticipating the loss of water through evaporation and losses of sodium through sweating.

Sodium is not stored in the body in significant amounts, which means that it's best to supplement it little and often. The most common form of supplementation for sodium is sodium chloride, more commonly known as salt. Sodium chloride contains 40 percent sodium. It has been estimated that a ruminant requires about 0.5 g Na/ day/100 Kg B.W.; 2.5 g K/day/100 Kg B.W. and 2.5 gm Cl/day/100 Kg B.W. for maintenance only. Offering salt to animals in blocks or free-access rock salt in troughs can work really well and it allows the animals to regulate how much sodium they need.

Sulphur occurs in the body in both organic and inorganic forms. Mammals are incapable of synthesizing the organic forms of sulphur from sulphate. Sulfur is necessary for the production of amino acids cysteine, cystine and methionine in ruminant animals, which are manufactured by the microorganisms in the animal's forestomach, called the rumen. Cysteine contains a disulphide bridge which is easily reduced to give two molecules of cystine. This disulphide bridge is very important in protein structures, particularly for example, in alpha keratin, and in immunoglobulins. Methionine and cysteine are important constituents of wool proteins. Sheep and goats typically require more dietary sulfur than cattle due to the large amounts of sulfur they require to grow hair and wool.

Sulphur is also a constituent of several biologically important molecules; thiamine, biotin, lipoic acid and coenzyme A. The liver is the principal site of sulphur metabolism. The transmethylation reaction allows the synthesis of lipoproteins phospholipids and cholesterol esters necessary for transport of lipids in blood. One thus understands why deficiency of sulphur containing amino acids has such serious consequences; accumulation of fat in liver, slowing of protein synthesis, perturbation of the oxidation reduction reactions. Sulphur deficiency brings about a rapid emancipation of the animals and prevents the growth or the alpha keratin rich tissues (horns, nails and hairs).

Cobalt

The only known physiological function of cobalt in mammals is as the catalytic center of the vitamin B_{12} coenzyme. Cobalt deficiency has been observed in ruminants, particularly cattle and sheep, in many areas of the world. All the effects of deficiency appear to reflect failure of synthesis by the rumen microorganisms of vitamin B_{12}, of which cobalt is a constituent. There have been no reports of the production of cobalt deficiency in non ruminant animals, all of which require dietary vitamin $B_{12.}$

Magnesium

Magnesium (Mg^{2+}) is essentially an intracellular element. Bone is the main magnesium store and during deficiency bone magnesium is progressively released into circulation. In ruminants reticulo-rumen is the main site of magnesium absorption whereas in non ruminants most of Mg is absorbed through the small intestine.

Magnesium is basically an enzyme activator.

Another important function of magnesium is as a competitor for Ca^{2+} binding sites in the excitation secretion coupling process.

The major deficiency symptoms of Mg^{+2} include impaired growth with hypoproteinemia ostensibly due to decrease in protein synthesis: tetanic seizures due to inhibition of cholinesterase of the neuromuscular junction and also disturbance in calcium pump of the sarcoplasmic reticulum.

The retention and the plasma level of Mg are controlled through renal excretion, but endocrine involvement in homeostasis has not been demonstrated either for urinary excretion or for intestinal absorption.

Iron

Iron is an essential component of haemoglobin in the red blood cells. A deficiency of iron and consequently haemoglobin and red blood cells causes anaemia. The young growing animals or adult animals infested with parasites or subjected to haemorrhages or during pregnancy are very susceptible to iron deficiency.

Iron is stored in most tissues but especially in liver, spleen and bone marrow. The major storage form is ferritin and hemosidderin.

Haemoglobin is mainly concerned with oxygen transport in the body. Iron binding proteins (transferrin, ferritin and hemosiderrin) are widely distributed in the body. Another iron binding protein, lactoferrin can be isolated from milk and leukocytes.

The rate of haemoglobin synthesis and the production of new red blood cells is controlled by a glycoprotein hormone, *erythropoietin* which is produced mainly in the kidney and is present in the circulating blood. The trigger of erythropoietin secretion is the low oxygen content of the arterial blood, which ensures a *regulatory feedback* of red blood cell production. Erythropoietin is high in the blood of cattle and human beings residing at high altitude.

Zinc

Zinc is an essential trace element for both plants and animals. After iron, zinc is the second most abundant trace metal in the human body. About 7 percent of ingested zinc is absorbed from the digestive tract. Zinc is more concentrated in leukocytes and pituitary but all tissues contain zinc. More than three fourths of excreted zinc passes out with the faeces and less than one-fourth is excreted in the urine.

Functions : Dietary zinc has been shown to mobilize vitamin A from liver hepatocytes into blood through retinol binding protein for utilization by different tissues.

Zinc is required for the activity of > 300 enzymes, covering all six classes of enzymes. Zinc ion is an essential cofactor for the observed biological function of these metalloenzymes.

The zinc dependent enzyme alcohol dehydrogenase is involved in the reversible conversion of retinol and retinal in the process of vision. Greater alcohol dehydrogenase activity in the intestinal tissue as a result of zinc supplementation is important for greater conversion of β-carotene to vitamin A in the intestinal wall and in the retina in the process of vision.

Zinc deficiency may occur because of inadequate intake or availability, malabsorption or increased rates of loss from the organism. Zinc deficiency is mainly seen in dogs and pigs, sometimes in ruminants and horses. Decreased zinc availability has been seen in certain dog foods containing excessive levels of phytate which interferes with zinc absorption.

In ruminants, there is alopecia, crusts and scales on face, neck and distal extremities and mucocutaneous junctions. Low zinc status leads to lower quality milk and increased incidence of mastitis. The deficiency of zinc causes parakeratosis, in growing swine. The condition is characterised by a crusty proliferation and cracking of the skin. This condition has also been reported in cattle. Alopecia in various body regions has been reported in buffaloes suffering from zinc deficiency. In ruminants, zinc supplementation can increase reproductive performance by increasing conception rate.

Serum zinc levels may have good diagnostic value. Normal levels are 80-120 μg/dL (12.2-18.2 μmol/L) in sheep and cattle.

Zinc containing enzymes in the animal body include Carbonic anhydrase, Alcohol dehydrogenase, Glutamic dehydrogenase, Lactic dehydrogenase, Carboxypeptidase.

Trace Elements

Notwithstanding the minute quantities of copper, cobalt, zinc, manganese and other elements in the body, they are indispensable for life. They are frequently referred to as trace elements. These elements make up less than 0.01% of the body of a mammal. These elements occur in such small amounts that though early investigators could demonstrate their presence in the body, analytical methods were not sufficiently accurate for a precise analysis. These elements, therefore, were mentioned as occurring in trace amounts and they became known as trace elements.

Inadequate trace mineral nutrition is obviously limiting livestock production in several parts of the world. Mineral supplementation represents low input/high output nutrients for greatly increasing livestock production.

Some of the trace elements are essential for the activity of certain enzymes. For example magnesium is important for carboxylase enzyme activity, zinc in carbonic anhydrase and iron in catalase and peroxidases. Copper functioning in the synthesis of haemoglobin, is stored in the liver, especially in young animals. It is found in many oxidases. Copper is stored in and transported in the plasma by means of a blue copper protein ceruloplasmin. Deficiency of cobalt leads to anaemia. This may find its explanation in that cobalt is a constituent of vitamin B_{12}. Lack of manganese disturbs the reproductive function in both the male and female. It is also important in enzyme reactions.

Selenium : Selenium is necessary for growth and fertility in animals, and for the prevention of a variety of disease conditions occurring due to deficiency of vitamin E. These diseases include muscular dystrophy (white muscle disease) in lambs, calves and foals. In addition selenium deficiency has been known to cause a disease called **Degnala disease**. Selenium has long been recognized for its toxic effect on farm animals.

The general biochemical role of selenium is in protecting tissues against oxidative damage. Their tremendous effect on metabolism is possible because of their activity as part of the metabolic catalysts, enzymes. The catalyst is a substance which is required in small amounts but can increase the rate of the reaction tremendously. The vitamins are a part of the helpers of the body catalysis (enzymes) called coenzymes.

Summary

- Digestive system ensures a continual supply of water, electrolytes and nutrients needed for sustaining life processes.
- Digestion usually consists of two elements: a mechanical/physical stage, e.g. mastication, churning, emulsification, in which no chemical bonds are broken and no enzymes are required; and a chemical stage requiring enzymes in which complex food molecules are broken down by hydrolysis into a state in which they can be absorbed.
- Ruminants such as cattle, sheep, and goats are herbivores. They have large microbial fermentation chambers where the plant materials are partially broken down before the food reaches the true stomach.
- Non ruminant herbivores, such as horses, are called hindgut fermenters. They have an extremely well developed and expansive fermentation chamber (the cecum) at the junction of the small and large intestines that allows microbes to help break down plant materials.
- Unlike monogastric animals, ruminants, via their microbial flora, can effectively use nonprotein nitrogen (NPN) to meet some of their dietary protein requirements.
- Structure and function of the stomach is the major difference between monogastrics and ruminants.

9

Respiration

The primary role of the respiratory system is to provide O_2 to the tissues for metabolic needs and remove the CO_2 formed by them. Body needs oxygen to oxidise the food nutrients and derive energy. In this process carbon dioxide is produced in the body, which is toxic and must be removed quickly and efficiently. The oxygen utilization & carbon dioxide production takes place within the mitochondria of cells of the various tissues. The transport of O_2 and CO_2 to and from the cells of various tissues is done by the blood. But the actual uptake of oxygen from the air and discharge of CO_2 into the environment takes place at the level of lungs. This exchange of O_2 and CO_2 between the organism and the environment is defined as respiration. Air is moved in and out of the lungs by their bellows action (ventilation). It is then distributed within each lung, so that alveoli are adequately ventilated and also perfused by the blood. In addition to exchange of gases, some amount of ammonia and ketone bodies are also excreted through the lungs.

Respiration entails two processes: the external respiration and internal respiration. The internal respiration or tissue respiration refers to the utilization of O_2 and production of CO_2 by the tissues.The external respiration includes supply of O_2 to the tissues from the environment and excretion of CO_2 released by the tissues into the atmosphere.The process of external respiration involves three major events:

- **Pulmonary ventilation**, i.e. exchange of gases between the environment and lungs. It includes mechanics of respiration.
- **Pulmonary diffusion** refers to transfer of gases from alveoli to the blood by diffusion across the respiratory membrane. Oxygen and carbon dioxide are exchanged between the gas mixture in the alveoli and the blood in the pulmonary capillaries (gas transfer).
- **Transport of gases** from the blood to the body cells and back. The exchanged gases are transported in the blood to the tissue.

Pulmonary physiology is concerned with the processes necessary for the exchange of oxygen and carbon dioxide between cells of the body and the external environment These processes include 1) gas transport properties of the blood, 2) mechanics of breathing, 3) O_2 and CO_2 exchange across the alveoli of the lungs, and 4) regulation of breathing

Functional Morphology of The Respiratory Apparatus

The respiratory system in mammals includes the tissues and organs associated with pulmonary ventilation and pulmonary respiration (air passages) which comprises mainly lungs and musculoskeletal system. The chief organs of the respiratory system are right and left lungs. The oxygen in the atmospheric air reaches the lungs by passing through a series of respiratory passages, which also serve for the removal of CO_2 from the alveoli to the atmosphere. The respiratory system also includes a pump that ventilates the lung. This pump consists of the chest wall and respiratory muscles.

The respiratory passage is composed of the nasal passages, pharynx, bronchi, bronchioles and alveoli of the lungs (other parts of passage). The muzzle, which holds the nostrils, is made up of the nose and lips on most domestic animals. The nostrils are the external openings of the respiratory tract through which air passes during the breathing process. The horse's muzzle and nostrils are soft and expandable, allowing for large amounts of air to pass when needed.

Nasal cavities: The nasal cavities are lined with a mucous - secreting, pseudostratified ciliated epithelium. Nasal cavity is divided in half by the nasal septum and vomer bone. The nasal valve is the narrowest point in the nasal cavity and is a major contributor to nasal resistance. The mucus and the cilia trap the particulate matter contained within the air. Thus the air passing through the nasal cavities is filtered, warmed and moistened. The nasal cavity is also the site of receptors for the sense of smell.

Pharynx : Pharynx is a common passageway for the respiratory and digestive system. The pharynx ensures that the food or liquid does not enter the respiratory system during swallowing.

Larynx : The larynx serves as a valve for the respiratory passageway separating the upper respiratory system from the lower respiratory system. The larynx forms the communicating channel between the pharynx and the trachea and functions during breathing, vocalization and deglutition. The larynx is composed of cartilage and muscle and is covered with a mucous membrane. The mucous membrane covers the vocal ligament, forms the vocal folds and lines the lateral ventricles, forming the laryngeal saccules.

Trachea : Air passes through the nasal cavities pharynx into the trachea or windpipe, which is a tubular structure. The trachea is surrounded by three-quarter rings of cartilage, except on the side next to the esophagus. Here the cartilage is replaced by connective tissue which is less rigid and permits easier passage of food down the esophagus.

The upper end of the trachea is modified to form the larynx or voice box, which contains the vocal cords. The opening between the pharynx and the larynx is the glottis, guarded by a flap of fibre cartilage, the epiglottis. The muscles of the larynx can vary the shape and size of the glottis and close it altogether. The action of these muscles are important in phonation as well as in preventing objects from the respiratory passageway.

The Lungs: The trachea divides into-two branches, the bronchus. Each bronchus enters a lung and divides into smaller and smaller branches, the bronchioles. The bronchi have rings of cartilage and the larger bronchioles have plates of cartilage that hold them open. The small bronchioles lack cartilage but have highly developed smooth muscle, circularly arranged.

Each terminal bronchiole leads into a small sac, formed by a grape-like cluster of microscopic sacs called alveoli.

Each inspiration draws air down this system of passages to its destination in the alveoli where the gas exchange occurs. Microscopically, the alveoli are composed of a single layer of epithelial cells, covered by a thin layer of elastic connective tissue.

The alveoli are surrounded by capillaries that arise from branches of the pulmonary artery and feed into the branches of the pulmonary vein. The membranes separating the air in the alveoli from the blood in the capillaries are thin. The major function of the lung is gas exchange- uptake of oxygen and elimination of carbon dioxide.

The other set of structures associated with respiration (skeletal and muscular) consists of ribs, intercostal muscles, diaphragm and accessory muscles.

The respiratory conducting passages are divided into the upper respiratory tract and the lower respiratory tract. The upper respiratory tract includes the nose, pharynx, and larynx. The lower respiratory tract consists of the trachea, bronchial tree, and lungs. These tracts open to the outside and are lined with mucous membranes. In some regions, the membrane has hairs that help filter the air. Other regions may have cilia to propel mucus.

Mechanics of Breathing

Ventilation, or breathing, is the movement of air through the conducting passages between the atmosphere and the lungs. The air moves through the passages because of pressure gradients that are produced by contraction of the diaphragm and thoracic muscles. Pulmonary ventilation is commonly referred to as breathing. It is the process of air flowing into the lungs during inspiration (inhalation) and out of the lungs during expiration (exhalation).

Pulmonary ventilation involves three different pressures:

- Atmospheric pressure: Atmospheric pressure is the pressure of the air outside the body.
- Intra Alveolar (intrapulmonary) pressure: Intra Alveolar pressure is the pressure inside the alveoli of the lungs.
- Intrapleural pressure:Intrapleural pressure is the pressure within the pleural cavity. These three pressures are responsible for pulmonary ventilation. The changes in intrapulmonary pressure are changed by changes in intrapleural pressure which in turn are brought about by changes in the size of thoracic cavity. Expansion of the thoracic cage leads to fall in the intrapleural pressure and decrease in the thoracic cavity leads to rise in intrapleural pressure. Changes in size of the thoracic cavity are brought about by the actions of respiratory muscles.

Pulmonary ventilation is accomplished by two processes: Inspiration or inhalation refers to the inflow of atmospheric air into the lungs. This obviously occurs when the intrapulmonary pressure falls below the atmospheric air pressure.Expiration or exhalation refers to the outflow of air from the lungs into the atmosphere. This occurs when the intrapulmonary pressure rises above the atmospheric air pressure.

In order to reach the alveoli, fresh atmospheric air must flow along an extensive system of large and small tubes. However, gases flow from one region to another only if a pressure difference exists. The lungs themselves contain elastic fibres in the connective tissue that binds the air sacs together, but they contain no muscle. The lungs cannot pump air into and out of it. Any such pumping mechanism would necessitate thick muscular walls to the lungs, which would impede the rapid exchange of gases. The lungs and the heart lie in an airtight cavity, the thoracic cavity. This is bounded by the sternum in front, the spinal column behind and the ribs that connect them. The thoracic cavity is closed off above by the dome shaped diaphragm.

During inspiration, the thoracic cavity increases in size in all three dimensions. Contractions of the skeletal muscles of the diaphragm flattens the dome of the diaphragm, increasing the thoracic cavity from top to bottom. The contraction of the external intercostal muscles connecting the ribs, also increase in the size of the thoracic cavity. This increase in the volume of the thoracic cavity results in a negative pressure, forcing the air to enter through the only passage available, namely the lungs.

Expiration is a decrease in size of the thorax and lungs with air outflow. As the air fills the lungs, the elastic fibres in the connective tissue are stretched and develop tension. The muscles of the diaphragm and the external intercostal muscles also relax during expiration, thereby decreasing the volume of the thoracic cavity and increasing the pressure inside it. The positive pressure inside forces the air out of the lungs, up the trachea and out through the nasal cavities.

Expiration is a purely passive process in contrast to inspiration, which is an active process requiring energy expenditure for the contraction of muscles.

Pulmonary Blood Vessels

The pulmonary artery carries blood from the right ventricles of the heart. It divides into right and left branches which pass into the respective lungs. These arteries arborize, following the pattern of the bronchi and supply the gross structure of the lung and alveoli.

The air in the alveolus is separated from blood in the capillary by (1) the alveolar wall, (2) the capillary wall and in some cases (3) an interstitial layer between the alveolar and capillary walls. Drainage is from the capillaries into small veins that ultimately unites to form the pulmonary veins that empty into the left auricle.

In addition to forming the connection between the arteries and veins, capillaries have a vital role in the exchange of gases, nutrients, and metabolic waste products between the blood and the tissue cells. Substances pass through the capillary wall by diffusion, filtration, and osmosis. Oxygen and carbon dioxide move across the capillary wall by diffusion. Fluid movement across a capillary wall is determined by a combination of hydrostatic and osmotic pressure. The net result of the capillary microcirculation created by hydrostatic and osmotic pressure is that substances leave the blood at one end of the capillary and return at the other end.

Respiration Rate

A breath is one complete respiratory cycle that consists of one inspiration and one expiration.Respiration rate is the number of breaths per minute. Respiration occurs at a relatively fixed frequency in various species of domestic animals. Normal respiratory rate of adult human beings varies from 12 to 20. A respiration rate under 12 or over 25 breaths per minute while resting is considered abnormal.Respiration is perhaps the easiest vital sign to obtain since no contact with the animal is required in order for it to be measured. In contrast, respiration is also the most variable of all the vital signs, and the most affected when the animal is excited or in pain. It is not uncommon for respiration rates to double or triple with pain or anxiety. To measure Respiration / breathing rate, count the number of times the chest expands in 15 seconds and multiply by four. You can do this either by watching your pet or resting your hand on the ribs. The respiratory rates in cycles per minute for domestic species.

The respiratory rate at rest varies considerably among animals of the same species. Faster rates are normally found in young animals. Exposure of cattle to thermal heat stress leads to physiological responses such as the elevation of rectal temperature, respiration rate and pulse rate with concomitant declines in feed intake and production.

An instrument called a spirometer is used to measure the volume of air that moves into and out of the lungs, and the process of taking the measurements is called spirometry.

The respiratory rate is controlled by respiratory center in the brain.The respiratory rate is increased along with tidal volume by almost any respiratory stimulus such as **exercise**.

Transport of Blood Gases

Blood serves to transport the respiratory gases. Oxygen, which is essential for the cells, is transported from the alveoli of the lungs to the cells. Carbon dioxide, which is the waste product in cells is transported from cells to lungs.Transport of oxygen from the lungs to the tissues occurs due to constant circulation of blood and diffusion of O_2 that occurs in the direction of concentration gradient. Because of poor solubility the of oxygen in water content of plasma, amount of oxygen transported physically soluble form in blood is very negligible. Most of the O_2 in blood is carried in a loose and reversible combination with hemoglobin. The combination of oxygen and hemoglobin is oxygenation and not oxidation as it is only a physical combination of oxygen and hemoglobin. Oxygen combines with hemoglobin in blood and is transported as oxyhemoglobin. Transport of oxygen in this form is important because, maximum amount (97%) of oxygen is transported by this method.

Normal atmospheric air has a composition of roughly 79 percent nitrogen, 20 percent oxygen and a variable amount of carbon dioxide, rare gases and water vapour making up the remaining one percent. Air expired from the lungs will contain approximately 79 percent nitrogen, 16 percent oxygen, four percent carbon dioxide and will be saturated with water vapour. The essential difference between expired and inspired air is an exchange of four percent of oxygen for four percent carbon dioxide.

Hemoglobin accepts oxygen readily whenever the partial pressure of oxygen in the blood is more. Hemoglobin gives out oxygen whenever the partial pressure of oxygen in the blood is less. Oxygen carrying capacity of hemoglobin is the amount of oxygen transported by 1 gm of hemoglobin and it is 1.34 mL/g.

The expired air in the alveoli is separated from the blood in the pulmonary capillaries by a thin membrane consisting of the epithelial lining of the alveoli and the endothelial lining of the capillaries. Diffusion of oxygen and carbon dioxide takes place across this alveolar membrane which results in a change of 'venous blood' to 'arterial blood'.

The rate of gas exchange is influenced by several factors including the permeability of the membrane, the area of surface in contact, the relative partial pressure of gases in blood and alveoli, and the volume of blood exposed to the alveoli.

Oxygen is taken up by the venous blood and carbon dioxide is released by it to be carried to the external environment along with the expired air. The oxygen taken up by the blood is transported in the form of a combined oxygen haemoglobin complex.

Oxygen Dissociation Curves

The amount of oxygen that can be taken up by a sample of blood or by aqueous solution of haemoglobin at varying oxygen pressures, can be plotted on a standard graph paper with the percentage of haemoglobin saturation as the ordinate and the oxygen pressure in millimeters mercury as the abscissa.

The curves are basically similar over a wide range of animal species. The dissociation curve of O_2 from Hb is somewhat sigmoid in shape. The curve clearly shows that the actual amount of oxygen combining with Hb is a function of partial pressure of oxygen. The movement of carbon dioxide into and out of the blood is of importance to determine the combining capacity of oxygen with haemoglobin at a given pressure . The pH ,temperature and the concentration of 2,3 - diphosphoglycerate affect the oxygen-hemoglobin dissociation curve. The decrease in O_2 affinity of hemoglobin when the pH of blood falls is called the Bohr effect.

A dusky bluish discoloration of the tissue due to a higher concentration of reduced hemoglobin is called cyanosis. Peripheral cyanosis is when there is a bluish discoloration to your hands or feet. It's usually caused by low oxygen levels in the red blood cells or problems getting oxygenated blood to your body. Sometimes cold temperatures can cause blood vessel to narrow and lead to temporarily blue-tinged skin. Warming or massaging the blue areas should return normal blood flow and color to the skin.

The Binding Equilibria of Haemoglobin

Haemoglobin binds oxygen in a characteristic manner in order to function as a carrier of oxygen in the erythrocyte, from the oxygen rich gas phase of the lung to the oxygen-poor peripheral tissues.

Because of the ability of the haemoglobin to bind oxygen, whole blood can absorb some 21 ml of gaseous oxygen per 100 ml, whereas blood plasma alone can absorb only about 0.3 ml of oxygen by physical solution.

A plot of percent saturation of haemoglobin against oxygen partial pressure is sigmoidal. The sigmoidal oxygen binding curve of haemoglobin means that haemoglobin has relatively low affinity for binding the first one or two oxygen molecules but once they are bound, the binding of the subsequent oxygen molecules is greatly enhanced. Conversely, the loss of one oxygen molecule from fully oxygenated haemoglobin causes the rest to dissociate more readily when the oxygen pressure is decreased.

Effect of pH

The position of the haemoglobin oxygen equilibrium is also affected by the pH. The higher the pH of the haemoglobin solution at a given partial pressure of oxygen, the greater the percent saturation with oxygen. This reversible effect results because when haemoglobin is oxygenated, it ionizes, to set free one protein according to the equation.

$$HHb^{+} + O_2 \longrightarrow HbO_2 + H^{+}$$

in which HHb^{+} is a protonated subunit of a deoxyhemoglobin molecule. Since this reaction is freely reversible, increasing the concentration will cause the equilibrium to shift to the left, toward decreased saturation whereas decreasing the concentration will cause the equilibrium to shift to the right, toward increased saturation. This effect of pH on the oxygen-haemoglobin equilibrium is called the Bohr effect.

The partial pressure of oxygen and the pH are the two most important factors regulating the function of haemoglobin in the transport of oxygen. In the lungs, where the partial pressure of oxygen is high (about 100 mm Hg) and the pH also relatively high, haemoglobin tends to become almost maximally saturated with oxygen, about 96 percent. In the interior of the peripheral tissues, where the oxygen tension is low (about 45 mm Hg) and the pH also low (due to the high concentration of CO_2 formed as the end product of respiration) the haemoglobin binds oxygen less strongly and will thus unload some of its oxygen to the respiring cell mass, until the haemoglobin is only about 65 percent saturated. Haemoglobin thus cycles between 65 and 96 percent saturation with oxygen, in its function as an oxygen carrier.

Foetal and neonatal oxygen transport

From conception until birth, the embryo and fetus depend on the mother for a supply of oxygen and nutrients and for removal of carbon dioxide and other metabolic byproducts. The embryo exchanges these substances by diffusion through the uterine fluids. As the conceptus increases in size, the specialized exchange organ, known as the placenta, becomes essential. The placenta brings maternal and fetal blood into close apposition over a large surface area that is provided by a network of capillaries.Fetal oxygen transport is assisted by fetal hemoglobin, which has a high affinity for oxygen. The fetus depends on the placenta for the exchange of gas, nutrients, and metabolic byproducts. The efficiency of gas exchange at the placenta depends on the species-variable arrangement of fetal and maternal blood vessels. In ruminants the placenta has rows of discrete circular-to-oval cotyledons that are attached to approximately 100 highly vascularized caruncles in the uterine epithelium. Countercurrent flow of maternal and fetal blood provides the most efficient exchange and allows equilibration of fetal and maternal arterial gas tensions. Concurrent flow of fetal and maternal blood allows fetal vessels to equilibrate with the maternal venous gas tensions. In crosscurrent and pool types of equilibrators, fetal capillaries loop down to maternal vessels or into a pool of maternal blood.The fetal circulation mixes oxygenated and deoxygenated blood at several points, so the fetus exists in a state of hypoxemia. The lung develops in three stages, and pulmonary surfactant must be present at birth. At or shortly after birth, umbilical vessels rupture, pulmonary vascular resistance decreases, and the foramen ovale and ductus arteriosus close.

The fetal circulation is not a passive system and is capable of considerable regulation, particularly as the fetus matures. Fetal hypoxia can stimulate vasodilation in the heart and brain and vasoconstriction in the gut, kidneys, and skeletal tissues. The fetal pulmonary circulation constricts vigorously when the fetus is hypoxic. This constriction diverts more blood through the ductus arteriosus to the systemic tissues.

Dissociation Curves, Pressures, Recoil Tendency

Oxygen is transported throughout the body in red blood cells, which contain an oxygen-binding protein called haemoglobin. Oxygen dissociation curves show the relationship between oxygen levels (as partial pressure) and haemoglobin saturation. Oxygen dissociation curve is an important tool for understanding how blood carries and releases oxygen. More specifically it relates between the – Percentage of Oxygen carrying capacity of Haemoglobin and Partial pressure of Oxygen.

Hb in 2 forms –deoxyHb and oxyHb – In DeoxyHb- globin units are tightly bound(TENSE CONFIGURATION) –which has reduced affinity of Hb molecules to Oxygen. When 1st oxygen is bound- the bonds holding globin chains are released producing RELAXED CONFIGURATION Which exposes more oxygen binding sites leading to high fold affinity to oxygen binding.In other words, when hemoglobin has no bound oxygen, nor bound carbon dioxide, it has the unbound conformation (shape). The binding of the first oxygen molecule induces change in the shape of the hemoglobin that increases its ability to bind to the other three oxygen molecules.

The oxygen–hemoglobin dissociation curve plots the proportion of hemoglobin in its saturated form on the vertical axis against the prevailing oxygen tension on the horizontal axis. The oxygen dissociation curve of adult haemoglobin is a sigmoid curve.

At pressures above about 60 mmHg, the standard dissociation curve is relatively flat, which means that the oxygen content of the blood does not change significantly even with large increases in the oxygen partial pressure. Although binding of oxygen to hemoglobin continues to some extent for pressures about 50 mmHg, as oxygen partial pressures decrease in this steep area of the curve,. the oxygen is unloaded to peripheral tissue readily as the hemoglobin's affinity diminishes. The partial pressure of oxygen in the blood at which the hemoglobin is 50% saturated, typically about 26.6 mmHg for a healthy person, is known as the P50.

P50 is a conventional measure of hemoglobin affinity for oxygen. In the presence of disease or other conditions that change the hemoglobin's oxygen affinity and, consequently, shift the curve to the right or left, the P50 changes accordingly. Increased P50 indicates a rightward shift of the standard curve, which means that a larger partial pressure is necessary to maintain a 50% oxygen saturation. This indicates a decreased affinity. Conversely, a lower P50 indicates a leftward shift and a higher affinity.

Elasticity and compliance

Elasticity: tendency to return to initial structure after being distended.In order to inflate the lungs during inspiration, each breath must overcome both the natural resistance of the airways and the tendency of the lungs to collapse (elastic recoil, attributable to tissue elasticity and the surface tension within the alveoli). The chest wall and the thoracic cage play a role in the mechanics of breathing. The chest wall has a natural tendency to expand but is also elastic. This outward pull of the chest wall opposes the elastic recoil of the lung itself, preventing the lung from collapsing.

Elastic recoil means the rebound of the lungs after having been stretched by inhalation. With inhalation, the intrapleural pressure (the pressure within the pleural cavity) of the lungs decreases. Relaxing the diaphragm during expiration allows the lungs to recoil and regain the intrapleural pressure experienced previously at rest. Elastic recoil is inversely related to lung compliance.Elasticity occurs because of the elastin in the elastic fibers in the connective tissue of the lungs, and because of the surface tension of the film of fluid that lines the alveoli.

Compliance

The **compliance** of a system is defined as the change in volume that occurs per unit change in the pressure of the system. In layman terms, compliance is the ease with which an elastic structure can be stretched. Compliance is, therefore, basically a measurement of the elastic resistance of a system. Pulmonary compliance is the total compliance of both lungs, measuring the extent to which the lungs will expand (change in volume of lungs) for each unit increase in the trans-pulmonary pressure (when enough time is allowed for the system to reach equilibrium). A balloon has a high compliance because a small pressure increase inside the balloon will greatly expand the balloon. A rigid tube has a low compliance because a small pressure increase inside the rigid tube will not result in a significant increase in the volume of the rigid tube.

The expansibility of thorax and the total compliance is reduced in several diseased conditions such as abnormal thorax, pneumothorax, pleural effusion, paralysis of respiratory muscles, fibrotic pleurisy and deformities of thorax.

Exchange of gases in lungs and tissues

Peripheral gas exchange is also known as 'internal respiration', as it involves the respiratory processes that occur within the tissues of the body rather than the lungs. Internal respiration involves gas exchange between the bloodstream and tissues, and cellular respiration. Gas exchange in tissues is a result of tissue surface area, gas partial pressure gradients, and the blood perfusion of those tissues.

Tidal volume: Tidal volume is the amount of air which flows in and out of the lungs with each respiration, during quiet breathing. This volume may be considered as the average volume inspired or expired during a single respiratory cycle. In a healthy, young human adult, tidal volume is approximately 500 mL per inspiration or 7 mL/kg of body mass. Tidal volume of different species of animals.

With maximal inspiration and expiration, this value can be increased several fold.

Vital Capacity : Vital capacity is the largest possible respiratory volume. It is the volume of air which flows during the deepest possible inspiration.

Inspiratory Reserve Volume : The extra air that can be taken in after a normal inspiration is known as inspiratory reserve volume.

Expiratory Reserve Volume : The extra air that can be forced out after a quick expiration is the expiratory reserve volume.

Residual Volume: Residual volume is the volume of air left in the lung after all of the expiratory reserve volume has been forced out. Residual air cannot be expelled by exhaling but only by collapsing the lungs by injections of air into the intrapleural spaces.

Total Lung Capacity : Total lung capacity is the residual air plus the vital capacity.

How to Determine Whether A Young is Born Dead or Alive

From its lung : Lungs of a living animal or an animal which was born alive, will contain the minimal volume, hence will float in water. The lungs of the fetus or animal born dead are solid, because there is no air within them and will sink in water. This is sometimes a useful test in determining whether or not a newborn animal has taken a breath following birth.

Respiratory dead space : Respiratory dead space may be defined as the volume of gas that is inspired or expired but takes no part in the gas exchange. This may be due to the volume of the conducting airways (anatomical dead space) or the part which does not take part in gas exchange within the respiratory zone (physiological dead space).

Types of Respiration

Respiration is of two types.

1. **Internal respiration** (gaseous exchange between cells and fluid medium i.e. gas exchange at cellular level).
2. **External respiration** (gaseous exchange at lung or alveolar level).

Eupnea: Is the state of ordinary quiet breathing. It is assumed to be effortless.

Dyspnea: Is a condition of laboured breathing as evident from facial expressions or other behavioural traits.

Hyperpnea : Is a condition of breathing in which the rate or the depth, or both, are increased.

Polypnea : Is a rapid shallow panting type of respiration. The predominant change is an increase of respiratory frequency. Polypnea occurs during heat stress in goat, sheep, dog etc and is a physiological mechanism to dissipate excess heat from the body during heat stress. Tachypnea and Polypnea are technically similar, but in the strictest clinical sense, polypnea is used to mean panting, and so is used more frequently in veterinary science than in human health sciences (panting is increased respiration rate, usually associated with an attempt to lose excess heat). Tachypnea means the rate of respiration has increased above normal. Tachypnea is caused by a buildup of carbon dioxide in the lungs, which causes a buildup of carbon dioxide in the bloodstream.

Apnea : signifies cessation of breathing.

Morphological Adaptations and Pigment Synthesis

Domestic animals acclimated to high altitudes have increased vital capacity and pulmonary ventilation. Most birds and mammals at high altitudes synthesize more haemoglobin than at sea level.

Oxygen Consumption of Domestic Animals

Rate of oxygen consumption is influenced by activity, temperature, nutrition, body size, stage in life cycle, season and time of the day.

Role of Pleural Liquid in Lungs

Pleural effusion, sometimes referred to as "water on the lungs," is the buildup of excess fluid between the layers of the pleura outside the lungs. The pleura are thin membranes that line the lungs and the inside of the chest cavity and act to lubricate and facilitate breathing. Normally, a small amount of fluid is present in the pleura.

Role of Pulmonary Surfactants in Lungs

Surfactant is an agent that decreases the surface tension between two media. Its main function is to reduce the surface tension at the air/liquid interface in the lung. This is achieved by forming a surface film that consists of a monolayer which is highly enriched in dipalmitoylphosphatidylcholine and bilayer lipid/protein structures closely attached to it. Surfactant is a secretory product, composed of lipids and proteins. It is essential for efficient exchange of gases and for maintaining the structural integrity of alveoli. Alterations in surfactant homeostasis can result in surfactant insufficiency which may be responsible for diseases like respiratory distress syndrome, lung proteinosis, interstitial lung diseases and chronic lung diseases.

The pulmonary surfactant is produced by the alveolar type-II (AT-II) cells of the lungs. Phosphatidylcholine and phosphatidylglycerol are the major lipid constituents and SP-A, SP-B, SP-C, SP-D are four types of surfactant associated proteins. The lipid and protein components are synthesized separately and are packaged into the lamellar bodies in the AT-II cells. Lamellar bodies are the main organelle for the synthesis and metabolism of surfactants. The synthesis, secretion and recycling of the surfactant lipids and proteins is regulated by complex genetic and metabolic mechanisms. The lipid-protein interaction is very important for the structural organization of surfactant monolayer and its functioning.

Neural and Chemical Regulation of Breathing

Breathing is controlled by the central neuronal network to meet the metabolic demands of the body. Breathing is regulated by the complex actions of the various muscles of the respiration. The muscles of the chest, diaphragm, thorax and those within the lungs function in an integrated manner. Respiration is a reflex process. The rhythm of inspiratory and expiratory movements depends upon both extrinsic and intrinsic mechanisms for control.

Chemical control of respiration :The intrinsic or chemical control of respiration ensures that respiration is adequate to meet the needs of the body.

Neural control of respiration : Nervous mechanism that regulates the respiration includes:

1. Respiratory centers
2. Afferent nerves
3. Efferent nerves.

Respiratory Centers

Respiratory centers are group of neurons, which control the rate, rhythm and force of respiration. Within the pons there are two paired respiratory centres, the pneumotaxic centres and the apneustic centres, which influence respiratory rate and rhythm. Within the medulla there are two additional centres, the inspiratory center and the expiratory center.

Many aspects of the act of breathing are integrated at the cord level, but the origin of the rhythmicity and the setting of the limits of the tidal volume and respiratory frequency are dependent upon the neuronal pools in the medulla oblongata.

The information from the peripheral receptors, chemosensitive areas in the brain and from higher nervous centres including the cerebral cortex is synthesized by the respiratory centres. The respiratory centres send out efferent impulses via the phrenic and intercostal nerves setting the breathing pattern.

The cranial nerves and the upper part of the brain above pons does not regulate respiration, as the animal continues to breathe regularly even if these areas or nerves are cut or damaged.

Apneustic and Pneumotaxic Center

The apneustic center and the pneumotaxic center lie in the pons. The pneumotaxic center sends periodic inhibiting response which converts the continuing discharge activity of the inspiratory center into a rhythmic pattern.

Inspiratory and Expiratory Centres

Both the inspiratory and expiratory centres lie in the medulla. Inspiratory stimulus when stimulated causes deep inspiration, due to contraction of the muscles of the thorax, and the diaphragm. Expiratory center when stimulated, causes the cessation of inspiration and the contraction of the expiratory muscles follow.

The pneumotaxic center, the inspiratory center and the expiratory center make up a feedback circuit between the medulla and the pons.

Respiratory center is located in medulla. It is divided in 4 major collections of neurons:

1. Dorsal respiratory group (DRG)
2. Ventral respiratory group (VRG)
3. Pneumotaxic center
4. Apneuestic center

Central Control of Respiration in Mammals

Role of Vagus *(Hering Breuer reflex)* : The vagus nerve carries affarent impulses that originate in receptors in the lung tissue which are sensitive to stretch. The Hering–Breuer inflation reflex, named for Josef Breuer and Ewald Hering, is a reflex triggered to prevent over-inflation of the lung. Pulmonary stretch receptors present on the wall of bronchi and bronchioles of the airways respond to excessive stretching of the lung during large inspirations.

Chemical Control of Respiration

Chemical mechanism of regulation of respiration is operated through the chemoreceptors. **Chemoreceptors** are the sensory nerve endings, which give response to changes in chemical constituents of blood. The activity of the respiratory center can be modified chemically. The most important of them are the partial pressures of carbon dioxide and oxygen. A high partial pressure of carbon dioxide provides a constant chemoreflex stimulus to the central nervous system, thereby, increasing the rate and depth of respiration. A decrease in the partial pressure of carbon dioxide depresses the rate and depth of respiration.

A decrease in PO_2 below about 65 mm causes the respiration rate and depth to increase.

The chemical control of breathing is brought about by specialized receptors present in the carotid and aortic bodies. The carotid body sends impulses to the respiratory centres of the medulla via the carotid sinus nerve.

Diffusion, Perfusion, Hypoxia

Respiration ensures that cells, tissues, and major organs of the body receive an adequate supply of oxygen and that the carbon dioxide, a waste product, is efficiently removed; the exchange of oxygen and carbon dioxide occurs via diffusion across cell membranes. Diffusion is the process of something moving from high concentration to low concentration. Diffusion continues until equilibrium is reached. The exchange of gases (O_2 & CO_2) between the alveoli & the blood occurs by simple diffusion: O_2 diffusing from the alveoli into the blood & CO_2 from the blood into the alveoli. Diffusion requires a concentration gradient. So, the concentration (or pressure) of O_2 in the alveoli must be kept at a higher level than in the blood & the concentration (or pressure) of CO_2 in the alveoli must be kept at a lower lever than in the blood. This is achieved by breathing - continuously bringing fresh air (with lots of O_2 & little CO_2) into the lungs & the alveoli.

Partial Pressure is the individual pressure exerted independently by a particular gas within a mixture of gasses. The air inspired by animals during respiration is a mixture of gasses: primarily nitrogen, oxygen, & carbon dioxide. That part of the total pressure generated by oxygen is the 'partial pressure' of oxygen, while that generated by carbon dioxide is the 'partial pressure' of carbon dioxide. A gas's partial pressure, therefore, is a measure of how much of that gas is present (e.g., in the blood or alveoli).

The partial pressure exerted by each gas in a mixture equals the total pressure times the fractional composition of the gas in the mixture. So, given that total atmospheric pressure (at sea level) is about 760 mm Hg and, further, that air is about 21% oxygen, then the partial pressure of oxygen in the air is 0.21 times 760 mm Hg or 160 mm Hg. Because of the differences in partial pressures of oxygen & carbon dioxide in the systemic capillaries & the body cells, oxygen diffuses from the blood & into the cells, while carbon dioxide diffuses from the cells into the blood.

Ventilation (V) refers to the flow of air into and out of the alveoli, while perfusion (Q) refers to the flow of blood to alveolar capillaries. Ventilation is 50% greater at the base of the lung than at the apex. Perfusion is also greater at the base of the lung due to gravity pulling blood down towards the base. Alveolar dead space occurs when some alveoli are not perfused.

Individual alveoli have variable degrees of ventilation and perfusion in different regions of the heart. Collective changes in ventilation and perfusion in the lungs are measured clinically using the ratio of ventilation to perfusion (V/Q). Changes in the V/Q ratio can affect gas exchange and can contribute to hypoxemia.

Oxygen is essential for normal aerobic metabolism in mammals. The key reaction occurs in the mitochondria of cells and involves combining a fuel (eg, sugars, fats) with oxygen to produce energy (converting adenosine 5′-diphosphate to adenosine 5′-triphosphate) along with CO_2 and H_2O. Hypoxia is the presence of lower than normal oxygen content and pressure in the cell. Causes of hypoxia include hypoxemia (low blood oxygen content and pressure), impaired oxygen delivery, and impaired cellular oxygen uptake/utilization. Depending upon the cell type, its metabolic demands, and its ability to adapt to hypoxia, the response to various levels of hypoxia can range from substantial adaptation to cell death.

Frictional Resistance to Air Flow, Airways Smooth Muscle Contraction

Airway resistance is an essential parameter of lung function and results from the frictional forces of the airways, which oppose airflow. In order to breathe the animal must overcome and work against the frictional resistance generated by the tissues and flow through the breathing tubes (airways). Resistance to flow in the airways depends on whether the flow is laminar or turbulent, on the dimensions of the airway, and on the viscosity of the gas.

Resistance during laminar flow may be calculated via a rearrangement of Poiseuille's Law.

Respiratory Muscle Work, Panting

Breathing is an active process - requiring the contraction of skeletal muscles. The primary muscles of respiration include the external intercostal muscles (located between the ribs) and the diaphragm (a sheet of muscle located between the thoracic & abdominal cavities). The external intercostals plus the diaphragm contract to bring about inspiration.

Contraction of external intercostal muscles > elevation of ribs & sternum > increased front- to-back dimension of thoracic cavity > lowers air pressure in lungs > air moves into lungs

Contraction of diaphragm > diaphragm moves downward > increases vertical dimension of thoracic cavity > lowers air pressure in lungs > air moves into lungs:

To exhale

relaxation of external intercostal muscles & diaphragm > return of diaphragm, ribs, & sternum to resting position > restores thoracic cavity to pre inspiratory volume > increases pressure in lungs > air is exhaled

As the external intercostals & diaphragm contract, the lungs expand. The expansion of the lungs causes the pressure in the lungs (and alveoli) to become slightly negative relative to atmospheric pressure. As a result, air moves from an area of higher pressure (the air) to an area of lower pressure (our lungs & alveoli). During expiration, the respiration muscles relax & lung volume decreases. This causes pressure in the lungs (and alveoli) to become slight positive relative to atmospheric pressure. As a result, air leaves the lungs.

Panting, also called tachypnea, is rapid shallow breathing. Panting is a controlled increase in respiratory frequency in concert with a decrease in tidal volume, which increases ventilation of the upper respiratory tract while preserving alveolar ventilation.

The increase in upper respiratory tract ventilation increases evaporative heat loss. Panting, a method of cooling, used by many mammals, and most birds, accomplished by means of the evaporation of water from internal body surfaces. As the animal's body temperature rises, its respiration rate increases sharply; cooling results from the evaporation of water in the nasal passages, mouth, lungs, and (in birds) air sacs.

Pigs and sheep are considered panting mammals, although wallowing for pigs and sweating for sheep can be major avenues of heat loss during extreme heat stress. Among livestock, poultry are the best examples of true panting animals.

Many animals respond to a hot environment by resorting to an increase in respiration rate and, in some cases, by open-mouth panting. The increased respiration rate is usually accompanied by reduced tidal volume, an increase in alveolar volume, a decrease in the arterial partial pressure of carbon dioxide and an increase in respiratory minute volume.

Adaptation of Respiration During Muscles Exercise

The oxygen requirements of the cardiac and skeletal muscles is greatly increased during exercise. This increased oxygen requirement is obtained from the inspired air partly by an increase in the ventilation rate and partly by circulatory adjustments. The circulatory adjustments are as follows:

(i) Increase in blood flow which occurs through an increase in cardiac output and blood pressure. The cardiac output can increase as a result of an increase in heart rate or an increase in stroke volume or an increase in both rate and stroke volume.

(ii) Preferential distribution of blood flow to working muscles.

(iii) Increase in the amount of oxygen transferred to the active tissues from each unit volume of blood traversing the capillary beds.

High Altitude Hypoxia

High altitude (above 9000 feet) has decreased atmospheric pressure which decreases the oxygen partial pressure in the ambient air. This means that although the relative percentage of oxygen is unaltered, the number of molecules of O_2 present per breath decreases. The state of sub-optimal O_2 availability due to decreased ambient barometric pressure is termed as hypobaric hypoxia. Since O_2 is a primal requirement for life processes, its inadequate bio-availability to tissues or organs leads to deficiencies in biological processes such as energy production, biosynthesis and breakdown of cellular/tissue components, cognition, mental coherence, etc.

The molecular and physiological adjustments to compensate for reduction in bio-available O_2 is termed as 'acclimatization' which is of utmost importance. Environmental hypoxia ultimately affects the oxygen delivery to tissues.

At high altitude, due to the fall in ambient O_2 partial pressure, the alveolar partial pressure of O_2 falls; this further reduces its gradient against the partial pressure of O_2 in deoxygenated blood leading to reduced diffusion of O_2 into the arterial blood. Similarly, as the pressure differential between venous CO_2 and alveolar CO_2 decreases, the driving force for the removal of CO_2 diminishes and thus a higher amount is retained in the arterial blood at high altitude.

The immediate effect of exposure to high altitude hypoxia is faster respiration rate, i.e., pulmonary hyperventilation. Improvement in arterial oxygen content occurs by increase in haematocrit, haemoglobin and erythrocyte levels during hypoxia exposure. This boost in oxygen-carrying capacity is a direct outcome of erythropoietin secretion from the kidneys into the blood stream. Erythropoietin triggers erythropoiesis, i.e., red blood synthesis, in the bone marrow . Acute acclimatization is associated with diuresis, i.e., increased urine excretion. This facilitates loss of body water leading to reduced plasma volume thereby effectively increasing the proportion of red blood cells (RBCs) per unit volume of blood, a phenomenon called haemoconcentration. Haemoconcentration is an efficient way to increase oxygen carrying capacity of a given volume of blood.

Hormonal responses play very important regulatory functions during high altitude exposure. Under this, the role of renin– angiotensin–aldosterone axis as an important regulator of diuretic response.

High-altitude research is conducted on walk-in human and animal decompression chambers which nearly simulate the high-altitude environment and are equipped with real-time physiological monitoring equipments as well. The chamber essentially contains an airtight enclosure which is depressurised at a constant rate using a vacuum pump. Here the rate of depressurising is regulated to simulate the 'rate of ascent to high altitude' and similarly the release of vacuum is regulated to simulate the 'rate of descent to high altitude'.

Non-respiratory Lung Functions

The primary function of the lungs is gas exchange. However, the lungs perform several important non-respiratory functions that are vital for normal physiology. These nonrespiratory functions of the lung include its own defense against inspired particulate matter, the storage and filtration of blood for the systemic circulation, the handling of vasoactive substances in the blood, and the formation and release of substances used in the alveoli or circulation.

Secondary Functions of the Respiratory System

- The nasal passages also have the ability to maintain olfaction which helps in the ability to sense predators in animals. The receptors for the sense of smell are present in sensory epithelium located in the nasal passages. The sense of smell, also called the olfactory sense,is very important to many animals.
- The respiratory system has tremendous ability to accommodate increased oxygen demand of skeletal muscles during intense exercise eg in horses which can run in excess of 30 miles per hour. The lower respiratory tract also aids in thermoregulation through evaporative heat loss. The respiratory evaporation of water is an important means to maintain homeothermy in the face of heat stress in deserts.
- The respiratory system contributes to the process of acid–base control by its ability to influence the amount of CO_2 in the blood.
- Lung also functions in the metabolism of bioactive amines (pulmonary circulation), production of surfactant and maintenance of pulmonary defence mechanisms.

• Immune Function

- Immune function within the lung is mediated by pulmonary alveolar macrophages (PAMs) and a variety of immune mediators. Amoeboid PAMs engulf the particles that reach the alveoli. The macrophages are particularly effective against bacteria and ensure that the alveolar region of the lung is effectively sterile. **Pulmonary alveolar macrophages**. Being actively phagocytic cells they ingest the inhaled bacteria and small particles. They thus play an important role in defence system.
- Immunoglobulin-A (IgA) is secreted in the bronchial secretion and protects against respiratory infections.

- Ciliary escalator action is an important defence system against the air-borne infection. The dust particles in the inhaled air are often laden with bacteria. While passing through the repeatedly branched bronchial tree the dust particles and the bacteria are caught in the mucous layer present at the mucosal surface of respiratory passages and are moved up towards pharynx by the rhythmic upward beating action of cilia and swallowed.

Cough is a vital defensive physiological function frequently observed both in people and small animals. The cough reflex prevents aspiration of foreign or noxious material and preserves the health of the respiratory system by inducing a rapid and forceful removal of harmful substances, such as inhaled foreign particles, pathogens or excessive bronchial secretions from the upper airways. The laryngeal, tracheal and bronchial mucous membranes contain vagal afferent terminals, which act as irritant receptors. Stimulation of these receptors by chemical or mechanical stimuli (excessive mucus, inadvertently inhaled foodstuff, etc.) produces a bout of coughing, which helps in expulsion of foreign material.

Absorption of certain drugs can be carried out in the nasal passages.Certain drugs that rapidly pass through the alveolar capillary barrier by diffusion are administered by inhalation, e.g. anaesthetic gases, aerosol and other bronchodilators.

The lung is ideally positioned to filter out particulate matter such as clots, fibrin clumps, and other endogenous and exogenous materials from entering the systemic circulation.

The lung, with its unique ability to distend and recruit pulmonary vasculature, acts as a reservoir of blood, fine tuning preload to the left heart to optimize cardiac output.

Pulmonary epithelium forms the first line of defence against inhaled particles.

The airway epithelial cells secrete a variety of substances such as mucins, defensins, lysozyme, lactoferrin, and nitric oxide, which non-specifically shield the lung from microbial attack.

The large surface area of the alveoli is perfectly suited for gas exchange, but can also serve as a portal of entry for inhaled toxic agents.

Pulmonary neuroendocrine cells (PNECs) secrete a wide variety of amines (e.g. serotonin) and peptides (e.g. bombesin) and play a significant role in cell growth, differentiation, and branching morphogenesis in the developing lung.

Pulmonary metabolic capacity is easily saturated, but pulmonary endothelial binding of some drugs alters their pharmacokinetics.

Thus the lung is responsible for several important non-respiratory functions, vital for maintenance of normal physiology.

Respiration in Birds

Birds must be capable of high rates of gas exchange because their oxygen consumption at rest is higher than that of all other vertebrates, including mammals, and it increases many times during flight. The unique anatomy and physiology of birds enable some to fly at altitudes of 32,000 feet without supplemental oxygen, to dive underwater for many minutes, and to live at environmental extremes from the frozen deserts of the polar regions, to the heat and humidity of the tropics, to the dry heat of the earth's deserts. The respiratory system of birds facilitates efficient exchange of carbon dioxide and oxygen via continuous unidirectional airflow and air sacs.

The avian respiratory system is physically distinct from the mammalian respiratory system, both in structure and in its ability to exchange gas as efficiently as possible. The bird's respiratory system consists of paired lungs, which contain static structures with surfaces for gas exchange, and connected air sacs, which expand and contract causing air to move through the static lungs.

Birds have relatively small lungs and nine air sacs that play an important role in respiration. Avian lungs are unique in that the air flows in only one direction, rather than in and out as in other vertebrates. As a consequence of the continual, unidirectional airflow, the lungs of birds are more completely ventilated than the lungs of mammals. Supplementing the lungs is an elaborate system of interconnected air sacs in birds, not present in mammals. In birds, the lungs are rigid and their volume does not change during respiratory cycle.

The nine flexible air sacs that act like bellows to move air through the rigid lungs and air sacs do not take part in the actual oxygen exchange, but do greatly enhance its efficiency for the high metabolic rate found in birds. Some air sacs extend to the proximal end of the extremities and skull.

Birds lack a diaphragm and the thoracic and abdominal cavity and forms a continuous body cavity. The nine air-sacs are one inter clavicular sac, two cervical sacs, two anterior thoracic sacs, two posterior thoracic sacs and two abdominal sacs.

Summary

- The primary role of the respiratory system is to provide O_2 to the tissues for metabolic needs and remove the CO_2 formed by them.
- Respiration entails two processes: the external respiration and internal respiration. The internal respiration or tissue respiration refers to the utilization of O_2 and production of CO_2 by the tissues.The external respiration includes supply of O_2 to the tissues from the environment and excretion of CO_2 released by the tissues into the atmosphere.
- Blood serves to transport the respiratory gases. Oxygen, which is essential for the cells, is transported from alveoli of lungs to the cells. Carbon dioxide, which is the waste product in cells, is transported from cells to lungs.
- Surfactant is essential for efficient exchange of gases and for maintaining the structural integrity of alveoli.
- The oxygen requirements of the cardiac and skeletal muscles is greatly increased during exercise. This increased oxygen requirement is obtained from the inspired air partly by an increase in the ventilation rate and partly by circulatory adjustments.

- The immediate effect of exposure to high altitude hypoxia is faster respiration rate, i.e., pulmonary hyperventilation. Improvement in arterial oxygen content occurs by increase in haematocrit, haemoglobin and erythrocyte levels during hypoxia exposure.
- Nonrespiratory functions of the lung include its own defense against inspired particulate matter, the storage and filtration of blood for the systemic circulation, the handling of vasoactive substances in the blood, and the formation and release of substances used in the alveoli or circulation.

10

Structure and Functions of the Kidney

Substances which are in excess of the body and/or are harmful need to be removed constantly. This function is carried out by the excretory organs which include skin, gastrointestinal tract and kidney. Skin excretes water and salts in the form of sweat. Gastrointestinal tract removes undigested food material as well as some heavy metals in the form of faeces. Kidneys are the main excretory organs which together with a pair of ureters, a urinary bladder and urethra constitute the excretory system. Renal function is essential for homeostasis. The urinary system produces, stores, and eliminates urine. The kidneys play a vital role in the excretion of waste products and the regulation of electrolytes, maintenance of acid–base balance, regulation of blood pressure, and production of several hormones. Kidneys perform the following functions.

- Excretion of metabolic waste products. In addition to the metabolic wastes, the kidneys also excrete foreign substances from the body, such as drugs, pesticides and other chemicals ingested in food.
- Regulation of water and inorganic ion balance
- Regulation of acid-base balance.
- Regulation of volume and composition of the body's internal environment.
- Hormonal function- As an endocrine gland, kidneys produce and secrete renin, calcitriol and erythropoietin

The basic function of the kidneys is to filter blood, reabsorb what is needed, and excrete what is not. By secreting urine the kidney serves as the outstanding guardian of the milieu interieur.

The main functions of the kidney in the maintenance of body homeostasis are listed below.

1. Maintenance of osmotic balance.
2. Maintenance of body fluid volume.
3. Maintenance of electrolyte concentration.
4. Regulation of acid-base balance
5. Regulation of blood pressure
6. Erythropoiesis

7. Removal of waste products including nitrogenous end products of protein metabolism primarily urea, creatinine and ammonia.
8. Removal of foreign substances and/or their metabolic end products.
9. Retain nutrients

Endowed with a relatively huge blood supply, the renal glomeruli filter about 200 litres per 24 hours of protein free fluid from the blood in human being (i.e. 50-60 times the plasma volume). This filtrate, which contains the soluble non protein components of the plasma, is submitted to extensive reabsorption by the renal tubules. The relative control on the reabsorption process by the kidney is the key mechanism by which the kidney is able to maintain the composition of the milieu interieur. The kidney of a 20 kg dog filters approximately 80 liters of fluid in 24 hours. Out of this 79.5 liters is reabsorbed, and only 0.5 liter to be excreted as urine.

During passage through the renal tubules, the extensive reabsorption of important nutrients such as glucose and amino acids takes place and waste products such as urea is filtered out. The reabsorption of water gets increased when the water supply to the animal is reduced e.g. during heat stress. Kidney control the concentration of most of the constituents of body fluids. In case of birds, the primary end product of protein metabolism is uric acid instead of urea. So, the major excretory product through urine in case of birds is uric acid. Progressive decline in kidney function in humans can lead to serious illness and ultimately death if not treated by dialysis or transplantation.

Kidney also releases several hormones like calcitriol (active metabolite of vitamin D), erythropoietin (involved in red blood cell production), renin (blood pressure control) and prostaglandins, which have the capacity to influence cells and alter their physiological processes.

The kidney regulates water recovery and blood pressure by producing the enzyme renin. It is renin that starts a series of reactions, leading to the production of the vasoconstrictor angiotensin II and the salt-retaining steroid aldosterone.

Kidney- Functional Morphology ofNephron

The kidneys are a pair of bean shaped organs in the abdominal cavity. The longitudinal section of the kidney shows the outer darker region called cortex and the inner paler region called medulla.

The kidney is composed of basic units called nephron. There are about 2.5 million nephrons in a horse kidney, above 1 million in pig kidney and 0.5 million nephrons in a sheep kidney.The average nephron number in human kidney is approximately 900,000 to 1 million per kidney. There is a loss of nephron (glomeruli) due to age-related glomerulosclerosis. Glomerulosclerosis refers to scarring or hardening of the glomeruli -- blood vessels located in the kidneys.

The nephron is composed of a 'Malpighian body or Bowman's capsule'. The Bowman's capsule consists of a single layer of epithelial cells surrounded by a basement membrane. A small artery enters into each Bowman's capsule or Malphighian body, where it splits up into a bundle or tuft of capillaries, the glomerulus. The first step in urine formation is the passage of fluid from the glomeruli into the capsule.

It is through the walls of the glomerular capillaries that fluid is forced out by the blood pressure. The capsule is continued into a long U shaped tube. The part immediately following it is called the proximal tubule. Thus the glomerular filtrate enters from the capsule to the tubule which leads from the Malphighian body. Within the tubule the glomeruli filtrate is modified both by reabsorption and by tubular secretion to form the final urine.

In the proximal part of the tubule many solutes such as salts and glucose as well as water are extensively reabsorbed.

The proximal tubule is continued into the distal tubule through a loop called the loop of Henle. The Henle loop dips down towards the medulla while the Bowman's capsule and the proximal tubule lie in the cortex region. The process of changing the tubule fluid into urine is continued in the distal tubule.The loop is the particular structure in the nephron that is responsible for the formation of urine which is more concentrated than blood plasma.

Nephron is the functional unit of the kidney. The nephron has the following functions- Filtration, Reabsorption, Secretion and Excretion.

The number of nephrons is constant within the species i.e. the larger breeds of dog contain a similar number of nephrons as in the smaller breeds of dog. Epithelial lining of the bladder is transitional epithelium. There are 2 types of nephrons (depending upon their location)

1. Cortical nephrons : Do not have loop of Henle (ascending thin limb)
2. Juxtamedullary nephrons : Have loop of Henle (100% in dog and cat, 3% in pigs and about 25% in human)

Juxtamedullary nephrons are more important for developing and maintaining the osmotic gradient from low to high in the outer medulla to inner medulla respectively.

Loop of Henle . Three parts viz;

1. Descending thin limb
2. Ascending thin limb (It is not permeable to water, moderately permeable to urea and highly permeable to NaCl)
3. Ascending thick limb

Collecting duct – Three parts viz;

1. Cortical collecting duct
2. Outer medullary collecting duct
3. Inner medullary collecting duct

Two basic processes required for the formation of urine are ultrafiltration and active transport.

In ultrafiltration, pressure forces a fluid through a semipermeable membrane that withholds protein & similar large molecular solutes to pass.

Active transport is the movement of solute against its electrochemical gradient by processes requiring the expenditure of metabolic energy.

Juxtaglomerular Apparatus

The collecting tubule passes from the cortex back downwards through the medulla, paralleling the loops of Henle. Then it empties into the pelvis of the kidney.

Hormonal and Autacoid Control of Renal Circulation

The kidneys receive appreciable quantities of blood, which amount to over 20% of the **cardiac output** in adults. Compared with other tissues, the kidneys have a particularly rich supply of blood. The much higher blood flow to the kidneys ensures adequate delivery of plasma to be filtered by the glomeruli, a physiological process necessary for the regulation of body fluids. Therefore, a change in renal blood flow changes the glomerular filtration rate (GFR) and, consequently, the volume and composition of body fluids.

The following systems contribute to the regulation of renal blood flow: (1) the sympathetic nervous system, (2) hormones and autacoids, and (3) the renin–angiotensin system.

Many hormones and autacoids modulate the vascular tone of the renal blood vessels and, in turn, renal blood flow. Autacoids or "autocoids" are biological factors (molecules) which act like local hormones, have a brief duration, and act near their site of synthesis. Depending on the physiological function of these hormones or autacoids, they may constrict or dilate the renal blood vessels.

Neural Regulation of the Kidney

Renal nerves regulate renal blood flow, GFR, and salt and water reabsorption by the nephron. The nerve supply to the kidneys consists of sympathetic nerve fibers that originate in the celiac plexus. No parasympathetic innervation occurs. Sympathetic nerves innervate the renin-producing granular cells of the afferent arterioles. Renin secretion is stimulated by increased sympathetic activity. Nerve fibers also innervate the proximal tubule, loop of Henle, distal tubule, and collecting duct; activation of these nerves enhances Na+ reabsorption by these nephron segments.

Neural control is exercised principally via the juxta glomerular apparatus, which regulates the amount of blood that passes through the glomerulus.

Kidney Metabolism

The kidney have an extremely high rate of respiratory metabolism and also show considerable metabolic flexibility. As sources of fuel they can utilize blood glucose, free fatty acids, ketone bodies and also amino acids, degrading them ultimately via acetyl-CoA and the tricarboxylic acid cycle. From two-third to four-fifths of the total energy generated by the kidney is utilized in the formation of urine.

Factors Determining Filtration Pressure

The basic function of the nephron is to clean, or clear the blood plasma of unwanted substances as it passes through the kidney. The substances that must be cleared include particularly the end products of metabolism such as urea, creatinine, uric acid and **urates**. In addition many other substances such as sodium ions, potassium ions, chloride ions and hydrogen ions tend to accumulate in the body in excess quantities; it is the function of the nephron to clear the plasma of these excesses as well.

Nephrons are composed of different segments that perform specific functions. The walls of the nephron are made of a single layer of cube-like cells, called cuboidal epithelial cells, and their ultrastructure changes depending on the function of the segment they are in. For example, the surface of the cells facing the lumen of the proximal convoluted tubule are covered in microvilli (tiny finger-like structures). This type of surface is called a brush border. The brush border and the extensive length of the proximal tubule dramatically increase the surface area available for reabsorption of substances into the blood enabling around 80% of the glomerular filtrate to be reabsorbed in this segment. Another notable feature of these cells is that they are densely packed with mitochondria (the cell's energy generators). The mitochondria ensure a good supply of energy is available to fuel the active transport systems needed for efficient reabsorption.

The kidney is able to perform its excretory function by virtue of the following three processes.

- **Glomerular filtration**
- **Tubular reabsorption**
- **Tubular secretion**
- **Glomerular Filtration**

The fluid that filters through the glomerulus into Bowman's capsule is called glomerular filtrate, and the membrane of the glomerular capillaries is called the glomerular membrane.

The glomerulus acts as an ultrafilter, separating from the plasma, a solution which contains all of the solutes of plasma except the proteins. The hydrostatic pressure in the glomerular capillaries provide the driving force for the filtration process. The capillaries in the glomerulus are approximately 100-1000 times more permeable than that of the capillaries in the limbs.

The pores in the glomerular membrane prevent filtration of all particles with diameters greater than 70 ^{O}A (such as plasma proteins).

The composition of the glomerular filtrate is the same as that of blood without the cells and proteins.

Determination of Glomerular Filtration rate (GFR) and Renal Plasma Flow (RBF)

The quantity of glomerular filtrate formed per minute in all nephrons of both kidneys is called the glomerular filtration rate. The glomerular filtration rate in man has been estimated to be 125 ml./min. Determination of glomerular filtration rate (GFR) is a valuable, yet underused, diagnostic tool for evaluating renal function in dogs and cats. As a result of glomerular filtration, an ultra-filtrate of plasma is formed, which is known as 'glomerular filtrate'. It appears in the Bowman's capsule. Two theories have been proposed for Autoregulation of Renal Plasma Flow and Glomerular Filtration Rate.

1. Myogenic theory

Increased blood pressure ⟶ Expansion of artery ⟶ It respond by contracting ⟶ GFR and glomerular hydrostatic pressure decreased and vice-versa.

2. Juxtaglomerular theory

Angiotensin-Renin system

Measurement of Glomerular Filtration Rate

Glomerular filtration can be measured accurately by substances which are freely filtered in the glomerulus but are not secreted or reabsorbed by the kidney tubules. The other requirement for such substances include that it must be inert. The marker should be:

1. Freely filtered at glomerulus
2. Must not be reabsorbed from tubular lumen
3. Must not be secreted from the tubular epithelial cells.

GFR has been successfully determined with a variety of substances that are principally excreted by glomerular filtration including endogenously produced creatinine and exogenously introduced creatinine, inulin and iohexol.

Inulin (fructose polysaccharide) – most commonly used

Creatinine is a nitrogenous by-product of muscle metabolism (used in some species only because in other species it is secreted by renal tubules, it is successfully used in case of dog, cat, sheep, cattle.

Iodixanol / iohexol- Iodixanol is an isotonic, nonionic, contrast medium that has been used to measure GFR in cattle.

The glomerular filtrate formed each day can be several times the whole body fluid content. Over 99% of this filtrate is usually reabsorbed in the tubules, while the remainder passes into the urine.

Measurement of Renal Plasma Flow

Renal plasma flow or effective renal plasma flow is the volume of blood plasma delivered to the kidneys per unit time. Paramino hippuric acid is most commonly used for measurement of Renal Plasma Flow (RPF). The decrease in renal blood flow with age without a parallel decrease in blood pressure could be explained by either the presence of intraluminal vascular pathology or by increased renal vascular resistance caused by arteriolar vasoconstriction. During pregnancy, there is an increase in the flow of blood to various organs including a 50–80% increase in effective renal plasma flow which results in a corresponding 40–65% increase in the glomerular filtration rate

State-of-the-art gamma cameras and computers have allowed the development of methods for estimating GFR and RPF without collecting blood or urine samples.

Reabsorption mechanisms for glucose, protein, amino acids, electrolytes; ammonium mechanism

The nephrons in kidneys are specifically designed to maintain body fluid homeostasis. Tubular reabsorption is the process that moves solutes and water out of the filtrate and back into the bloodstream. This process is known as reabsorption, because this is the second time they have been absorbed; the first time being when they were absorbed into the bloodstream from the digestive tract after a meal.

The fluid that filters through the glomerulus and Bowman's capsule (glomerular filtrate) is very similar to blood plasma without the proteins. Several substances filtered by the glomerulus get absorbed by the tubules, either actively or passively in order to maintain their concentrations in the blood. Tubular reabsorption mechanisms in the nephrons of kidneys return the water and solutes that the body needs, back into the extracellular fluid and circulatory system.

Passive Reabsorption

The movement of any substance across the kidney membrane which can be explained entirely by gradients of concentration, and/ or gradients of electrical potential, is considered passive movement. The movement of urea from the tubular lumen to peritubular fluid is an example of passive reabsorption.

The glomerular filtrate entering the tubules of the nephron flows:

1. Through the proximal tubule
2. Through the loop of Henle
3. Through the distal tubule and
4. Through the collecting tubule into the pelvis of the kidney.

Along the course, substances are selectively reabsorbed or secreted by the tubular epithelium and the resultant fluid entering the pelvis is urine.

Absorption of Water

Water is reabsorbed so that only a limited amount of urine (One to few litres in different domestic animals) is formed per day by varying the extent of water reabsorption. Incidentally, the kidney compensates for the changes in the plasma volume. During excessive hydration, the renal output of water is increased. During prolonged dehydration, the daily excretion of urine is much reduced. The volume of the urine is specifically adjusted to the needs of water balance.

It is estimated that 7/8th of water which enters the proximal tubules from the glomeruli is reabsorbed. This absorption of water is passive and is secondary to the active reabsorption of 7/8 of the sodium filtered.

Active Reabsorption

Absorption of Glucose

Glucose is completely reabsorbed in the proximal tubule. The absorption of glucose is active, in the sense ATP is required for it. Any interference with ATP synthesis will hamper glucose reabsorption. Na^+ is also absorbed actively in the first portion of the renal tubule, but some of it later passes back into the urine again by secondary exchange with other cations.

The transport of Na^+ and K^+ is an especially important process in the kidney, which must help to regulate the concentration of these vital cations in the blood. Ouabain, a specific inhibitor of the Na^+ K^+ - ATP ase, inhibits the rate of oxygen consumption of kidney cell suspensions upto 65 to 70 percent, indicating that the active transport of Na^+ and K^+ by the Na^+ K^+ - ATP ase requires most of the ATP energy generated by respiration of the kidney. The inward directed Na^+ gradient so generated is used for the active transport of both glucose and amino acids which are believed to enter epithelial cells cons transport with Na^+.

Tubular Maxima

Glucose is reabsorbed only up to a certain concentration in the blood. If the concentration of glucose in the plasma is increased beyond a certain level, glucose starts appearing in the urine. This maximum which represents the capacity of the tubules to transport glucose, is designated as glucose 'Tubular Maxima' (Tm). Phosphate, creatinine, sulphate, uric acid, ascorbic acid, calcium and magnesium also gets actively reabsorbed in the tubules.

Tubular Secretion

Tubular secretion refers to a process whereby substances are actively transported from the peritubular capillaries to the tubular urine. There are specific active transport processes for the secretion of each group of chemical compounds. Substances secreted by the renal tubules are often poorly filterable at the glomerulus; in many instances these compounds are bound to plasma proteins and cannot cross the glomerular membranes.

Uric acid secreted by the kidney of birds, is the chief method of eliminating nitrogenous waste in these species.

One of the most important aspects of tubular secretion, is the excretion of H+ by the renal tubules. This process is of paramount importance in maintaining the proper pH of the body fluids and the acid base balance of the individual. Ruminants kept on an alkaline ash diet produce an excess of base during digestion. This extra base is excreted mainly by the kidneys in the form of HCO^-.

Thus, the urine that is eventually formed is composed of filtered substances and secreted substances. It is calculated that each millilitre of final urine is formed by the concentration of some 50 to 100 ml of glomerular filtrate.

Reabsorption and Secretion of Individual substances in Different Segments of the Tubules

Normally substances of nutritional value to the body such as glucose, proteins, amino acids, acetoacetate ions and the vitamins, are completely or almost completely reabsorbed by active processes in the proximal tubules of the kidney. Therefore, almost none of these substances remains in the tubular fluid entering the loop of Henle.

Proteins

Whatever proteins which happen to get filtered are reabsorbed through the brush border of the proximal tubular epithelium by pinocytosis. During this the protein attaches itself to the membrane and this portion of the membrane then invaginates to the interior of the cell. Once inside the cell the protein is probably digested into its constituent amino acids which are then actively absorbed through the base and sides of the cell into the peritubular fluids.

Salts

The herbaceous diet of the ruminants presents a special problem because of its high potassium content. This does not result in higher levels of potassium in the extracellular fluids of ruminants than in non ruminants. The potassium ingested is excreted in the urine by glomerular filtration supplemented by direct secretion by the cells of the distal tubule of the kidney.

The duck and many species of wild birds, possess salt glands in the region of the eyes which act as an additional channel for the excretion of excess salt ingested e.g. from drinking sea water in gulls.

Hormonal Regulation of the Kidney

Hormonal control is exerted principally by the Antidiuretic hormone (ADH) also known as vasopressin which is stored in the posterior pituitary. Vasopressin or ADH is released in response to increased osmotic pressure of the circulating blood. Vasopressin causes retention of water by increasing permeability of renal collecting ducts. Water is absorbed from the urine, the urine becomes concentrated and its volume decreases. Vasopressin stimulates increased osmotic pressure of the water, which in turn produces decreased fluid excretion (although the quantity of chemical wastes other than water is not changed). A reduction in the circulating level of ADH would therefore result in an increased urine volume at the expense of fluid derived from the blood. An increase in ADH secretion occurs regularly in sheep during feeding and this explains the reduced urine flow (oliguria), which is known to accompany feeding.

During heat stress or disease, when the animal is called upon to conserve water, increased secretion of ADH/vasopressin will cause decrease in water excretion through urine. Animals vary in the degree to which they can produce a concentrated urine, sheep notably superior to cattle in this respect. Vasopressin/ADH deficiency causes a condition known as diabetes insipidus which is characterised by a large volume of hypotonic urine.

Vassopressin is stored in the posterior pituitary and released into the bloodstream in response to stimulation of osmoreceptors or baroreceptors

Aldosterone

The kidneys secrete the enzyme renin and renin acts in concert with angiotensin-converting enzyme to form angiotensin II which acts on the adrenal cortex to increase the secretion of aldosterone. Aldosterone increases the retention of sodium from the urine via action on the renal collecting duct. Aldosterone, secreted by the adrenal cortex, acts on the kidney tubules. Aldosterone , a mineralocorticoid hormone, is synthesized by the adrenal zona glomerulosa and it plays an important role in normal fluid and electrolyte balance of the body. Aldosterone increases the rate of reabsorption of sodium into the blood from the tubular fluid. Since the sodium reabsorption is accompanied by water reabsorption , considerable changes in fluid volume can follow changes in the circulating level of aldosterone.

Angiotensin II directly stimulates sodium reabsorption in the proximal tubules, the loops of Henle, the distal tubules, and the collecting tubules. One of the direct effects of angiotensin II is to stimulate the sodium-potassium ATPase pump on the tubular epithelial cell basolateral membrane. A second effect is to stimulate sodium-hydrogen exchange in the luminal membrane, especially in the proximal tubule. Thus, angiotensin II stimulates sodium transport across both the luminal and the basolateral surfaces of the epithelial cell membrane in the tubules. These multiple actions of angiotensin II cause marked sodium retention by the kidneys when angiotensin II levels are increased.

Glomerulotubular Balance

The ability of the tubules to increase reabsorption rate in response to increased tubular load is known as glomerulotubular balance. Glomerulo tubular balance refers to the phenomenon whereby a constant fraction of the filtered load of the nephron is reabsorbed across a range of Glomerular Filtration Rates (GFR). If the GFR spontaneously increases, the rate of water and solute reabsorption in the tubule proportionately increases,thus maintaining the same fraction of the filtered load being resorbed. Glomerulotubular balance helps to prevent overloading of the distal tubular segments when GFR increases.Glomerulotubular balance acts as a second line of defense to buffer the effects of spontaneous changes in GFR on urine output. The first line of defense includes the renal autoregulatory mechanisms especially tubuloglomerular feedback which helps to prevent changes in GFR.

The autoregulatory and glomerulotubular balance mechanisms prevent large changes in fluid flow in the distal tubules.

Counter Current Mechanism

This mechanism exists to establish and maintain high osmolality in the interstitial fluid of the renal medulla.

Kidney comprises of 2 countercurrent mechanisms

1. Countercurrent multiplier (Loop of Henle)
2. Countercurrent exchanger (Vasa recta)

Countercurrent multiplier (Loop of Henle)

- Transport of tubular solute form lumen of ascending thick limb of loop of Henle, with retention of water in the tubule, dilutes the tubular fluid.
- The osmotic gradient is amplified or multiplied vertically by countercurrent flow in the descending thin limb (permeable for water not for solutes).

- Water diffuses from the lumen of the descending thin limb to the peritubular fluid in response to the horizontal gradient established by transport activities of the ascending thick limb.
- ADH increases the permeability of inner medullary collecting duct, not only for water but also for urea.
- With no ADH there would be no water and urea reabsorption beyond the distal tubule, there could be continued NaCl reabsorption under the influence of aldosterone.
- For urea only the thin ascending limb of loop of Henle is permeable, thick ascending is impermeable.

Counter Current Exchanger

- It is a counter current system in which transport between the outflow and the inflow is entirely passive.
- **Vasa recta** act as counter current exchanger. Vasa recta is permeable to water and solutes through out their length.

Endocrine Function of the Kidney

The kidney also acts as a source of many hormones.

- **Erythropoietin**- Peritubular capillaries of the kidney secrete erythropoietin. It stimulates the bone marrow and causes erythropoiesis. Erythropoietin is secreted whenever there is hypoxia. Chemically it is a glycoprotein with 165 amino acids.
- **Thrombopoietin**
- **Renin**- Renin was the first kidney hormone, to be discovered in 1939. It is secreted from the intracellular granules of juxtaglomerular cells.A decrease in the blood pressure in the afferent renal arterioles results in an increased rate of renin secretion. Renin is a proteolytic enzyme which acts on a plasma globulin to produce angiotensin. Angiotensin, in turn, acts on the adrenal cortex resulting in an increased rate of aldosterone secretion.
- **1,25-Dihydoroxycholecalciferol**
- **Prostaglandins**
- **Kinins**- The renal kinins convert alpha 2 globulin into bradykinin in the presence of enzyme kallikrein. Bradykinin is a vasodilator substance.
- **Urogastrone** which inhibits gastric motility

Methods of Studying Renal Functions

The common urinary disorders and renal failure needs to be assessed for their severity. The common urinary disorders include anuria, oliguria, polyuria and increased urinary frequency.

Renal failure refers to the deterioration of renal functions resulting in a decline in the glomerular filtration rate (GFR) and rise in urea and non-nitrogenous substances in the blood.

Renal function tests are carried out to assess the functional capacity of the kidneys. They may include analysis of urine and blood, renal clearance tests, radiology and renal imaging and renal biopsy.

The urine is generally examined for volume, specific gravity, osmolality, pH, microscopic examination and bacteriological findings. Blood is generally examined for blood urea and plasma creatinine as an index of glomerular function. In severe glomerular damage, the blood urea and plasma creatinine begins to rise. Renal function and impairment has been diagnosed by serum biochemistry viz. elevated blood urea nitrogen concentration, elevated serum creatinine concentration, hyperphosphatemia, hyperkalemia or hypokalemia and hypoalbuminemia. Urine creatinine has been used as a gold standard for screening renal disorders.

Current conventional tests of kidney damage and function in blood (serum creatinine and urea nitrogen) and urine (urine protein creatinine ratio and urine specific gravity) are widely used for diagnosis and monitoring of kidney disease. In general, the presence of high- and intermediate-molecular weight proteins in the urine are indicative of glomerular damage, while low-molecular weight proteins and enzymes in the urine suggest tubular damage due to decreased reabsorption of proteins, direct tubular damage, or both. GFR is the rate of blood flow to the kidneys and it serves as an indicator of the kidney's functioning capacity to filter the fluid plasma and excrete creatinine and other waste elements from the body.

Kidney stones (also called renal calculi, nephrolithiasis or urolithiasis) are hard deposits made of minerals and salts that form inside kidneys. Kidney stones can affect any part of the urinary tract — from kidneys to bladder. If the kidney stones become lodged in the ureters, it may block the flow of urine and cause the kidney to swell and the ureter to spasm. Most kidney stones are calcium stones, usually in the form of calcium oxalate. Stones can form in any part of the urinary tract in dogs and cats, but unlike in humans, stones of the kidney are less common and do not often cause significant disease, although they can contribute to pyelonephritis and chronic kidney disease. Stones tends to occur frequently in domesticated cats, especially in those that are not very active, don't take in enough fluids, and don't urinate enough.

Ultrasound and radiographic screening are generally used to look for the increase or decrease from normal size of the kidneys,changes in echogenicity of kidney texture etc. Although abdominal ultrasonography has dramatically enhanced the ability to evaluate the kidneys in animals with renal disease, it provides no quantitative measure of renal function.

Shock wave lithotripsy involves using ultrasound (high-frequency sound waves) to pinpoint where a kidney stone is. Ultrasound shock waves are then sent to the stone from a machine to break it into smaller pieces so it can be passed in urine.

Dialysis

The term dialysis in physiological sense refers to the diffusion of solutes from an area of higher concentration to the area of lower concentration through a semipermeable membrane. This principle has been used to dialyse the blood of patients with renal failure especially those developing uraemia. Dialysis is a medical process of removing wastes and excess water from the blood by diffusion and ultrafiltration. When kidney function fails, dialysis must be done to artificially rid the body of wastes and fluids. This is a vital process to keep patients alive. In some cases, the patients undergo artificial dialysis until they are eligible for a kidney transplant.

In veterinary medicine two types of dialysis are generally performed especially in small animals.1. Peritoneal dialysis and 2. Hemodialysis or artificial kidney.

Animals which have acute rises in blood urea nitrogen and plasma creatinine concentration may be treated with many interventions coincided with treating specific causes. The most common treatment is conventional fluid therapy. The high techniques will include hemodialysis and peritoneal dialysis.Peritoneal dialysis is an effective modality for the treatment of acute and chronic renal failure, specific intoxications, electrolyte abnormalities, and fluid overload. The hemodialysis uses vascular access by using double lumen catheter introduced into the jugular vein.Hemodialysis can be used with effective removal of nitrogenous waste within a short time period.

Renal Transplantation

Renal transplantation is the final answer to all the problems in cases with chronic renal failure in human beings. It reverses metabolic and excretory abnormalities. Kidney transplantation has so far only been performed with any degree of success on cats and **dogs**, most usually cats as they are particularly prone to kidney diseases.

Kidney transplantation is the only potentially curative treatment for chronic renal failure. Cats receiving transplanted kidneys have been known to survive as long as 6 years or more after surgery. The implanted kidney functions normally and should provide a much improved quality of life for the transplant recipient. Renal transplantation reverses metabolic and excretory abnormalities. Lifelong immunosuppression, consisting of a combination of cyclosporine and prednisolone is necessary to prevent allograft rejection.

Urine Concentration

The urine concentrating mechanism plays a fundamental role in regulating water and sodium excretion. When water intake is large enough to dilute blood plasma, a urine more dilute than blood plasma is produced; when water intake is so small that blood plasma is concentrated, a urine more concentrated than blood plasma is produced. Initially the countercurrent multiplication mechanism was the theory to explain the concentration of urine in the kidney.

The mechanisms for the independent control of water and sodium excretion are mostly contained within the renal medulla. The renal medulla produces concentrated urine through the generation of an osmotic gradient extending from the cortico-medullary boundary to the inner medullary tip. Identification and localization of key transport proteins for water, urea, and sodium which play an important role in urine concentration mechanism has been carried out.

Micturition

The urinary bladder, a hollow muscular sac, is a temporary reservoir for urine. Micturition is defined as the periodic complete emptying of the urinary bladder, under voluntary control. Urine is stored in the urinary bladder before voiding (Micturition). Micturition involves nervous, muscular and mechanical mechanisms in coordination . Micturition or the expulsion of urine from the bladder is a reflex activity stimulated by distension of the bladder from the constant inflow of urine by the ureters. The bladder gets distended with the gradual inflow of urine, till the pressure is high enough to stimulate the reflex centres in the spinal cord, which in turn causes contractions of the smooth muscle wall of the bladder by sacral parasympathetic nerves. The micturition response involves reflex pathways, but is under voluntary control in humans. The micturition reflex is a completely automatic cord reflex, but it can be inhibited or facilitated by the centres in the brain which include a facilitatory center in the upper pons and a facilitatory centre in the hypothalamus. Inhibitory controls are also there at the level of superior colliculus and in the cerebral cortex.

Composition of Urine

A comparison of the composition of blood plasma and urine emphasises the manner by which water and important electrolytes and metabolites are conserved while wastes are eliminated in the urine. Composition of the urine is variable in consonance with the requirement of whole body fluid homeostasis. Urine is composed of several excretory substances formed during body metabolism dissolved in water. Several inorganic salts which are ingested in excess of body requirements and need to be removed are also present in urine. Essential nutrients like glucose, amino acids and fatty acids are not normally present in the urine, because any excess of these vital nutrients is taken care of by the liver and adipose tissue, which can store excess of these. The amount of urine excreted varies considerably. Some of the factors which may affect the volume of urine excreted include the amount and quality of food intake, work, ambient temperature, season and amount of water consumed by the animal.

Physical Characteristics of Urine

Color – The color of the urine varies from clear to yellowish. The color is influenced by diet, drugs, and health state. The color of urine is due to pigment called urochrome, which is a combination of urobilin and urobilinogen with a peptide. The intensity of the color usually varies with urine concentration; thus, concentrated urine is dark yellow, and dilute urine is pale yellow.

Abnormal constituents may alter the color of urine. Bilirubin or its degradation products may give urine a darker yellow color than normal. Hemoglobin or hematuria may impart a red or brown color, and myoglobin a reddish brown appearance.

Odor – The odor of urine is slightly aromatic and it is influenced by diet, drugs, and health state.

Turbidity : Turbidity of urine varies among species and among samples in the same individual. Horse urine is normally markedly turbid because of calcium carbonate content and mucus originating from glands in the renal pelvis. Cow urine becomes turbid on standing because of calcium carbonate crystals. Dog and cat urine is often clear but may be turbid in the absence of abnormalities.

The degree of turbidity or cloudiness is usually influenced by excess amounts of cellular debris and casts but can also be secondary to proteinuria, crystals, or contamination with vaginal discharge.

pH and Volume of Urine: The pH of the urine can vary between 4.8 and 8.0. By excreting excess acid or base, the kidneys help to maintain a constant hydrogen ion concentration in the body. The kidneys also regulate the volume of the blood and the overall osmotic pressure of the body fluids by the amount of water and salt excreted.

Normally urine contains 95 % water. Rest 5% are usually solutes mainly urea, uric acid and creatinine.

Urea : The major component of the urine is urea. Urea is the waste product of protein breakdown. The amount of urea in urine is dependent on the amount of protein in the diet, but some excretion of urea will take place in the complete absence of dietary protein, which is the amount produced by the breakdown of tissue protein. This amount of nitrogen (mostly as urea) excreted in the absence of dietary protein is called endogenous urinary nitrogen.

Uric acid: Uric acid is formed during the metabolism of nucleic acids.

Creatinine: Creatinine is the waste product of creatine, which occurs in muscles as high energy storage product, creatine phosphate.

Renal Clearance

Renal Clearance (RC) - the rate at which the kidney can remove a substance from the blood

RC = U/P X V

U/P = concentration of substance in urine (mg/ml)

concentration of substance in plasma (mg/ml)

V = rate of the formation of urine (ml/minute)

(normal = 1 ml/minute)

Excretion of Nitrogenous End Products

When carbohydrates, fats and proteins are utilized as fuels for the liberation of energy, water and carbon dioxide are produced. The water enters the body fluids of the animal, and its fate becomes inseparable from the general problem of water balance. The CO_2 is removed via the respiratory cycle. There remains a third major excretory product, the nitrogen containing part, which is split off from the amino acids during their metabolism. This nitrogen containing part is ammonia which formed during the process of deamination of amino acids. Ammonia is the waste produced by metabolism of nitrogen-containing compounds like proteins and nucleic acids. Thus the basic need in nitrogenous excretion is therefore the elimination of ammonia. The deamination is carried out with the help of enzymes which may be oxidative eg amino acid oxidases or non oxidative hydrolytic enzymes which deaminates specific amino acids eg glutamic dehydrogenase.

The ammonia formed cannot be stored and is toxic if large amounts are produced in the body and present in the body. This is eliminated from the body in the form of more complex nitrogenous substances which are normally either urea or uric acid. Ruminants can use urea as a protein source. On a low protein diet, these animals eg camel, sheep etc., recycle part of the urea produced through the salivary glands and hence can reduce their urea excretion quite considerably. The concentration of ammonia in the blood of most domestic animals does not normally exceed 0.1 mg/100 cm^3.

Urea is much less toxic than ammonia and is slightly more soluble in water than ammonia. Its high solubility means that water must be used to eliminate it from the body but the amount required will be much less than for an equivalent amount of ammonia because its relative lack of toxicity allows it to be concentrated to a much greater extent.

Animals which excrete ammonia as the main end product of amino acid metabolism are said to be ammoniotelic animals. When urea is the main end product, they are called ureotelic animals and where uric acid is the final excretory product they are called uricotelic animals. In actual practice, most animals produce a mixture of nitrogenous wastes.

Urea Cycle

Urea metabolism is an important way to excrete ammonia, which is a waste product of proteins. The diet and the breakdown of endogenous tissues, particularly of skeletal muscle, are important sources of protein. Urea is synthesized from ammonia through a cyclic process called 'urea cycle or ornithine cycle'. The urea cycle is a cycle of biochemical reactions that produces urea from ammonia. The urea cycle takes place primarily in the liver and, to a lesser extent, in the kidneys. The urea cycle is a compartmentalized cycle, with reactions occurring in both the cytoplasm and the mitochondrion. Before the urea cycle begins ammonia is converted to carbamoyl phosphate. The reaction is catalyzed by carbamoyl phosphate synthetase I and requires the use of two ATP molecules. The first three enzymes in this cycle, N-acetylglutamate synthase (NAGS), carbamoyl phosphate synthetase I (CPSI), and ornithine transcarbamylase (OTC) function inside mitochondria, and the latter three, argininosuccinic acid synthase, argininosuccinic acid lyase (ASL), and arginase, act in the cytosol.

Carbamyl phosphate condenses with ornithine to yield citrulline in the ornithine transcarbamylase (OTC) reaction. In the hepatic cytosol, citrulline reacts with aspartate to form argininosuccinate, catalyzed by argininosuccinate synthetase. Argininosuccinate lyase cleaves argininosuccinate to form fumarate, which is oxidized in the tricarboxylic acid cycle, and arginine, which is hydrolyzed to urea and ornithine via hepatic arginase.

Although the steady-state concentration of ammonia in the liver is extremely small, it is a major metabolite arising in one major and diverse minor reactions. Urea concentration in the blood is around 20-30 mg/100 ml. The concentration of urea in the blood has been reported to be an indicator of protein status of the animals. Such a synthesis requires a considerable cost of chemical bond energy. The urea cycle is best known to occur in mammalian liver. Organisms that cannot easily and quickly remove ammonia usually have to convert it to some other substance, like urea or uric acid, which are much less toxic. Insufficiency of the urea cycle occurs in some genetic disorders (inborn errors of metabolism), and in liver failure. The result of liver failure is accumulation of nitrogenous waste, mainly ammonia, which leads to hepatic encephalopathy.

The diffusion of water from the proximal tubule to the interstitial space is accompanied by diffusion of urea, where as 65% of the filtrate water may be reabsorbed from proximal tubule, only 30-40% of the urea is reabsorbed at that location, indicating that epithelium of proximal tubule is not as permeable for urea as it is for water.

Uric acid production and Metabolism

Uric acid production and metabolism are complex processes involving various factors that regulate hepatic production, as well as renal and gut excretion of this compound. Uric acid is the end product of an exogenous pool of purines and endogenous purine metabolism. The exogenous pool varies significantly with diet, and animal proteins contribute significantly to this purine pool. The endogenous production of uric acid is mainly from the liver, intestines and other tissues like muscles, kidneys and the vascular endothelium.Uric acid is a $C_5H_4N_4O_3$ (7,9-dihydro-1H-purine-2,6,8(3H)-trione) heterocyclic organic compound with a molecular weight of 168 Da. Many enzymes are involved in the conversion of the two purine nucleic acids, adenine and guanine, to uric acid. The normal reference interval of uric acid in human blood is 1.5 to 6.0 mg/dL in women and 2.5 to 7.0 mg/dL in men. Humans cannot oxidize uric acid to the more soluble compound allantoin due to the lack of uricase enzyme. Normally, most daily uric acid disposal occurs via the kidneys. Elevated serum levels of uric acid have been shown to play an important role in many disease states including **gout** and articular degenerative disorders as well as vascular inflammation and atherosclerosis. **Gout** is a common metabolic disorder that results in abnormal accumulation of urates in domestic birds. Gout is caused by raised levels of uric acid in the blood (hyperuricaemia), which may be due either to

- Overproduction of uric acid,
- To impaired destruction of uric acid because of deficient enzymes systems or
- To its decreased excretion, either due to impaired filtration or altered excretion in the tubules as may occur in drug therapy like aspirin, mercuric salts etc.

Avian gout is a consequence of kidney damage which can occur from a number of potential causes leading to the accumulation of uric acid/urates in the renal tubules and serous coats of the heart, the liver, the mesentery, the air sacs or the peritoneum. The causes of avian gout are varied, ranging from management and/ or nutrition-related, to pathogens and/or the presence of mycotoxins in feed. Anti-inflammatory drug diclofenac has been blamed for disappearance of vultures in the Indian subcontinent, possibly due to uric acid accumulating in the birds' blood and crystallizing around their internal organs—a condition called visceral gout.

Uraemia

Urine contains a diverse range of substances that are either waste products or substances ingested in excess. The importance of the kidneys in maintaining body fluid composition is clear when we look at what happens when we consider the impact on the body when our kidneys start to fail. Retention of waste products causes disturbances in multiple organ systems including cardiovascular, hematological, gastrointestinal, neurological, skeletal, hormonal, respiratory, skin and reproductive systems. Loss of water and electrolyte homeostasis lead to elevated extracellular body fluid volume, which may produce edema and hypertension, reduced phosphate excretion, loss of bone calcium, and symptoms of lethargy, nausea, diarrhoea and vomiting.

Chronic renal failure refers to a slow, insidious deterioration of kidney functions resulting in uraemia. Uraemia develops when more than 75% of nephrons are damaged. Common causes of chronic renal failure are mainly due to kidney diseases: polycystic kidney, pyelonephritis. Uraemia is the condition of having high levels of urea in the blood. Urea is one of the primary components of urine. Uraemia is indicative of deterioration of renal function.Uraemia is associated with fluid, electrolyte, and hormone imbalances and metabolic abnormalities. Uraemia more commonly develops with chronic kidney disease but it also may occur with acute kidney injury.

Diuretics can help restore normal urination and remove waste from the body. Antiemetics can treat severe vomiting. Dialysis or surgery may be needed in cases where the kidneys have suffered severe damage. However, even with treatment, the mortality rate for dogs who suffer from uraemia is as high as 50 percent.

Diabetes insipidus is a rare disorder that causes you to feel very thirsty (despite drinking a lot), and to produce large amounts of urine. It is usually caused by a malfunction in the production of antidiuretic hormone (ADH), a hormone that prevents the production of dilute urine (i.e., retains water in the body). This can happen for a number of different reasons, including damage to the pituitary; e.g., caused by a tumour, surgery, or an infection, that disrupts the normal production, storage and release of ADH. However, it may also occur due to a defect in the tubules themselves that prevents them from responding to ADH, or during pregnancy, when a placental enzyme destroys ADH in the mother.

Summary

- Renal function is essential for homeostasis.
- Kidneys are the main excretory organs which together with a pair of ureters , a urinary bladder and urethra constitute the excretory system.
- Vasopressin causes retention of water by increasing permeability of renal collecting ducts.

- The kidneys secrete the enzyme renin and renin acts in concert with angiotensin-converting enzyme to form angiotensin II which acts on the adrenal cortex to increase the secretion of aldosterone. Aldosterone increases the retention of sodium from the urine via action on the renal collecting duct.
- Hormonal control of the kidney is exerted principally by the Antidiuretic hormone (ADH) also known as vasopressin which is stored in the posterior pituitary.
- The urine concentrating through a countercurrent mechanism plays a fundamental role in regulating water and sodium excretion.
- Urine is stored in the urinary bladder temporarily till voided through micturition. Micturition is defined as the periodic complete emptying of the urinary bladder which involves nervous, muscular and mechanical mechanisms in coordination

11

Fluid and Water Balance

A large proportion of the body of mammals including domestic animals, is made up of water. This water is an essential attribute for the life of the animals. Animals deprived of food but provided water will survive much longer than the animals provided with food but deprived of water. Water is the basis of the liquid environment of the cells, which Claude Bernard called the milieu interieur, and Cannon the fluid matrix. Homeostasis refers to the relatively stable state inside the body of an animal. Animal organs and organ systems constantly adjust to internal and external changes in order to maintain this steady state. Homeostatic mechanisms keep the body in dynamic equilibrium by constantly adjusting to the changes that the body's systems encounter. Osmoregulation is the process of maintaining salt and water balance (osmotic balance) across membranes within the body. The fluids inside and surrounding cells are composed of water, electrolytes, and nonelectrolytes.

Water's most important biophysical qualities are its solvent properties, its ionization and its heat of vaporization. Water is essential for metabolic processes, as most of these reactions must occur in aquatic environments. Water provides the medium for the transport of nutrients from their sites of absorption to the site of metabolism. Water also provides the medium for the transport of waste products from their sites of production to their sites of final excretion. Together with the main electrolytes, water forms an excellent buffering medium. Moreover, water is an essential substrate or end product of many biological reactions. Water due to its high latent heat of evaporation or fusion is an excellent insulator for the loss of body heat and is essentially required for the loss of heat to maintain body temperature, through the evaporation of water from the skin and the respiratory tract. Water also acts as a vehicle for the transportation of nutrients, hormones, waste products and gases etc.

The body's homeostatic control mechanisms ensure that a balance between fluid gain and fluid loss is maintained. The hormones ADH (antidiuretic hormone, also known as vasopressin) and aldosterone play a major role in this.

Body water is derived from several sources which include the water drunk, intake of water through food and metabolic body water. Water is lost from the body through several routes which include loss of water through the feces and urine, evaporation of water from the skin and respiratory tract. In recent years the pressure over the water resources has been increased due to population growth, climatic change, economic development and increased demand of industries and agriculture sector. So, in coming years, the water demand for livestock may compete with those of the humans and water required for crop production.

Water as a solvent

Water is the solvent of body fluids in which numerous inorganic or organic solutes are dissolved, and normally accounts for approximately 60% to 70% of the body weight (depending on the amount of fatty tissue present and age of the animal). Fatty tissue has a lower water content than other tissues. Similarly older animals have less water as compared to the young animals.

Water moves passively across membranes of the body. It constantly diffuses from areas of higher to lower water concentrations, a process commonly referred to as osmosis.

Potassium, magnesium, sulfate, phosphates, protein, amino acids, cholesterol, phospholipids and neutral fat are normally found in higher concentrations in intracellular than in extracellular fluids. Sodium, chloride, calcium, bicarbonate and glucose are normally found in higher concentrations in extracellular fluids (i.e. plasma and interstitial fluid).

The concentration of water in the body varies from one tissue to another, being least in the dentine of teeth and greatest in the grey matter of the brain. The amount of water in the body also varies considerably with the age of the animal. The younger animals contain considerably more water than the older animals. This effect is mostly due to an increase in the fatty tissues in the body, which contains relatively much less water, as the relative composition of tissues of the body other than fat remains relatively constant. The proportion of water in ruminants is higher as compared to nonruminants.

The water content is particularly low in adipose tissue. The consequence of this is that, for a given body weight, the body fluids represent a smaller percentage of the body weight in fat than in thin (lean) animals. Since the proportion of bone and other non-fatty tissues is fairly constant, the water content of an animal is a good indirect estimate of its fat content. Because this determination is of major interest for animal husbandry purposes, linear regressions relating total body water content to fat content have been derived for various methods and species. Body water can be estimated by dilution techniques using urea, antipyrine etc and by using radioisotopic dilution technique using tritiated water. Thus water is indispensable for all biochemical and physiological processes.

Total Body Water

Total body water content depends upon the body condition of animals.

50 % within cell 15 % in interstitial space 5 % in blood plasma

Fat tissue is exceptional in its low water content of 10% or less.

Water Intake and Outgo

Water is available to the animal from three sources.

1. **Water drunk by the animal.**-Drinking water is an important requirement of livestock and lack of a sufficient source of water can become a limiting factor in productivity of the animals. It has been estimated that direct watering requirement of livestock is about 5 billion cubic meters a year based on a norm

of 18-30 litre per capita per day. A lactating cow can drink about 18-30 litres per day but can go upto 95 litres per day. Water drunk or intake by the animal is affected by the environmental temperature or heat load.

Zebu cattle may have a lower intake of water than European breeds.Similarly Young calves generally have higher intakes of water per kilogram of dry matter consumed than by older cattle. During the last 4 months of pregnancy, cows may consume 30 percent more water than when dry and open.

2. **Water contained in the food stuffs**.- Water contained in the feed is extremely variable. It may range from a low of 5 percent in dry grains to about 90 percent in young, fast-growing grasses.
3. **Metabolic body water** i.e. water produced *de novo* by oxidative metabolism in the body. The catabolism of 1 kg of fat, carbohydrate, or protein produces 1190, 560, or 450 g of water, respectively. Metabolic body water becomes important when the animal is in negative energy balance or say when body fat or tissue protein is getting utilized for maintenance of the body functions.

Water derived from these sources is balanced by loss of water in urine and faeces, in expired air from the respiratory tract and by evaporation from the skin. In ruminants the loss of water through feces is substantial, approximately equal to urinary losses. The high-fiber nature of ruminant diets requires proportionately more water to carry the ingesta through the gastrointestinal tract than for nonruminants. The ability to reabsorb water in the lower gut and excrete drier fecal pellets instead of wet, loose feces is presumably one mechanism of water conservation.

Water loss from the respiratory tract is extremely variable, depending on relative humidity and respiration rate. Expired air is over 90 percent saturated; hence, under conditions of low relative humidity, respiratory losses are high. Conversely, losses are low when inspired air is near saturation.

Cutaneous evaporation of water is the major means of heat loss in cattle and sheep at high temperatures. There are large differences among species in the importance of sweating with domestic livestock ranked in the descending order of horses, donkeys, cattle, buffaloes, goats, sheep, and swine. Swine and poultry are examples of species that depend more on the respiratory than cutaneous route for water loss.

Control of Water Intake

Thirst is an osmoregulatory mechanism to increase water input. The control of water intake is mainly a function of the medial lateral hypothalamus, but the participation of other regions of the brain is necessary for the integration of the system. The natural signals are blood plasma osmotic pressure (which acts on the hypothalamus), blood pressure (stretch receptors in the right atrium) and increased body temperature (hypothalamus). The response to these signals is the induction of thirst and the secretion of antidiuretic hormone (ADH) from the neurohypophysis. The urge to drink results from a complex interplay of hormones and neuronal responses that coordinate to increase water input and contribute toward fluid balance and composition in the body.

Urinary Excretion of Water and Its Hormonal Control

If an animal is deprived of water, the rate of water excretion in the urine decreases; and conversely if an excess of water is ingested, urinary volume will rise. The excretion of water by the kidney is controlled primarily by the antidiuretic hormone (ADH) of the posterior pituitary gland. The release of ADH from the posterior pituitary gland is believed to be caused primarily by changes in the osmo concentration of the plasma.

Transport of Water Across Gut Membrane

The absorption of water from the gut is very efficient. The transport of water across the mucosa cannot be attributed to hydrostatic and osmotic pressure differences, but depends upon metabolic processes. Glucose is required to induce water transport against an osmotic gradient : without glucose there is only a passive transfer of water; the fact that water is never transported alone suggests that water transfer is driven by osmotic forces resulting from active transport of some ions.

Loss of Water from The Body

Water is lost from the body through the following routes.

- Faeces
- Urine
- Skin
- Respiratory tract

The loss of water from the skin and respiratory tract varies considerably with the environment and species. Loss of water through these routes is higher at high environmental temperature. However some species are better sweaters than others. Dogs, for example, lose almost all the water required for thermoregulation through the respiratory passage as it contains little or no sweat glands.

Special Features of Water Metabolism in Camel

Most domestic animals including camels are required to strike a balance between the water intake and water outgo. Camels are exposed both to the heating effect of the sun and to relatively dry air for extended periods. In order to preserve the body water, the camel shows a wide variety of adaptations. During such exposures the water loss through the urine is reduced considerably. Camel is resistant to water losses to the magnitude of 30%. As a result, the camel can go without drinking for periods for perhaps 6 to 8 days under desert conditions that would be fatal in a single day to a man without water. The ability of the body to store water is rather limited. Camel is reputed to store water during the times of opulence in the hump and the stomach but these views have been refuted by several studies. Schmidt Nielson states that camels, like other mammals, drinks to replenish lost water and to restore the normal water content of the body and there is no evidence that it over drinks in anticipation of future needs.

Body Fluids

A major proportion of the body is made up of fluid. The fluid compartments of the body are distinguished into two parts.

1. *Intracellular fluid :* It provides the medium in which metabolic reactions take place.
2. *Extracellular fluid :* It serves to nourish the cells and remove waste products.

The water in the body acts as a constituent of the body fluids. These body fluids are distributed in different compartments of the body. Thus extracellular fluid is further composed of two components. The blood plasma and the interstitial fluid. The plasma and the cellular elements of the blood fill the vascular system and together they constitute the total blood volume. In the adult domestic animal the amount of body water is about 70% of the body weight, 50% of the body weight is intracellular fluid, 15% is interstitial fluid and 5% plasma. However, it is important to remember that the fluids in different compartments are in dynamic equilibrium with one another and there is a continuous interchange of fluid between the different compartments.

The volume and composition of body fluids are altered as a result of certain diseases, during adaptation to high attitude or heat and in many stressful situations.

Regulation

Under normal conditions body fluid regulation is affected mainly by hormonal mechanisms involving particularly the secretions of the adrenal and posterior pituitary glands.

Interstitial Fluid

The main difference between plasma and interstitial fluid is the much smaller quantity of protein in the interstitial fluid. This arises from the relative impermeability of the capillary walls to plasma proteins.

Intracellular Fluid

The intracellular fluid is quite different from the extracellular fluid. There is considerably more protein within the cells. The main electrolyte in the intracellular fluid is potassium instead of sodium. Magnesium is also important to a lesser extent and its importance stems from the fact that it serves as an essential cofactor in many intracellular reactions occurring within the cells.

Measurement of Body Fluid Volumes

Body water : Total body water can be determined directly by drying the whole animal and measuring the loss of weight. However this method is inconvenient and necessitates the death of the animal.

The method most commonly used to estimate total body water is based on the **dilution technique**. The dilution technique involves the injection of a compound into the body which is distributed in all compartments of the body containing water, which is freely permeable, non toxic and can be determined easily. Unfortunately while the compound is being distributed throughout the fluid compartment, it may also be excreted or metabolized and corrections must be made for these losses occurring during the distribution time.

The best compounds for measurement of total body water are heavy water (deuterium oxide) and radioactive water (tritium oxide). Isotopically labelled water distributes itself in a fashion identical to the normal water of the body. Other compounds used include antipyrine, sulfanilamide, thiourea and urea.

Blood Volume

It is not possible to determine the volume of blood in the body merely by bleeding an animal to death. A considerable amount of blood is left in the vessels even after the animal dies of haemorrhage. Clotting and vasoconstrictor mechanisms retain a large amount of blood in the vessels. Some people attempted to wash out the blood retained in the vessels after bleeding. The amount of wash fluid was subtracted from the total volume. However, this method suffers from the defect that the animal must be killed. Moreover, the blood volume data so obtained are not necessarily both accurate and precise.

Indirect methods using dilution techniques have been used quite successfully. Evans blue dye (T-1824) or radioactive iodine (^{131}I) are substances which have been most commonly used for this purpose.

Extracellular fluid: Dilution techniques using inulin have been most commonly used but sucrose, thiocyanate, thiosulphate and others have also been useful.

Intracellular fluid volume: Intracellular fluid volume cannot be calculated directly but rather it must be calculated as the difference between total and extracellular fluid volume.

Fluid Therapy

Fluid Therapy is the administration of fluids to a patient as a treatment or preventative measure. It can be administered via intravenous, intraperitoneal, subcutaneous and oral routes.

Dehydration is defined as the condition when the body is in negative water balance as a result of excessive output of water in excess of intake. Dehydration leads to decrease in body water content. Oral rehydration therapy (ORT) is a simple treatment for dehydration associated with diarrhea, particularly gastroenteritis/gastroenteropathy,for any causes. ORT consists of a solution of salts and sugar which is taken by mouth. For most mild to moderate dehydration mostly in young animals the favorite treatment in an emergency department is ORT over intravenous replacement of fluid. Rational fluid therapy must appreciate the pathophysiology of the diseases causing derangement of fluid balance.

Intravenous (IV) fluid administration is probably the most frequently used therapy in veterinary hospitals. Continuous IV fluid administration in hospitalized patients have long been considered fundamental in the management of critically ill animals. When used appropriately, IV fluids can improve outcomes in the most critically ill animals. GI emergencies are among the most common reasons for prescribing fluid therapy in small animals. Outpatient or subcutaneous crystalloid supplementation to correct fluid deficits caused by vomiting, diarrhea, and lack of oral water intake is common practice in veterinary medicine. During surgical procedures, fluid requirement increases by increased evaporation, fluid shifts and/or excessive urine production indicating fluid therapy.

The fluids are administered to animals to achieve the following therapeutic objectives.

- To restore the volume of body fluids to its normal level.
- To correct the acid base balances
- To correct electrolyte balance
- To provide nutritional supplementation

Isotonic solutions are commonly used as intravenously infused fluids in patients. Most isotonic solutions do not provide calories or free water. Examples of isotonic solutions are 0.9% sodium chloride, commonly called normal saline (NS), and lactated Ringer's (LR). Ringer's lactate solution (RL), also known as sodium lactate solution and Hartmann's solution, is a mixture of sodium chloride, sodium lactate, potassium chloride, and calcium chloride in water. It is used for replacing fluids and electrolytes in those who have low blood volume or low blood pressure. Lactated Ringer's solution has been used as a resuscitation standard for treatment of hypovolemia and hemorrhagic shock.

Dextrose – Often indicated for cattle in early lactation with severe ketosis, hepatic lipidosis, or hypoglycemia. Glucose as a 5% solution can be administered at a slow rate for several days.

Indications for Fluid Therapy

1. Fluid therapy is indicated either when there is a loss of fluid In cases of moderate to severe dehydration
2. Electrolytes abnormalities,
3. Hypotension
4. Hypovolemia
5. Decreased oxygen delivery

Dehydration

Dehydration is defined as an excessive loss of body fluid. Dehydration may result due to lack of drinking water under moderate environmental conditions, or due to severe diarrhoea, vomiting etc. The first sign of dehydration is a tendency to seek and drink water. Most animals will not eat during moderate or severe dehydration and hence part of the body weight loss is loss of tissue substance used for energy metabolism.

Many factors influence the water requirements for livestock including level of activity, lactation, rate of weight gain, pregnancy, diet and environment temperature. Inadequate water supplies can result from evaporation in summer heat, freezing in winter or poor management. Dehydration can be lethal, especially in young or depleted animals, and can promote secondary health problems such as acidosis and kidney failure in otherwise healthy animals. In dehydrated animals the mouth, tongue, nose or nostrils and eyes will be dry.

Skin pinch test :The classic sign for dehydration is skin tenting. If you take a pinch of skin over the animal's shoulders and pull up gently, the skin should snap back into place when released. As the animal gets more dehydrated, the skin goes back in place more and more slowly.

Test capillary refill time: Pull back the animal's lip and press your finger against the gum. The resultant pale, whitish spot should turn pink again instantly. If it doesn't, this slow capillary refill time could indicate dehydration.

Most animals will not eat during moderate or severe dehydration except donkey and camel. Donkey will eat before drinking and the camel continues to eat in a normal fashion despite what would be considered severe dehydration for other animals.

Animals are always faced with the problem of slow dehydration. Any serious dehydration involves the loss to both water and electrolytes. The first sign of dehydration is a tendency to seek and drink water and decrease in urine volume. This is generally seen when there is 1-2% of body weight loss as water. Dehydration to the extent of 10% of body weight is considered severe. A dog deprived of water under moderate condition will lose about 10% of its body weight in 5 days. If we look at the eyes, besides being dry, the eyes of dehydrated animals appear sunken and dull. In dairy cattle, milk production decreases dramatically or ceases altogether in dehydration.

Water Concentration Mechanisms

Several animals can survive better than others when deprived of water for long periods. Such animals are better adapted to lack of water. Desert camel and donkey are two examples of species adapted for such conditions. Cattle appear to have no special water conservation mechanism but there are important differences. Zebu cattle can dissipate larger quantities of heat by evaporation of larger quantities of water from their body surface than European cattle. Partly this is due to more and larger sweat glands in Zebu cattle as compared to European cattle.

Camels and donkeys can survive a water deficit more because they conserve more water. Both camel and sheep produce relatively dry faeces and can reduce their excretion of urine considerably. During the day, when the heat stress is greatest, the camel permits its body temperature to rise thereby storing heat and saving the water which would have been required to dissipate the heat. In the camel the summer fur, which is most prominent on the dorsal surfaces of the animal, is very effective in reducing heat gain and therefore relieves the animal of the necessity of using water to dissipate that heat. Another important point is that camels are able to rehydrate quickly.

Diffusion

Diffusion is the process by virtue of which molecules move from higher concentration to lower concentration. The ratio of diffusion of gases through porous bodies are inversely proportional to the square root of their densities. For example, the lower the density higher will be the rate of diffusion. A membrane does not stop the process of diffusion, if it is permeable to the particles of the dissolved substances. The process of diffusion is caused by the kinetic motion of the molecules. Blood when passes through the capillaries, continual exchange occurs between the plasma portion of the blood and the interstitial fluid in spaces surrounding the capillaries. Since the capillaries are porous a large amount of fluid can diffuse back and forth between the blood and tissue spaces.

Donnan Equilibrium

The plasma protein has net negative charge and therefore tends to bind cations, such as Na^+ and K^+, thus holding an extra amount of less cations in the plasma along with the plasma proteins. On the other hand negatively charged ions (anions) tend to have a slightly higher concentration in interstitial fluid, compared with the plasma because the negative charges of the plasma protein repel the negatively charged anions.

Donnan equilibrium concerns the distribution of diffusible solutes separated by a membrane that is freely permeable to water and electrolytes but totally impermeable to one species of ion confined to one of the two compartments. In this situation, the diffusible solutes become unequally distributed among the two compartments. Donnan's equilibrium is fundamental to many situations in physiology such as kidney tubules and red blood cells.

Suppose NaCl is dissolved in pure water in a compartment which is separated from water in a second compartment through a semipermeable membrane. After a short while the Na^+ and Cl^- ions will diffuse from compartment I to compartment II until the concentration of Na^+ and Cl^- becomes equal on both sides of the membrane.

Suppose some sodium salt is added to compartment I which contains an anion to which the membrane is impermeable. In such a situation, the distribution of Na+ ions and Cl^- ions again change and a new equilibrium is set up to satisfy the requirements of physical principles. One of the conditions which must be satisfied is that there must be electroneutrality in both the compartments.Thus compartment I will now have Na^+ Cl^- ions as earlier and Na^+ and X^- (non diffusible ions) be added. Thus there are more Na^+ ions in compartment I. Since only Na^+ and Cl^- can be transferred from compartment I to II not the X^-, these two diffuse from I to II in such a way that the following equation is satisfied.In such a situation, the diffusible cation Na^+, becomes more concentrated in the compartment in which the non diffusible anion is added, whereas the diffusible anion becomes less concentrated in this compartment than in the other.

A Gibbs Donnan equilibrium arises in biology when a solution containing charged protein molecules and salts is separated from one containing only salts, by a membrane which allows the salts to cross easily but which is impermeable to proteins.

The consequence is that the diffusible ions take up a distribution such that (a) a potential occurs across the membrane so that (at body pH) the protein side becomes negative (b) there are more diffusible ions on the protein side of the membrane than on the other side and so the osmotic differential between the sides is due partly to the protein and partly to the excess of diffusible ions on each side of the membrane is equal. The Gibbs Donnan equilibrium is important in the red cells.

Acid Base Balance and H+ Regulation, Correction and Evolution of Imbalances

The water and other solutes contained in the body fluids occur in the form of **ions**. Among these ions H^+ is the most important for determining the acid base status of the fluids. The unit for measurement of acidic or basic nature of a solution is known as pH. pH is defined as the negative logarithm of hydrogen ion concentration. The pH of any solution may vary from 1 to 14. The pH of water (pure) is 7. Solutions having pH less than 7 are called acidic. The solutions having pH more than 7 are alkaline in nature. The pH of the extracellular fluids is usually 7.4.

Acid is defined as any substance that can donate a proton. Base is a substance that can accept a proton.

Ampholytes refer to the substances that can act both as acids and bases. Water is the best example of ampholyte.

Buffer solution is one that resists a change in pH on the addition of acid or alkali. The ability to prevent large change in pH is an important property of most biological systems. The cytoplasmic fluids which contain dissolved proteins, organic substances and inorganic salts resists excessive change in pH. The blood plasma is a highly effective buffer solution almost ideally designed to keep the range of pH of blood within 0.2 pH units of 7.2 to 7.3; outside this range is not compatible with life. Acid base balance in the body means the regulation of pH of the body fluids. Only slight changes in pH from normal values can cause marked alterations in the rates of chemical reactions in the cells, some being depressed and others accelerated. For this reason the regulation of hydrogen ion concentration is one of the most important aspects of homeostasis.

The normal pH of arterial blood is 7.4, while the pH of the venous blood and of interstitial fluids is about 7.35 because of extra quantities of carbon dioxide which form carbonic acid in these fluids. The importance of buffers is biological fluids is best understood from recognising that many of the metabolites constantly being produced and utilized in the cell are weak acids. The maximum catalytic action of enzymes in the body cells is also pH dependent. A small change in pH may greatly reduce their activity.

An animal is said to have **acidosis** if the pH of the blood is less than 7.4 and alkalosis if the pH of the blood rises above 7.4.

Body Defences Against Changes in pH

Body has several mechanisms to resist the changes in the pH of body fluids.

1. **Buffer systems**: Many buffer systems are present in the body fluids that immediately combine with any acid or alkali and thereby prevent excessive changes in hydrogen ion concentration.
2. **By altering the rate of pulmonary ventilation**: If the hydrogen ion concentration does change measurably, the respiratory center is immediately stimulated to alter the rate of pulmonary ventilation. As a result the rate of carbon dioxide removal from the body fluids is automatically changed, and this causes the hydrogen ion concentration to return towards normal.

3. **By changes in the urinary pH :** When the hydrogen ion concentration changes from normal, the kidneys excrete either an acid or alkaline urine, thereby also helping to readjust the hydrogen ion concentration of body fluids back towards normal.

Total Osmotic Pressure

If pure water is placed on one side of a semipermeable membrane (e.g. bladder wall) and an aqueous solution is placed on the other side, the water passes through the membrane into the solution. This phenomenon is termed osmosis (from Greek for 'push'). The tendency to move through the semipermeable membrane is called osmotic pressure.

Osmotic pressure is the pressure developed by diffusion of a liquid or solvent through a membrane. The solvent passes from the dilute to the more concentrated solution through the membrane separating the two solutions. Osmotic pressure is defined as the pressure that must be applied to the solution side to stop fluid movement when a semipermeable membrane separates a solution from pure water. Osmotic pressure of the blood has values approximating 300 mOsm /L.

Osmotic pressure is a colligative property of a solution related to the number of osmotically active particles dissolved therein, not their size, molecular weight or chemical composition. Colligative properties are properties of solutions that depend on the ratio of the number of solute particles to the number of solvent molecules in a solution, and not on the nature of the chemical species present.

The osmotic pressure is proportional to the concentration of the solute and also to the absolute temperature, (degree Kelvin, K^{o}). Semipermeable membrane is one which allows the movement of the solvent but not of the solute.

Thus a solution of sugar separated from pure water by a semipermeable membrane will permit only the movement of water into the sugar solution but it will not permit the movement of sugar out of it. Thus there will be a net movement of water into the sugar solution (osmotic flow) through the membrane from the solution of lower solute concentration to the solution of higher solute concentration. Osmotic flow provides the basis for net water movement across many biological membranes and epithelia.

The sum of the concentrations of solutes in a solution is sometimes obtained by measuring the colligative properties of the solution (e.g. by measuring the depression of freezing point). The osmolarity so measured is expressed as osmoles or milliosmoles. These units are, in theory, equivalent to the molarity of a solution of an ideal non dissociating solute exhibiting the same colligative properties.

Osmotic pressure is a consequence of the total number of particles, dissolved in a solution. A 1 molar (1M) solution of glucose has the same number of particles as does a 0.5M solution of sodium chloride, or, more correctly, of sodium and chloride ions. Every molecule of sodium chloride dissociate into one Na^+ ion and one Cl^- ion, whereas the glucose does not dissociate. The logic can be extended further. Magnesium chloride ($MgCl_2$) dissociates to one Mg^{2+}ion and two Cl^- ions, for a total of three. Thus a 0.33M solution of MgCl2, a 0.5M solution of NaCl, and 1 M solution of glucose are all said to be isosmotic. The three solutions each contain the same number of particles.

Potassium is the most abundant cation in the intracellular fluid and it plays a vital role in the maintenance of normal cell functions. Thus, potassium homeostasis across the cell membrane is very critical because a tilt in this balance can result in different diseases that could be life threatening. Potassium is one of the most important minerals in the body. It helps regulate fluid balance, muscle contractions and nerve signals. What's more, a high-potassium diet may help reduce blood pressure and water retention, protect against stroke and prevent osteoporosis and kidney stones. Hypokalemia most often is associated with excessive potassium losses from the gastrointestinal tract as the result of vomiting or diarrhea. Hypokalemia occurs relatively frequently in domestic animals and may result from depletion of the body's potassium stores or from a redistribution of potassium from the ECF into the ICF space.

Insulin, the most important hormonal regulator of internal potassium balance, lowers plasma potassium by promoting the cellular uptake of the cation, specifically in skeletal muscle and liver.

Aldosterone is best known for its effect on transporting tissue, increasing potassium secretion in distal segments of the nephron and colon. Aldosterone concentrations are regulated by the renin-angiotensin system.

In metabolic acidosis, the excess hydrogen ions are buffered in the cell and electroneutrality is maintained by movements of intracellular potassium into the extracellular fluid. Respiratory acidosis and alkalosis do not significantly change potassium balance.

The activities of some genes have been identified to regulate potassium homeostasis. Notable among the genes are mammalian with-no-lysine K (WNK) kinases which are a family of four serine-threonine protein kinases, WNK1–4.

Electrolyte and Water Imbalances

Electrolyte imbalance, or water-electrolyte imbalance, is an abnormality in the concentration of electrolytes in the body. An electrolyte is a substance that conducts electricity when dissolved in water. They are essential for a number of bodily functions. Electrolytes play a vital role in maintaining homeostasis in the body. They help to regulate heart and neurological function, fluid balance, oxygen delivery, acid–base balance and much more. Electrolyte imbalances can develop by consuming too little or too much electrolyte as well as excreting too little or too much electrolyte.

Disturbance in acid base balance

Order of Response in Acid Base Disturbance

- First response – Reaction with buffers
- Second response – Compensation (respiratory or renal that may be complete or incomplete)
- Third response – Correction (complete or incomplete)

Metabolic Acidosis

Decreased HCO_3 results in the fall of all buffer bases of ECF and RBCs.

For each H^+ excreted, one HCO^- ion will be restored to the plasma.

Metabolic Alkalosis

Causes

- Persistent vomiting
- K^+ deficiency (H^+ excretion increases)
- Oxidation of ingested/injected salts of organic acids such as lactate or citrate
- Injection of bicarbonate solution

Respiratory Acidosis

Respiratory acidosis is a condition that occurs when the lungs can't remove enough of the carbon dioxide (CO_2) produced by the body. Excess CO_2 causes the pH of blood and other bodily fluids to decrease, making them too acidic. Symptoms and signs are a result of high CO_2 concentrations and low pH in the CNS and any accompanying hypoxemia.

The rise in PCO_2 represents a rise in carbonic acid and buffer reactions occur with the non-bicarbonate bases. Hb is the most important of these bases and reaction with it will be

$H_2CO_3 + Hb^- \longrightarrow HCO^-_3 + HHb$

This interaction between blood buffers results in an appreciable rise in plasma HCO^- concentration. Such reactions between blood buffers are known as interaction reaction. This buffer action ameliorates the fall in pH caused by the rise in carbonic acid.

Respiratory Alkalosis

- Respiratory alkalosis occurs when the levels of carbon dioxide and oxygen in the blood are not balanced.
- Body needs oxygen to function properly. During inhalation oxygen is introduced in the lung. During exhalation , carbon dioxide is released which is a waste product. Normally, the respiratory system keeps these two gases in balance.
- Respiratory alkalosis occurs when you breathe too fast or too deep and carbon dioxide levels drop too low. This causes the pH of the blood to rise and become too alkaline.
- Caused by hyperventilation which can be due to panic attacks, anxiety, heart attack, pain, drug use, asthma, fever, chronic obstructive pulmonary disease, infection, pulmonary embolism, pregnancy etc.
- Hyperventilation directly caused by ammonia toxicity and indirectly by hypoxemia acts reflexly via the peripheral chemoreceptors.
- Renal compensation: Renal compensation for respiratory alkalosis involves a decrease in HCO_3 – reabsorption.It begins in a few hours and reaches its maximal capacity after several days.

Body Buffers

Buffers are chemical compounds that prevent marked changes in hydrogen ion concentration when either an acid or a base is added.

Bicarbonate Buffer System: A typical buffer system consists of a mixture of carbonic acid (H_2CO_3) and sodium bicarbonate ($NaHCO_3$) in the same solution. Carbonic acid is a weak acid. When a strong acid, such as hydrochloric acid is added to a buffer solution containing bicarbonate salt, the following reaction takes place.

$HCl + NaHCO_3 = H_2CO_3 + NaCl$

From this equation it can be seen that the strong hydrochloric acid is converted into the very weak carbonic acid. Therefore HCl lowers the pH of the solution only slightly.

On the other hand if a strong base such as sodium hydroxide is added to a buffer solution containing carbonic acid the following reaction takes place.

$NaOH + H_2CO_3 = NaHCO_3 + H_2O$

This equation shows that the hydroxyl ion of the sodium hydroxide combines with the hydrogen ion from the carbonic acid to form water and that the other products formed is sodium bicarbonate. The net result is exchange of the strong base NaOH for the weak base $NaHCO_3$.

Thus, the mixture of carbonic acid and sodium bicarbonate acts as a 'buffer' to prevent either a marked rise or fall in pH. Fortunately this buffer is present in all the fluids of the body, both extracellular and intracellular and it plays an important role in maintaining normal acid base balance.

The Phosphate Buffer System

Another buffer system, the phosphate buffer system acts in almost identically the same manner as the bicarbonate buffer system, but it is composed of the following two elements : $H_2 PO_4$ and HPO_4. This system is especially important in the tubular fluids of the kidney because phosphate usually becomes greatly concentrated in the tubules. The phosphate buffer is also extremely important in the intracellular fluids because the concentration of phosphates in these fluids is many times more than that in the extracellular fluid.

The Protein Buffer System

By far the most plentiful buffer of the body is the proteins of the cells and plasma. There is a slight amount of diffusion of hydrogen ions through the cell membrane and even more important carbon dioxide can diffuse readily through cell membranes and bicarbonate ions can diffuse to some extent. The diffusion of these two elements of the bicarbonate buffer system causes the pH of the intracellular fluids to change approximately in proportion to the change in pH in the extracellular fluids. Thus, all the buffer systems inside the cells help to buffer the extracellular fluids as well.

The method by which the protein buffer system operates is precisely the same as that of the bicarbonate buffer system. It will be recalled that a protein is composed of amino acids bound together by peptide linkages, but some of the different amino acids have free acidic radicals in the form of - COOH, and some have free basic radicals in the form of - NH_3OH. Therefore, proteins can combine with either acids or bases and thereby provide a very high degree of buffering. Haemoglobin is the second most important blood buffer.

Respiratory Regulation of Acid Base Balance

Because carbon dioxide combines with water to form carbonic acid, an increase in carbon dioxide concentration in the body fluids lower the pH toward the acidic side, whereas a decrease in carbon dioxide raises the pH toward the alkaline side. It is on the basis of this effect that the respiratory system is capable of altering the pH either up or down.

Balance between metabolic formation of carbon dioxide and pulmonary excretion of carbon dioxide: Carbon dioxide is continually being formed in the body by the different intracellular metabolic processes, the carbon in the foods being oxidized by oxygen to form carbon dioxide. This in turn diffuses into the interstitial fluids and blood and is transported to the lungs where it diffuses into the alveoli and is transferred to the atmosphere by pulmonary ventilation.

If the rate of metabolic formation of carbon dioxide becomes increased, its concentration as well as hydrogen ion concentration in the extracellular fluids is likewise increased. Conversely decreased metabolism decreases the carbondioxide and hydrogen ion concentration.

On the other hand, if the rate of pulmonary ventilation is increased, the rate of expiration of carbon dioxide becomes increased and this decreases both the amount of accumulated carbon dioxide and the hydrogen ion concentration in the extracellular fluids.

Effect of hydrogen ion concentration on alveolar ventilation: Not only does the rate of alveolar ventilation affect the hydrogen ion conc of body fluids, but in turn the hydrogen ion concentration affects the rate of alveolar ventilation. This results from a direct action of hydrogen ions on the respiratory center in the medulla oblongata, which controls breathing. The condition called respiratory acidosis occurs when blood pH falls as a result of decreased respiration. Such a condition can be produced by **asthma**, **pneumonia**, **emphysema** or **inhaling smoke**.

Role of Kidney in the Regulation of Acid Base Balance

Kidneys assist in the regulation of body pH by the following means.

Urinary pH and the Secretion of H^+ Ions

In the process of adjusting the hydrogen ion concentration of the extracellular fluid, the kidneys often excrete urine at pH as low as 4.5 or as high as 8.0. When acid is being excreted the pH falls, and when alkali is being excreted the pH rises. Even when the pH of the extracellular fluids is at the normal value of 7.4, a fraction of a millimole of acid is still being lost each minute. The reason for this is that about 50 to 100 millimole more acid must be removed continually. Because of the presence of this excess acid in the urine, the normal urine pH is about 6.0 instead of 7.4 i.e. the pH of the blood. A similar situation also exists in case of domestic animals too.

Electrolytes

Electrolytes such as sodium (Na), potassium (K) present in body fluids and perform a variety of functions, which include.

i. Nerve impulse conduction
ii. As cofactor to facilitate enzymatic reactions. Molybdenum is a factor of enzyme Xanthine oxidase
iii. Muscle contraction (mainly Ca^{++}, K^+ & Na^+)
iv. Carbon dioxide (CO_2) and Oxygen (O_2) transport

The extracellular fluid is rich in sodium, chloride and bicarbonate ions. The intracellular fluid is however rich in potassium, magnesium, phosphate and sulphate.

- The principal ICF solutes are K^+, Mg^{++}, organic phosphates and proteins.
- The principal ECF solutes are Na+, Cl- and HCO^- .
- Imbalance in the concentration of these solutes between ICF and ECF results for many of the clinical signs associated with the primary diseases.
- Some electrolyte imbalance, however, are potentially life threatening and require immediate treatment.

Acid Base Balance Chemical buffers of ECF. Principal buffers of ECF are

1. Bicarbonate buffer
2. Hb
3. Plasma proteins
4. Phosphate

Buffers Activity if strong acid is added to blood

Bicarbonate buffer	53%
Hb	35%
Plasma proteins	7%
Phosphate	5%

- Hb is second most important buffer of blood
- Buffer system consist of weak acid and its conjugate base
- Hb molecule present in part in form of proteinate ion (Hb^-)
- Phosphate buffers plays a minor role in the blood.
- Phosphate buffers are important intracellular buffers because of their greater intracellular concentration and because their pK of 6.8, is closer to the pH in the intracellular fluid than in the ECF.

Intracellular K+	Secretion of H+ in urine
More	Decrease
Less	Increase

Isohydric Principle

- As a result of this principle, addition of an acid or base to a solution containing several buffers will result in a change in the ratios of all the buffer pairs.
- By isohydric principle, a fall in HCO_3 concentration will result in a fall of all buffer bases of ECF and RBC. This condition of low blood concentration of buffer base is known as hypobasemia.
- The total amount of base in whole blood, including bicarbonate, Hb and other bases of lesser importance is known as buffer base (BB).
- Normal value of BB is 48 mEq/l of blood but this varies somewhat with Hb concentration.

Evaluation of Acid-base Status

Blood variables involved in assessment of acid-base disturbance are pH, PCO_2, plasma concentration.

Thirst

Thirst is defined as a conscious desire to drink. The function of the thirst mechanism is to ensure that water will be replenished promptly when a deficiency occurs. Thirst is regarded as a general sensation arising from lack of water in the body. True thirst arising from lack of water in the tissues persists until need is satisfied and must be distinguished from the false thirst of dryness of the mouth or throat. Dryness of the mouth and throat will always be present in general dehydration of the tissues, but moistening this region without restoring tissue water will at best afford temporary relief. Several theories have been propounded from time to time to explain the mechanism of thirst.

The classical theories include

Dry Mouth Theory

- **General sensation** (dehydration)
- **Thirst center theory**.

In 1950, Andersson and his colleagues at Stockholm, Sweden established the importance of diencephalon (medial hypothalamus) in thirst.

The volume of fluid ingested depends also on the amount of water absorbed from the gastrointestinal tract. The hypothalamus is known to be involved in the regulation of water intake. If the temperature regulating center in the anterior hypothalamus is warmed, as it is during exercise or in a hot environment, the animal will drink more than it does normally. Cooling the hypothalamus has the opposite effect and destruction of the anterior hypothalamus also results in reduced water intake.

Area along the anteroventral wall of the third ventricle that promotes ADH release also stimulates thirst. Located anterolaterally in the preoptic nucleus is another small area that, when stimulated, causes immediate drinking that continues as long as the stimulation lasts.All these areas together are called the thirst center.Anderson and

McCann (1955) have shown that the center controlling thirst and drinking behaviour is located in the medial hypothalamus. They permanently implanted electrodes in a certain region of the hypothalamus of goats. When electrical stimuli were applied to the conscious goat, the animal would immediately seek and drink water although no water deficit existed. These investigators were also able to inject minute amounts of hypertonic solutions in the same region of the hypothalamus and they found that this also caused the animal to drink. These results suggest that the cells of the hypothalamus are sensitive to changes in osmo concentration and that such osmotic stimuli cause thirst and drinking behaviour.

The Thirst Mechanism is controlled in the hypothalamus

- The hypothalamus detects changes and stimulates release of antidiuretic hormone
- ADH signals kidneys to reduce urine flow and return more water to the bloodstream
- Kidney releases angiotensin II (stimulated by secretion of renin) which constricts the blood vessels and causes retention of water

Water is also drawn out of salivary glands in the mouth to cause dryness.

There are three major reasons why dehydration leads to thirst:

1. When saliva production decreases, the mouth and throat become dry. Impulses go from the dry mouth and throat to the thirst center in the hypothalamus, stimulating that area.
2. When you are dehydrated, blood osmotic pressure increases, stimulating osmoreceptors in the hypothalamus and the thirst center in the hypothalamus is now further activated.
3. Decreased blood volume causes a decrease in blood pressure that is signaled by baroreceptors and stimulates the release of renin from the kidney. This causes the production of angiotensin II which stimulates the thirst center in the hypothalamus.

Formation and Excretion of Urine in Birds

The urinary organs of birds consist of paired kidneys and the ureters, which transport urine to the urodeum of the cloaca.Each kidney is divided into cranial, middle and caudal lobes. Each lobe is composed of lobules. Birds do not have a bladder or urethra. Birds conserve body water by producing urine osmotically more concentrated than the plasma from which it is derived. The excretory system of birds differ from mammals in several important aspects.

- Presence of two major nephron types
- Presence of a renal portal system
- The main excretory product of poultry birds is **uric acid** instead of urea.
- Post-renal modification of ureteral urine

Avian kidneys are characterized by having two major nephron types, reptilian and mammalian. The reptilian-type nephrons are located in the cortex and lack loops of Henle. Reptilian-type nephrons are not capable of concentrating urine. The mammalian-type nephrons have normal mammalian type structure and function. A renal portal system mechanism allows greater blood flow to the kidneys when the birds are frightened by diverting more blood to the renal portal system with the opening of the renal portal valve.

The main excretory product of poultry birds is uric acid. Birds convert toxic ammonia to uric acid instead of urea as in case of mammals. Xanthine oxidase is an enzyme which catalyzes the formation of uric acid from xanthine and hypoxanthine, which in turn are produced from other purines. Uric acid is a compound similar to purines found in nucleic acids. It is water insoluble and tends to form a white paste or powder. Conversion of ammonia to uric acid in birds requires more energy and is much more complex than conversion of ammonia to urea in mammals.

Uric acid is a more complex structure than urea, being a cyclic compound containing four nitrogen atoms in its molecule. It is virtually insoluble in water and therefore non toxic. In those animals in which it is the major excretory product, its lack of solubility allows it to be voided as a thick paste or a solid pellet and it is accordingly especially suitable for production by animals living in conditions in which water is scarce. Most birds are Uricotelic.

Disruption in the metabolic process of excretion of uric acid leads to gout. So gout can arise either due to production of uric acid over the capacity of kidneys to excrete it, or due to compromised kidney function failing to excrete the produced uric acid. Poultry Gout in India is still one of the major causes for huge mortality and morbidity in poultry, causing great monetary losses to the producers.

The excretory system in the domestic fowl consists of the two kidneys, each with a ureter that carries the urine produced by the kidneys to the cloaca where it leaves the body. When the kidneys are diseased or damaged and unable to carry out their functions efficiently, the animal becomes debilitated and death often occurs quickly. Its functions in the domestic fowl are to:

- maintain the electrolyte balance
- maintain the water balance
- eliminate metabolic wastes, particularly nitrogen products of metabolism (except carbon dioxide)

The Kidneys

The two reddish-brown kidneys of the domestic fowl, each generally with three lobes, are found immediately behind the lungs on each side of the vertebral column and closely associated with it. A relatively straight, narrow tube called the ureter, leaves the medial border of each kidney and opens into the cloaca adjacent to the deferent duct of the male or the oviduct of the female. The ureter connects to many funnel shaped structures from each lobe of the kidney.

Urinary System

The kidney, on close inspection consists of the renal cortex and the renal medulla. A microscopic examination of a section of kidney will show that it consists of a large number of renal tubules, or nephrons, each divided into cortical and medullary parts. Birds have two types of nephrons. A small number of 'mammalian-type' nephrons with a Loop of Henle (used to help concentrate the urine) found in the renal medulla and a much larger number of 'reptilian-type' nephrons without the Loop which are located in the renal cortex. The renal tubules extract the constituents of the urine from the blood that flows through the kidney.

- A renal tubule or nephron is composed of the:renal corpuscle which consists of a close network of blood capillaries almost enclosed in a capsule, called Bowman's Capsule. It is here that the necessary very close association with the blood occurs.
- proximal convoluted (spiral-like) segment leading from Bowman's Capsule
- the loop of straight tubule called the Loop of Henle (only in the mammalian-type nephrons).
- distal convoluted segment.
- collecting tubule that direct the urine into the ureter for elimination from the body.

Urine

Like almost all birds, the domestic fowl does not have a bladder as is found in most mammals and amphibians. The urine leaves the ureters and enters the cloaca where it is moved by reverse peristalsis into the large intestine, which permits excess water to be re-absorbed before elimination. This re-absorbed water is available for use by the bird and, to some extent, offsets the limited ability of birds to concentrate their urine as efficiently as mammals. The urine is in a thick pasty form with a very low water content but high in uric acid from nitrogen metabolism. It is usually passed as a paste and is deposited as a whitish or cream cap on some faecal stools.

When the kidneys are not functioning as efficiently as normal, or sometimes when a very high protein diet is provided, there will be large quantities of uric acid in the blood and the system may be unable to cope. The kidney tubules are likely to swell with accumulated urate deposits and when this happens, the white lines are clearly visible on the surface of the kidneys. The accumulation may lead to damage of the kidney cells which leads to nephritis. The high concentration of uric acid in the blood may result in filtration through the capillary walls which leads to visceral gout, which is when a whitish deposit is found on the surface of many visceral organs. Infectious bronchitis may produce these effects.

Systems of Clinical Evaluation of Acid Base Disturbance

1. Based on plasma HCO^- (pH- bicarbonate diagram)
2. Based on concept of base excess (Siggaard-Andersen nomogram)

Siggaard-Andersen nomogram would not provide further information, but the pH-bicarbonate diagram would be instructional in better visualizing the type of acidosis or alkalosis.

Other Methods of Evaluation of Acid-base Disorder

1. Blood gas analysis
2. Anion-gap method (useful in evaluation of metabolic acidosis) Anion gap = $[Na^+ + K^+] - [Cl^- + HCO^-]$

In case of diarrhea, loss of both Na^+ and HCO^- so no change in anion gap.

In renal diseases loss of HCO^- and gain of Cl^- anion gap.

so no change in r Hb and HCO^-

Important blood buffers

- Proteins and organic phosphates provide intracellular buffering.
- Usually in blood total cations exceed the total anions, so there is an anion gap.
- Anion gap increases in metabolic acidosis and vice versa.

Ionic Basis of Action Potential

1. Resting (polarized) state
   - Since at rest, K^+ permeability is greater than Na+ permeability, therefore, K^+ channels maintain resting membrane potential.
2. Depolarization
   - At the point of stimulation, when depolarization exceeds 7 mV, Na^+ channel activation occurs through 'm-gates' i.e. voltage gated Na^+ channels start to open at an increased rate.
   - When firing level (threshold level) is reached, the influx of Na^+ along its concentration and electrical gradient is so great (18-20 times) that it overwhelms the repolarization forces and run away depolarization results.
   - Opening of voltage-gated K^+ channels (n-gates), therefore, within 0.3 msec. of the threshold excitation K^+ leaves the cell along its concentration gradient.
3. Repolarization
   - Repolarization starts with K^+ efflux due to opening of voltage gated K^+ channels and decreases in further Na^+ influx.
   - The opening of voltage gated K+ channels is slower and more prolonged than the opening of Na+ channels.
   - Fast efflux of K^+ and slow influx of Na+ causes net transfer of positive charge out of the cell that serve to complete repolarization.
4. After depolarization
   - At the termination of the spike potential K^+ conductance is slow down and thus a few milliseconds are delayed in restoring the membrane potential. This last phase of slow K^+ efflux is known as after depolarization.

Threshold intensity = 1 / Duration of stimulus

5. After hyperpolarization

- With the disappearance of the after depolarization, though the resting membrane potential is achieved yet the resting ionic status is not established.
- It is achieved by the active Na^+ -K^+ pump mechanism which transports 3 Na^+ out the cell for every 2 K+ it transports inside the cell.

Local anesthetic Block Na^* channels and Prevent generation of action potential

Refractory Period

Types

1. *Absolute refractory period :* Firing level to 1/3rd of the completion of repolarization
2. *Relative refractory period :* From end of the absolute refractory period to the start of the after depolarization.

The action potential elicited during the relative refractory period has a lower upstroke velocity and a lower 'overshoot' potential than does the normal action potential.

Summary

- Water is essential for life as most of the metabolic reactions must occur in aquatic environments.
- Intravenous (IV) fluid administration is probably the most frequently used therapy
- Dehydration is defined as an excessive loss of body fluid. Dehydration can be lethal, especially in young or depleted animals, and can promote secondary health problems such as acidosis and kidney failure in otherwise healthy animals. In dehydrated animals the mouth, tongue, nose or nostrils and eyes will be dry.
- Electrolytes play a vital role in maintaining homeostasis in the body. They help to regulate heart and neurological function, fluid balance, oxygen delivery, acid–base balance and much more.

12

Cerebrospinal Fluid Synovial Fluid and Bone Metabolism

Animal body contains several fluids other than blood and lymph which have specialized functions for specific organs. Two of these fluids are cerebrospinal fluid and synovial fluid. The cerebrospinal fluids protects and supports brain and spinal cord function. Synovial fluid protects the functioning of the movement of the body by bone-muscular joints.

Cerebrospinal Fluid

The fluid contained in the central canal of spinal cord, sub arachnoid space and cerebral ventricles is known as cerebrospinal fluid. Cerebrospinal fluid (CSF) is a clear, colorless body fluid found in the brain and spinal cord. The volume of cerebrospinal fluid in the human brain is about 150 ml .

Table 12.1: Rate of CSF formation in various species

Species	Rate (μl/min)
Mouse	0.325
Rat	2.1-5 4
Guinea pig	3.5
Rabbit	10
Cat	20-22
Dog	47-66
Sheep	118
Goat	164
Calf	290
Monkey	41
Human	350-370

Modified from Davson and Segal (1996)
a Estimated by ventriculo-dstemal perfusion
b Calhoun et al (1967).

It is produced by the specialised ependymal cells in the choroid plexuses of the ventricles of the brain, and absorbed in the arachnoid granulations. Major part of cerebrospinal fluid is formed in the lateral ventricles. The choroid plexus are tufts of capillary projections present inside the four ventricles of the brain and are covered by pia mater and ependymal covering. The rate of formation of CSF is 0.3 μl per minute in human beings. It is present throughout the ventricular system except for the cerebral aqueduct, frontal horn of the lateral ventricle, and occipital horn of the lateral ventricle.

CSF acts as a cushion or buffer for the brain, providing basic mechanical and immunological protection to the brain inside the skull and regulates the chemical environment of the central nervous system. CSF also serves a vital function in cerebral autoregulation of cerebral blood flow. In addition, it also circulates nutrients and chemicals filtered from the blood and removes waste products from the brain. It is a vehicle for intracerebral transport

CSF is derived from blood plasma and is largely similar to it, except that CSF is nearly protein-free compared with plasma and has some different electrolyte levels. Cerebrospinal fluid has a low content of albumin and other proteins compared with plasma.The cerebrospinal fluid is generally alkaline in nature and its specific gravity is about 1.005. The cerebrospinal fluid contains 99 % water and small amount of solids which include proteins, amino acids, cholesterol, urea, uric acid, creatinine and lactic acid.The inorganic substances present in the cerebrospinal fluid are sodium, potassium, magnesium, chlorides, phosphates, bicarbonates and sulphates.

A sample of CSF can be taken via lumbar puncture. Lumbar puncture is carried out under sterile conditions by inserting a needle into the subarachnoid space, usually between the third and fourth lumbar vertebrae. Some anaesthetics and chemotherapy are injected intrathecally into the subarachnoid space, where they spread around CSF, meaning substances that cannot cross the blood-brain barrier can still be active throughout the central nervous system.

Examining the fluid, removed via lumbar puncture, can be useful in diagnosing many neurological diseases, including multiple sclerosis, systemic lupus erythematosus, and neurosarcoidosis.

The first experiments demonstrating the existence of the blood-brain/blood-CSF barrier were performed by Paul Ehrlich at the end of the 19th century: he injected aniline dyes (trypan blue) into the blood of experimental animals and noticed that all organs with the exception of the brain were stained. The blood-brain/blood-CSF barrier was compared with a second cell membrane surrounding the whole CNS.

Blood-cerebrospinal fluid barrier at the choroid plexus level not allow the movement of several substances from blood to the cerebrospinal fluid.

Synovial Fluids-Composition, Formation and Flow

Synovial fluid is a viscous fluid found in the cavities of synovial joints. The joint cavities are known as synovial cavities. These joint cavities are filled with a small amount of viscous fluid that lubricates & helps movement of the joints. The principal role of synovial fluid is to reduce friction between the articular cartilage of synovial joints during movement. The synovial fluid is secreted by the cells known as synoviocytes. Synovial fluid is an ultra-filtration of plasma and the exchange between plasma and synovial fluid is under the control of hydrostatic pressure difference. Synovial fluid is made of hyaluronic acid and lubricin, proteinases, and collagenases. The synovial fluid has a high concentration of hyaluronic acid. Hyaluronic acid is an important mucopolysaccharide or glycosaminoglycan found in the ground substance of synovial fluid of joints and vitreous humor of eyes. It is also present as a ground substance in connective tissues and forms a gel around. Hyaluronic acid serves as a lubricant and shock absorbent in joints.The synovial fluid also contains a glycoprotein lubricin synthesized by synoviocytes.

The functions of the synovial fluid include:

- **Reducing friction** - Synovial fluid lubricates the articulating joints.
- **Shock absorption** - As a dilatant fluid, synovial fluid is characterized by the rare quality of becoming more viscous under applied pressure. The synovial fluid in diarthrotic joints becomes thick the moment shear is applied in order to protect the joint and subsequently thins to normal viscosity to resume its lubricating function between shocks.
- **Nutrient and waste transportation** - The fluid supplies oxygen and nutrients and removes carbon dioxide and metabolic wastes from the chondrocytes within the surrounding cartilage.

Synovial tissue is sterile and composed of vascularized connective tissue that lacks a basement membrane. Cells found in normal synovial fluid are lymphocytes, monocytes/histiocytes, and synovial cells.: Chronic, low-grade inflammation of the synovium (synovitis) is a hallmark of osteoarthritis. Rheumatoid arthritis is an immune mediated inflammatory disease (IMID). Rheumatoid arthritis has been associated with class II major histocompatablity (MHC) antigens. One of the most important groups of mediators in rheumatoid arthritis are cytokines. The most prominent of these are TNF, IL-1, and IL-6. These cytokines, released in the synovial microenvironment have autocrine (activating the same cell), paracrine (activating nearby cells), and endocrine (acting at distant sites) effects and accounting for many systemic manifestations of disease. Soluble mediators of inflammation that may diffuse in from blood and/ or be formed locally within the joint cavity include prostaglandins, leukotrienes, metalloproteinases.

Joints

The musculoskeletal system is a system of bony levers operated by muscles. Any connection between different skeletal elements is called a joint. Bones in the skeleton articulate (xkaBnkj) at joints and are connected to one another by means of ligaments and cartilage.

Types of Joints

- Synovial Joints
- Cartilaginous Joints
- Fibrous joints
- Gomphosis joint

Cartilage is a tough and dense but elastic and compressible tissue.Bones are connected to each other by ligaments and cartilage which are important in movement around joints. Bones are moved by muscles acting directly on the bones or indirectly via the tendons. Tendons are closely packed parallel bundles of collagen fibers.

The hip, elbow, knee and thumb joints are all freely moving joints called synovial joints. The surface of the bones of synovial joints are covered with a thin layer of slick, articular cartilage called hyaline cartilage. The area between the adjacent bones is called the joint cavity. The membrane lining of the joint cavity secretes a lubricant called synovial fluid. The combination of hyaline cartilage coating the bone surfaces and synovial fluid lubricating these surfaces gives synovial joints durability with smooth movement and low friction.

The synovial joints can be further divided into different types like ball-and-socket joints, hinge joints, saddle-shaped , planer joints etc.

Carilaginous joints, the articulating bones are united by means of cartilage and very little movement is allowed. Mostly found in fetal growth. The cartilaginous joint is between the ribs and the breastbone (sternum) and Intervertebral disks between the bodies of adjacent vertebrae in the spine.

Cranial sutures are fibrous joints of the skull. In this the bones are close together with a very thin fibrous tissue in between.

A gomphosis joint is between the roots of the teeth and the bone of the jaws.

Most muscles are connected to bones via tendons. Ligaments are cords, bands, or sheets of collagenous bundles that extend between and bind the bones forming a joint.

Arthritis, often called degenerative joint disease (DJD), is a condition that afflicts many horses. Arthritis is not only painful, but makes it difficult for a horse to move about. The condition is normally characterized as a slowly developing chronic disease of the joint in which the joint surface (cartilage) wears down, resulting in pain and subsequent lameness.

Regulations of Bone Metabolism and Homeostasis

Bone-one of the strongest biological materials in existence-is the main supporting tissue of the body. Bones provide the rigid framework of the body of animals and man. The skeletal system serves three main functions.

(1) It supports and protects the soft tissues and organs of the body. They act as anchors for muscles, tendons and ligaments and as the rigid levers that muscles operate to produce movement.

(2) It helps to maintain, through homeostatic regulation, the constancy of the ionic environment within the organism.

(3) It helps in locomotion with the help of muscles and tendons. Bones act as essential mechanical components of the musculoskeletal system.

The physiological function of bones include

- Production of blood cells
- Reservoirs of calcium (essential for blood clotting and muscle contraction)
- Storage of fat

The varied mechanical and physiological functions of bones are intimately related to structure of bone tissue which is very dynamic tissue. In spite of its great strength, bone is a very light weight material. The skeleton constitutes about 20 of the weight of the human body.

The bone is a composite material, formed of protein (collagen) and mineral (hydroxyapatite). Bone is a living tissue which can repair and reshape itself in response to external stresses.

The ends of long bones is called the epiphysis: the long, compact shaft, the diaphysis where it joins the epiphysis, the metaphysis. The diaphysis is composed of a hollow cylinder which contained the medullary cavity and bone marrow . During postnatal life , erythropoiesis occurs mainly in the bone marrow. In the adult, bone contains on a wet weight basis approximately 25% water, 45 Percent ash and 30 percent organic matter. With increasing age, the ash content progressively increases as the water content decreases; the organic fraction remains relatively constant. Calcium constitutes about 37% of the ash content, and phosphorus about 18.5%.

Cells of Bone

There are three types of cells associated with specific functional aspects of bone tissue. These are (1) Osteoblasts (2) Osteoclasts (3)Osteocytes. Osteoblasts participate in the ossification process and are readily observed when a new bone is being formed. Osteoclasts are mainly found at sites where bone resorption is taking place. Osteocytes present in bone proper, maintain bone as a living tissue. Each cell type is interrelated and is derived from a common ancestor.

The hip, elbow, knee and thumb joints are synovial joints and surface of bones participating in synovial joints are coated with a hyaline cartilage. The area between the adjacent bones is the joint cavity filled with a lubricant called synovial fluid which resembles egg white in consistency. This fluid nourishes the cartilage cells of the joint.

Adult bones are basically divided into two types. Compact and spongy bone.

Resorption and osteogenesis happen concurrently to maintain bone integrity.

Three calcium-regulating hormones play an important role in producing healthy bone: 1) parathyroid hormone or PTH, which maintains the level of calcium and stimulates both resorption and formation of bone; 2) calcitriol, the hormone derived from vitamin D, which stimulates the intestines to absorb enough calcium and phosphorus and also affects bone directly; and 3) calcitonin, which inhibits bone breakdown and may protect against excessively high levels of calcium in the blood.

Parathyroid Hormone (PTH)

Produced by chief cells in the parathyroid glands in response to decreased serum calcium. In response, osteoclasts increase in number and resorb mineralised matrix to increase Ca in blood.

Calcitonin

Produced by C-cells in the thyroid glands in response to increased serum calcium. Inhibits osteoclasts.

In neonates, bone growth predominates and modelling is important. In adults, the formation of bone is balanced by resorption - remodelling. It continues throughout life under the influence of hormones and mechanical pressure. Bone resorption may exceed formation in pathological states (hormonal, trauma, nutritional) or in old age and disuse.

Growth hormone from the pituitary gland is also an important regulator of skeletal growth. It acts by stimulating the production of another hormone called insulin-like growth factor-1 (IGF-1), which is produced in large amounts in the liver and released into circulation. IGF-1 is also produced locally in other tissues, particularly in bone, also under the control of growth hormone. Growth hormone is essential for growth and it accelerates skeletal growth at puberty.

Thyroid hormones increase the energy production of all body cells, including bone cells. They increase the rates of both bone formation and resorption. Deficiency of thyroid hormone can impair growth in children, while excessive amounts of thyroid hormone can cause too much bone breakdown and weaken the skeleton.

Osteoporosis is by far the most common bone disease. Osteoporosis is "a skeletal disorder characterized by compromised bone strength, predisposing to an increased risk of fracture". Bone mineral density (BMD) is one of the best predictors of fracture risk and is determined by the amount of bone accumulated at the end of skeletal growth, the so-called peak bone mass, and by the amount of bone loss subsequently. Factors affecting bone growth have a profound effect on BMD, and can ultimately cause osteoporosis.

Heredity is the most important factor for strong bones. Many genes have been identified as influencing bone mass and strength.

Summary

- Cerebrospinal fluid is an ultrafiltrate of blood plasma and there is a blood brain barrier between the blood and the cerebrospinal fluid.
- Synovial fluid is a viscous fluid found in the cavities of synovial joints. The joint cavities are known as synovial cavities. These joint cavities are filled with a small amount of viscous fluid that lubricates helps movement of the joints.
- Synovial fluid is made of hyaluronic acid and lubricin, proteinases, and collagenases. The principal role of synovial fluid is to reduce friction between the articular cartilage of synovial joints during movement.

- Arthritis, often called degenerative joint disease (DJD), is a condition that afflicts many horses.
- Cartilage is a tough and dense but elastic and compressible tissue.Bones are connected to each other by ligaments and cartilage which are important in movement around joints.

13

Endocrine System

Endocrine glands are organs which secrete chemical substances called hormones into the bloodstream. Hormones are chemical substances that are produced in one tissue, released into the bloodstream, and carried to other tissues, where they act through specific receptors to bring about changes in cellular activities. The term hormone is derived from the Greek root meaning to excite.

A hormone is a chemical transmitter. It is released in small amounts from glands, and is transported in the bloodstream to target organs or other cells. Hormones are chemical messengers, transferring information and instructions from one set of cells to another. Chemically the hormones are either peptides, proteins or steroids

The organs/cells where these hormones bring about their actions are called target organs/cells. The target organs (hormone binding receptors) possess specific receptors for bringing about the action of these substances. Hormones are extremely potent and are produced in very small amounts. Endocrinology is the study of the structure and function of the endocrine glands and their secretory products, including the consequences of excessive or deficient production of these hormones. Endocrinology is the study of cell-to-cell signaling that occurs via hormones that travel through the bloodstream to influence target organs.

Hormones-biologically active substances secreted by glands.

Endocrine- hormones that have a biological effect far away.

Paracrine- hormones that have a biological effect nearby.

Autocrine- hormones that have a local effect

The coordination of metabolism in mammals is achieved by the neuroendocrine system. Several hormones are the product of nervous mechanisms hence the term neurosecretion is used and neurohumor for such substances. The term neurosecretion signifies the production and release of hormones by nerve cells that have the cytological characteristics of secretory cells. The endocrine system and the nervous system are complementary communication channels between the various cells in the body. Hormones regulate processes in which cell activity changes relatively slowly such as digestion, reproduction, growth and development. When immediate action is desired, the body employs the nervous system.

Hormone Functions

Growth and development: Thyroid, GH, Sex Steroids, Cortisol

Reproduction: Estrogen, Testosterone, FSH, LH, Thyroid

Homeostasis: Thyroid, Cortisol

Changes in environment: Cortisol, Thyroid, Aldosterone

Hormones act as a mode of transmitting information in the body in addition to the nervous system. Their mode of action is slow but more prolonged..

Hormones are secreted in very small amounts but their actions are profound. Early investigators were hampered by the non availability of suitable methods for their estimation. The availability of radioimmunoassay, radio-receptor assay, enzyme linked immunological assay have greatly facilitated research in the field of endocrinology.

Half-life of a hormone is the time required for the disappearance or decay of one-half of a hormone in the body. Different hormones have different half life. Protein hormones have a shorter half life as compared to steroid hormones. Oxytocin and vasopressin have a very short half life. The half life of steroid hormones is more because of the inability of the body to destroy the cyclo-pentano perhydro phenanthrene nucleus found in all steroid hormones. The protein hormones get destroyed due to the presence of specific proteases present in blood and tissues of the body.

Hormone Cell Interaction

Hormones activate a cellular response in the target cell by binding to a specific receptor in the target cell. The specificity of hormone action results from structural complementarity between the hormone and its receptor. A hormone receptor is a molecule that binds to a specific hormone. Receptors for peptide hormones tend to be found on the plasma membrane of cells, whereas receptors for lipid-soluble hormones are usually found within the cytoplasm.

After binding with hormones, the receptor can initiate multiple signaling pathways that ultimately lead to changes in the behavior of the target cells. The hormone activity within a target cell is dependent on the effective concentration of hormone-receptor complexes that are formed.

Subcellular Mechanisms-metabolism of Hormones

Steroid hormones function by affecting the rate of synthesis of specific proteins. The steroid enters the target cell, binds with a specific receptor in the cytoplasm. The steroid receptor complex is transported to the cell nucleus. In the nucleus, these nuclear steroid proteins complexes influence the rates of synthesis of specific RNAs by altering the template DNA available for transcription. Lipophilic hormones—such as steroid or thyroid hormones—are able to pass through the cell and nuclear membrane; therefore receptors for these hormones do not need to be, although they sometimes are, located in the cell membrane. Upon binding by the hormone the receptor undergoes a conformational change, and the receptor together with the bound hormone influence transcription, either alone or in association with other transcription factors.

Parahormones

There are several compounds whose action in animals is like that of hormones but which are not hormones by definition, because of their diffuse origin e.g. Angiotensin, Erythropoietin, Bradykinin , Prostaglandins etc.

Proteins and Polypeptide Hormones

These hormones bind to a specific receptor in the plasma membrane of the target cell, with resulting stimulation of membrane bound adenylate cyclase. The membrane bound adenylate cyclase stimulates the formation of cyclic-AMP from ATP which further modulates the hormone action by acting as a second messenger. The cyclic-AMP activates the protein kinase. The protein kinase phosphorylates several specific enzymes to render them active or inactive to bring about the desired effects. Thus cyclic-AMP activates glycogen synthase while inactivating phosphorylase kinase in skeletal muscle. The net result is the stimulation of glycogen breakdown and stopping of glycogen synthesis in the muscle.

Q: Which is a secondary messenger of the mechanism of hormone action?

(a) ATP (b) cAMP

(c) Proteins (d) lipids

Ans. (b) cAMP

Synthesis of Hormone

Biosynthesis of protein hormones : Protein hormones are initially synthesized as preprohormone. Then cleaved in RER (Rough endoplasmic reticulum) to form prohormones and in the golgi apparatus to form active hormones, which are stored as granules before being released by exocytosis.

Biosynthesis of steroid hormone

Steroid hormones are derivatives of **cholesterol** that are synthesized by a variety of tissues, most prominently the adrenal gland and gonads. The cholesterol precursor comes from cholesterol synthesized within the cell from acetate, from cholesterol ester stores in intracellular lipid droplets or from uptake of **cholesterol-containing low density lipoproteins**.

Biosynthesis of steroid hormones requires a battery of oxidative enzymes located in both mitochondria and endoplasmic reticulum. The rate-limiting step in this process is the transport of free cholesterol from the cytoplasm into mitochondria. Within mitochondria, cholesterol is converted to pregnenolone by an enzyme in the inner membrane called CYP11A1 which is controlled by cytochrome p 450 family II subfamily A member I, which is a protein coding gene. Pregnenolone itself is not a hormone, but is the immediate precursor for the synthesis of all of the steroid hormones.

- Steroids are synthesized from cholesterol.
- Cholesterol is synthesized by the liver.
- Steroids are not stored but released as they are synthesized.

- The first step in the synthesis of all steroid hormones from cholesterol involves cleavage of the side chain of cholesterol to form pregnenolone.
- The above step occurs within the mitochondrion.

Fate of hormones

Kidney and Liver are the major sites of hormone metabolism and degradation.The hormone metabolism culminates into either target cell uptake, metabolic degradation and/or urinary or biliary excretion.

Therapeutic use of hormones

Most of these hormones have been of therapeutic interest for several decades. The mode of administration of steroid hormones can be both oral or parenteral while protein hormones are active only when injected. Several of these hormones are used for increasing the production potential of meat animals, for improving the reproductive efficiency of domestic animals, hence are of direct economic importance to the farmers. Chemical characterization and their synthesis including their more potent analogues in several cases, have greatly facilitated their widespread application in the animal production and animal health strategies.

Methods of Study of Endocrine System

Measuring Hormone Concentrations

Hormones are present in the body in very very small concentrations so the methods for measurement of hormones in accurate concentrations were developed only after the development of radio isotope measurement techniques in the 1950s or so.

- Gas Chromatography–Mass Spectrometry. GC–MS is a method of detecting and measuring the amounts of a chemical, using the separation of chemicals by chemical properties and mass. This technique is very accurate, but can be expensive and sometimes more specific than is needed for many hormone studies compared to immunoassays, which are cheaper and better for high-throughput analyses. However, GC–MS is often used to initially validate hormone measures in immunoassays.
- High-Performance Liquid Chromatography. High-performance liquid chromatography or high-pressure liquid chromatography (HPLC) is a type of column chromatography used to separate, identify, and quantify hormone concentrations. A column is packed with chromatographic packing material called the stationary phase. The solvent and the extracted hormones are the mobile phase and are moved via a pump through the column to a detector. The detector records the retention times of the hormones in the sample. Retention time varies depending on the interactions between the stationary phase, the hormones, and the solvent used.
- Immunoassays. Immunoassays are very important for measuring hormone concentrations. Radioimmunoassay and enzyme-linked immunoassays tend to be the most utilized assays and are very sensitive, which is important because

hormones can be biologically active in concentrations as small as part per trillion!.

- Radioimmunoassay and Radio receptor Assay.- RIA was developed in the 1960s and 1970s and allows incredibly sensitive measures of hormone concentrations. The assay relies on a hormone specific antibody, which competitively binds the unknown hormone of interest with a known concentration of radioactively tagged hormone. The amount of bound radioactive hormone is compared with a standard curve, which allows one to calculate the unknown hormone concentration.
- Enzyme-Linked Immunoassay.- ELISA works the same way as RIA except that instead of radioactively tagging the known hormone, the hormone is tagged with a color-changing agent that can be measured using a spectrometer. This method does not involve handling radiation, which can be a logistical advantage over RIA.

Receptors- mechanism of Regulation

A hormone is a secreted chemical messenger that enables communication between cells and tissues throughout the body. Hormones are released into the bloodstream through which they travel to target sites.

The target cell has receptors specific to a given hormone and will be activated by either a lipid-soluble (permeable to plasma membrane) or water-soluble hormone (binds to a cell-surface receptor).Lipid-soluble hormones diffuse through the plasma membrane to enter the target cell and bind to a receptor protein.Water-soluble hormones bind to a receptor protein on the plasma membrane of the cell.

Receptor stimulation results in a change in cell activity, which may send feedback to the original hormone-producing cell. A hormone receptor is a receptor molecule that binds to a specific hormone. There are two main classes of hormone receptors. Receptors for peptide hormones tend to be cell surface receptors built into the plasma membrane of cells and are thus referred to as transmembrane receptors. An example of this is insulin. A lipophobic hormone binds to a transmembrane receptors on, or within, the plasma membrane, to initiate an intracellular signaling cascade.

Receptors for steroid hormones are usually found within the cytoplasm and are referred to as intracellular or nuclear receptors, such as testosterone. A lipophilic hormone that passes through the plasma membrane of a cell, binds to an intracellular receptor, and changes gene expression. Nuclear receptors function as transcription factors because they can bind to DNA and regulate gene expression. Nuclear hormone receptors are activated by a lipid-soluble hormone such as estrogen, binding to them inside the cell. Lipid-soluble hormones can cross the plasma membrane.

Hormone Signaling

The glands of the endocrine system secrete hormones directly into the extracellular environment. The hormones then diffuse to the bloodstream via capillaries and are transported to the target cells through the circulatory system. This allows hormones to affect tissues and organs far from the site of production or to apply systemic effects to the whole body.

Hormone-producing cells are typically specialized and reside within a particular endocrine gland, such as thyrocytes in the thyroid gland. Hormones exit their cell of origin through the process of exocytosis or by other means of membrane transport.

Cellular recipients of a particular hormonal signal may be one of several cell types that reside within a number of different tissues. This is so in the case of insulin, which triggers a diverse range of systemic physiological effects. Different tissue types may also respond differently to the same hormonal signal. As a result, hormonal signaling is elaborate and hard to dissect.

Hormones activate target cells by diffusing through the plasma membrane of the target cells (lipid-soluble hormones) to bind a receptor protein within the cytoplasm of the cell, or by binding a specific receptor protein in the cell membrane of the target cell (water-soluble proteins). In both cases, the hormone complex will activate a chain of molecular events within the cell that will result in the activation of gene expression in the nucleus.

The reaction of the target cells may then be recognized by the original hormone-producing cells, leading to a down-regulation in hormone production. This is an example of a homeostatic negative feedback loop.

All peptide hormones are hydrophilic and are therefore unable to cross the plasma membrane alone.

Chemistry of Hypothalamo-hypophyseal Hormones

The hypophysis is a small gland situated at the base of the brain. The hypophysis consists of anterior and posterior lobes and the pars intermedia, which differ from one another histologically , embryologically and functionally. The anterior portion, the neurohypophysis, is intimately connected with the hypothalamus in the brain through numerous nerve fibres forming the hypophysis and neurohypophysis.

The hypophysis cerebri or the pituitary gland is called the master gland of the body, as the several hormones secreted by the adenohypophysis and neurohypophysis, affect and control almost all the important body functions and other endocrine glands of the body. The secretions of the pituitary gland affect a wide range of psychological processes. The following hormones are known to be secreted from the hypothalamus.

1. Thyrotropin (TSH) Thyroid-stimulating Hormone (TSH)

Thyroid stimulating hormone stimulates the thyroid gland to secrete thyroxine and triiodothyronine. These hormones regulate the basal metabolic rate of the animal. TSH is also essential for normal reproductive functions. Thyroidectomy during gestation of female rats causes reduced litter size and other derangement. TSH is also required for normal testicular development. Thyroid hormones are especially important during fetal development.

Structure

Thyroid stimulating hormone is a glycoprotein with α and β subunits. The α subunit consists of 92 amino acid residues and two carbohydrate chains, similar to LH and FSH. The hormone specific subunit consists of 113 amino acid residues and a single carbohydrate chain. It has a molecular mass of 28000.

2. Adrenocorticotropin (ACTH)

Adrenocorticotropin stimulates the adrenal cortex to synthesize and release the glucocorticoids and mineralocorticoids. These two classes of steroid hormones are involved in the regulation of glucose metabolism and osmotic balance. In addition, fetal ACTH plays a critical role in the initiation of parturition by stimulating the release of luteolytic factor from the uterus.

Structure

ACTH is one of the smaller pituitary hormones consisting of 39 amino acid residues. It contains neither carbohydrate nor disulfide bonds. The amino acid sequences of porcine, bovine, ovine and human ACTH are known and porcine and human ACTH have been synthesized.

3. Luteinising hormone or Interstitial cell stimulating hormone (LH or ICSH)-

The LH is a glycoprotein hormone made up of α and β subunit. The half life of FSH is 60 minute.

4. Follicle-stimulating hormone (FSH) –

The FSH is a glycoprotein hormone made up of α and β subunit. The half life of FSH is 170 minute.

5. Prolactin

6. Melanin Stimulating Hormone

7. Growth hormone or Somatotropin (GH)

Somatotropin was first characterized in the 1920s when Evans and Simpson demonstrated growth promoting effects in rats treated with a crude extract from pituitaries. It was not until 1945, however, that ST was isolated from the anterior pituitary. Growth hormone (GH) is essential for postnatal somatic growth, maintenance of lean tissue at maturity in domestic animals and milk production in cows. Somatotropin or growth hormone is a protein hormone synthesized in and secreted from the anterior pituitary gland. Somatotropin contains 191 amino acids. There are variant forms of ST. bST is released from the pituitary as four variants. These variants have either a leucine or valine substitution at position 127 and an alanine (191 amino acid sequence) or a phenylalanine (190-amino acid sequence) at the NH2 terminus.

High yielding cattle and buffaloes have higher levels of growth hormone in their blood which indicates that growth hormone is concerned with milk production (Jindal,

1988). Growth hormone is known to increase the partitioning of nutrients towards milk production instead of fat deposition. This phenomenon is known as homeorhesis . Advances in biotechnology made possible the production of large quantities of recombinant bovine ST (bST).

Scientists at NDRI (Dr. R.S.Ludri and colleagues) used A recombinant form of bovine GH administered to dairy cows and buffaloes to increase milk production. This increase in milk production is likely mediated by GH stimulation of IGF-1 production, which then has two effects.It causes energy generated by absorption of nutrients from the diet to be repartitioned away from formation of triglyceride in adipose tissue and toward mammary gland production of proteins, lactose, and fats that will be incorporated into milk. This reduces adipose deposition and prevents dairy cows from becoming excessively fat in late lactation.

It inhibits apoptosis of alveolar cells. Normally, milk production declines over time due to the loss of alveolar cells by apoptosis. Growth hormone promotes a longer and higher level of milk production.

The secretion of these hormones is under the control of several release and release inhibiting factors secreted by the hypothalamus in response to neural or chemical responses originating from the body or the environment of the animal.

Target Organs

Hormone Release Factors

The hypothalamic releasing factors are physiological substances which will stimulate or inhibit the release of adenohypophyseal hormones. These substances are formed in the hypothalamus, pass via the hypophyseal portal system to influence the release of specific adenohypophyseal hormones.

The control of production and release of the releasing factors by the hypothalamus is modified by a hormone feedback system from the target glands of the tropic hormones. In addition to the feedback system control, stimuli from the external environment also affect anterior pituitary hormone release. In seasonal breeding animals such as ewe, bitch or mare the photoperiod most strongly influences the hypothalamus output of releasing factors. Many other external stimuli such as pain, emotional disturbance, restraint, anaesthesia, sexual excitation or milking influence the output of various releasing factors.

The hypothalamus thus plays an essential role in the control of the secretion of several anterior pituitary hormones. The key position of the hypothalamus in new endocrine regulation is mainly due to the fact that this region of the brain contain simultaneously the final elements of several afferent pathways (the receptors sensitive to feedback message) and the first elements of several afferent (or executive) pathways (the cells synthesising the releasing the inhibitory factors).

The release factors secreted by the hypothalamus are transported to adenohypophysis via special blood vessels, known as hypothalamo-hypophyseal portal system.

The various hypothalamic hormones that control the release of hormones from the adenohypophysis are listed below :

1. Growth Hormone Releasing Hormone (GHRH)
2. Growth hormone release inhibiting hormone (GHRIH)
3. Prolactin release hormone (PRH)
4. Prolactin release inhibiting hormone (PRIH)
5. Melanocyte stimulating hormone release hormone (MSHRH)
6. Melanocyte stimulating hormone release inhibiting hormone (MSHRIH)
7. Corticotropin (ACTH) releasing hormone (CRH)
8. Thyrotropin releasing hormone (TRH)
9. Gonadotropin releasing hormone (GnRH)

Somatomedins are a group of proteins produced predominantly by the liver when growth hormones act on target tissue. Somatomedins inhibit the release of growth hormones by acting directly on anterior pituitary and by stimulating the secretion of somatostatin from the hypothalamus. Somatomedin -C is another name of insulin-like growth factor 1 (IGF-1). Somatomedin A, is another name for insulin-like growth factor 2. A synthetic analog of IGF-1, mecasermin, is used in children for the treatment of growth failure. IGF-1 is produced throughout life. The highest rates of IGF-1 production occur during the pubertal growth spurt. The lowest levels occur in infancy and old age.

Neurohypophysis-Hormones of the Posterior Pituitary (Pars Nervosa)

Two hormones, namely vasopressin and oxytocin are released from the posterior pituitary Oxytocin and Vasopressin are manufactured in the hypothalamus, but released in the posterior pituitary gland. Both are produced primarily in the neurosecretory neurons specifically the neurons of the supra-optic and paraventricular nuclei of the hypothalamus. Oxytocin and vasopressin were isolated and synthesized by Vincent du Vigneaud in 1953, for which he received the Nobel Prize in Chemistry in 1955.

The hormones are stored in the pituitary in association with two proteins; neurophysin **I** and II, with molecular weights of 19,000 and 21,000 respectively. Each neurophysin is specific for its hormone. The secretion of these two hormones is under nervous control which further derives stimulus from various other stimuli of the body like osmotic pressure. Vasopressin, or Antidiuretic hormone (ADH) affects the reabsorption of water in the distal convoluted tubules of the kidney and is necessary for the formation of a concentrated urine. Vasopressin if injected in large and unphysiological amounts causes a marked rise in blood pressure owing to the constriction of the arterioles.

Oxytocin

All neuro-hypophysial hormones including oxytocin are nonapeptides with a disulfide bridge between Cys residues 1 and 6. Oxytocin causes *contraction of the smooth muscle of the uterus* in the pregnant female at the time of parturition and also *contraction of non pregnant uterus* during sexual intercourse to facilitate transport of sperm. The primary use of oxytocin is to induce the labor in animals suffering from weak or no contractions at parturition. In late pregnancy, uterine smooth muscle (myometrium) becomes sensitive to oxytocin and helps in childbirth and parturition. It enhances uterine contractions by increasing the permeability of sodium ions across muscle cells and helps to move the foetus into the birth canal.

It also causes *contraction of the smooth muscles of the mammary gland*, resulting in milk secretion. Oxytocin in fact contracts the myoepithelial cells of the alveoli and is important in milk ejection during *milking* in domestic animals and *breast feeding* in human beings. Therefore the major action of oxytocin is to cause *milk letdown*.

(Singh, M. (2011). Oxytocin: The Cuddle Hormone-A Review. *Agricultural reviews*, *32*(4)295-303.)

Vasopressin or Antidiuretic Hormone

Vasopressin and oxytocin are nonapeptides i.e. they consist of nine amino acids. Both are formed in the cell bodies of *hypothalamic supraoptic nucleus* and are transported along axons in the neurohypophysis, from where they are released into the blood. The neurohypophysis therefore serves as a storage and release organ for the hormones that are produced in the adjacent parts of the brain.

The single most important function of ADH is to conserve body water by reducing urine output. There are 3 types of receptors for ADH: V1A - V1B - V2.

In the absence of antidiuretic hormone, *diabetes insipidus* occurs. This is characterised by extreme diuresis.

Mechanism of antidiuretic hormone action starts with the binding of hormones to receptors in the basolateral membrane followed by the a activation of Adenyl cyclase and the generation of adenosine 3', 5' cyclic monophosphate (Cyclic-AMP). The c-AMP activates the cyclic- AMP dependent protein kinases which in turn affects the microfilaments and microtubules in some way to greatly increase the permeability of luminal membrane to water.

Pineal

The pineal gland originates as a neuroepithelial evagination protruding from the roof of the diencephalon. The pineal is conical in shape and lies within the posterior of corpus callosum and between the superior colliculi of the brain. Pineal is situated between superior colliculi in the diencephalon. It forms the posterior boundary of the third ventricle under the corpus callosum above the hypothalamus. Pineal has cells of two types namely the stromal cells – secretary and glial cells. Pineal gland contains highly permeable capillaries.

It is connected by a stalk to the posterior commissure and habenular commissure. The stalk contains some nerve fibres but the gland itself is largely non-neural, being composed of glia and secretory type cells. The metabolism of pineal is controlled by environmental lighting by an indirect pathway involving sympathetic nerves.

Hormones of Pineal

The mammalian pineal gland is a source of several biologically active hormones; *melatonin, serotonin (5-hydroxytryptamine), histamine, norepinephrine* and other indoles. Indole is an aromatic heterocyclic organic compound with formula C_8H_7N. It has a bicyclic structure, consisting of a six-membered benzene ring fused to a five-membered pyrrole ring.

Melatonin is the most potent among these and the pineal gland is the sole source of this indole in mammals. Melatonin is a neurohormone that is secreted from the vertebrate pineal gland. Pineal gland synthesizes melatonin from serotonin in the presence of an enzyme hydroxyindole-0-methyltransferase. This enzyme is present only in the pineal gland.

The enzyme serotonin-N-acetyltransferase is the rate limiting enzyme in melatonin synthesis. This hormone (melatonin) shows a circadian rhythm in its activity.

Melatonin was first isolated from the bovine pineal gland in 1958.Melatonin displays high lipid and water solubility, which allows it to diffuse easily through most cell membranes, including the blood-brain barrier. Its half-life is about 30 minutes, and it is cleared mostly through the liver and subsequently excreted in the urine as urinary 6-sulfatoxymelatonin.

Functions of Pineal

Role in circadian rhythm - Melatonin levels are higher during night and low during day time.- ie the hormone shows diurnal variation. Melatonin's main job in the body is to regulate night and day cycles or sleep-wake cycles.

Melatonin is involved in various mammalian reproductive functions and also acts as an antioxidant. Melatonin and its receptors play a crucial role in the regulation of the animal reproductive process, primarily in follicular development. Melatonin has shown to have a prominent role in follicular growth, oocyte maturation, luteinization and early development. Melatonin and its receptors are present in female and male organs, such as ovaries, heart, brain and liver. Melatonin has numerous effects on animal reproduction, such as protection of gametes and embryos, response to clock genes, immune-neuroendocrine reconciliation of seasonal variations in immune function, and silence or blockage of genes. Melatonin appears to govern most of its cellular action through its ability to bind to its G protein-coupled receptors, MT1 and MT2, and thereby enhancing G protein activity.

The pineal hormone melatonin controls reproduction of photoperiodic mammals and is an integral part of the circadian organization in birds. Melatonin is anti gonadotrophic in long day breeders like hamsters while it stimulates the reproductive process in short day breeders such as sheep. In sheep and other mammals, exposure to darkness stimulates melatonin synthesis while light suppresses it. Thus sheep through melatonin action ensures spring parturition by having a long gestation period (short-day breeders).

Induction of sleep -Darkness causes the body to produce more melatonin, which signals the body to prepare for sleep. Light decreases melatonin production and signals the body to prepare for being awake.

The concentration of Melatonin at night in cows' milk is about four times higher than in milk collected during the day. This fact has triggered in the marketing of designer milk products from evening milk or melatonin enriched milk. An organic milk, 'Slumbering Bedtime Milk' (Red Kite Farm, UK), was launched in the UK which is said to contain higher levels of melatonin than ordinary milk.

A melatonin-enriched milk produced in Switzerland, 'Nachtmilch', was banned by regulators, who considered sleeplessness to be an illness, thus the milk was regarded as a medicine. Melatonin is most commonly used for insomnia and improving sleep in different conditions. For example, it is used for jet lag, for adjusting sleep-wake cycles in people whose daily work schedule changes (shift-work disorder), and for helping people establish a day and night cycle.

Melatonin also acts as mood modifier, antioxidant, and anticancer agent. Melatonin is thought to be involved in osteoporosis prevention.

The egg production is associated with the length and intensity of the light received by the bird daily. Light has an impact on the pineal gland and helps in synchronization of circadian rhythm and inhibiting melatonin release. Short photoperiods early in life will reduce feed intake and limit growth. In caged housing, laying hens respond well to artificial lighting.

Thyroid

Thyroid is an endocrine gland situated at the root of the neck on either side of the trachea. The thyroid gland is unique in that it is the only tissue of the body which is able to accumulate iodine in great quantities and combine it into a hormone, thyroxine.

Functions

Thyroid hormones are required for most of the important body functions like growth, development, maturation and reproduction. Thyroid deficiency is known to produce cretinism in man and domestic animals. Gonadal impairment occurs as a result of thyroid hormone deficiency. At the cellular level, thyroid hormones have their effect upon nucleic acid and protein metabolism. Thyroid hormones have a profound effect on the basal metabolic rate (BMR) of man and animals.

The finding that radioactive thyroxine is very tightly bound by the chromatin of liver cells of the tadpole, might suggest that thyroxine functions by depressing specific genes. Thyroxine promotes an increased concentration of several respiratory enzymes like glycerol-3 phosphate dehydrogenase of mitochondria, a flavin dehydrogenase functioning in the glycerol phosphate shuttle.

Control of Thyroid Hormones Secretion-Neuroendocrine Control

The thyroid gland is controlled principally by an interaction between iodine availability — a requirement for thyroid hormone synthesis — and thyrotropin (TSH) from the pituitary gland. The secretion of thyroid hormone from the thyroid gland is under the control of thyroid stimulating hormone (TSH) from the anterior pituitary. The secretion of thyroid stimulating hormone is further regulated by the Thyrotropin Releasing Hormone (TRH) from the hypothalamus. The release of TSH release factors from the hypothalamus is controlled by the feedback mechanism by the concentration of thyroxine in the blood and other neuroendocrine factors. External stimuli transmitted by the nervous system modulate the activity of the hypothalamus.

Biochemistry of Thyroid Hormones

Two hormones are secreted from the thyroid namely-Thyroxine and Tri-iodothyronine. Thyroxine (3,5,3,5'-tetra-iodothyronine) was identified as a thyroid hormone in 1915, another, even more active compound, 3,5,3' - tri- iodothyronine, was isolated from thyroid tissue in 1952. Although five other organic iodine compounds have been isolated from thyroid tissue, only one 3,3'-di-iodothyronine has any significant activity in mammals. The term 'thyroid hormone' is generally reserved for thyroxine (T_4) and triiodothyronine (T_3).

Approximately one third of the total iodine in the thyroid is in the form of T_4 and usually less than 10 percent is in the form of T_3. The thyroxine and triiodothyronine are derived from the amino acid tyrosine.

Thus thyroxine and 3,5,3' - triiodothyronine are iodinated derivatives of tyrosine. Although thyroxine is produced in much larger quantities than triiodothyronine, the latter is 5 to 10 times more active.

Thyroxine in the blood is attached to a specific carrier glycoprotein, Thyroxine binding globulin (Mol. wt. 55,000).

Disorders of Thyroid Function

Goitre refers to any abnormal increase in the size of the thyroid gland. This is caused by **deficiency of iodine** in the diet Noninflammatory enlargements of the thyroid gland develop in all domestic mammals as well as birds which indicate goitre. Goiter is much more common in neonates and growing animals. Certain plants may produce goiter when ingested in sufficient amounts eg Soybeans, cabbage, rape, kale, and turnips etc.

Iodine is a part of the thyroid hormones thyroxine and triiodothyronine; thus, insufficient iodine reduces the ability of the thyroid to make these hormones. With reduced circulating thyroid hormone levels, the pituitary secretes more thyroid-stimulating hormone (TSH), which acts as a stimulus for hyperplasia of the thyroid gland and subsequent development of a goiter. Goitre in human beings especially children is characterized by retardation of growth and mental retardation. In domestic animals treatment of goitre include Pot.iodide 200mg/kg Bw orally may be repeated one or two times and application of tincture iodine locally on the inside of the flank.

Use of Antithyroid Compounds in Animal Production

The induced hypothyroidism by feeding of antithyroid compounds like (thiourea, thiouracil) has been advocated to increase the weight gain efficiency of meat producing animals. The idea is that the sluggishness and sleepiness induced by hypothyroidism would supposedly conserve energy and favour fattening.

Thymus

Thymus is a small organ situated just above the heart. The thymus is a small, irregular-shaped gland in the top part of the chest, just under the breastbone and between the lungs. It is located in an area of the body called the mediastinum. The thymus is part of both the lymphatic system and the endocrine system. Before birth and throughout childhood, the thymus is instrumental in the production and maturation of T-lymphocytes or T cells, a specific type of white blood cell that protects the body from certain threats, including viruses and infections. The thymus produces and secretes thymosin, a hormone necessary for T cell development and production.

The thymus is divided into 2 main parts – a right lobe and a left lobe. Each lobe is divided into smaller sections called lobules that give the thymus its bumpy appearance. Each lobule is made up of a centre part (called the medulla) and an outer layer (called the cortex). A thin covering (capsule) surrounds and protects the thymus. The thymus is mainly made up of epithelial cells, immature and mature lymphocytes and fat tissue. The thymus changes in size as the animal becomes old. It is large in newborns. It is biggest during puberty then slowly begins to shrink as adulthood approaches.

The thymus makes T cells (T lymphocytes) that travel throughout the body to help fight infection, disease and foreign substances. T cells derive their name from the location of their production ie the thymus.The thymus also makes hormones to help T cells develop and keep the immune system working properly.The thymus helps in immunologic response by the body. The primary function of the immune system is to protect the host from invasion by foreign organisms. Lymphocytes travel from the bone marrow to the thymus, where they mature into T cells. Once T cells mature, they are able to leave the thymus and enter the blood so they can help the immune system. T cells also travel to lymph nodes and the spleen where they continue to mature. But how does the immune system avoid mounting attacks against the host organism? Selection processes early in the developmental pathways for immune cells kill or suppress those immune cells that react strongly with self-antigens. Examination of the developmental pathways leading to the production of mature cytotoxic and helper T cells reveals the selection mechanisms that are crucial for distinguishing self from nonself. These selection criteria are quite stringent; approximately 98% of the thymocytes, the precursors of T cells, die before the completion of the maturation process.

Thymosin is the hormone of the thymus, and it stimulates the development of disease-fighting T cells.Thymosin is a 5-Da polypeptide hormone secreted by the thymus gland. Thymosin α1 stimulates the development of precursor T cells in the thymus to mature T cells.Thymosins are a group of small peptides with molecular weights of 1000–15,000Da, originally isolated from the thymus gland (Goldstein, 2007; Goldstein et al., 2005), although it is now known that the major thymosins [thymosin-α1, thymosin-β4 (Tβ4), thymosin-β10, thymosin-β15] are present in a variety of mammalian tissues.

Thymosin, a protein hormone of the thymus gland, has been purified from bovine thymus tissue. Thymosin is an acidic protein, and is free of carbohydrate, lipid, and nucleotides. Based upon amino acid analyses, sodium dodecyl sulfate polyacrylamide gel electrophoresis, and sedimentation equilibrium data, thymosin has a molecular weight of 12,000 ± 200.

The thymus gland will not function throughout a full lifetime, but it has a big responsibility when it's active—helping the body protect itself against autoimmunity, which occurs when the immune system turns against itself. Therefore, the thymus plays a vital role in the lymphatic system (body's defense network) and endocrine system.

Pancreas

The pancreas is a tubuloalveolar gland and has exocrine and endocrine tissues. The exocrine is the larger of the two parts and secretes pancreatic juice; a solution containing enzymes for carbohydrate, protein and triacylglycerol digestion. Pancreatic juice drains into the small intestine. Pancreas has 2 major types of cells

1. *Acini :* Secrete digestive juices
2. *Islets of Langerhans :* Secrete insulin and glucagon.

The pancreas is a discrete structure external to the intestine lying in the dorsal mesentery.

Four types of functional cell population in Islets of Langerhans and their secretions

The endocrine cells of the pancreas constitute only 2-3% of the total pancreatic mass and are located in clusters of cells called 'Islets of Langerhans'.

The pancreas has both exocrine and endocrine function. As an exocrine gland it produces and pours into the intestine a series of enzymes (or rather pro-enzyme) which act upon all three major types of food materials (carbohydrates, protein and fat) and are responsible for a great part of the digestive activities of the gut.

As an endocrine gland, pancreas is credited to secrete two major protein hormones concerned with the body metabolism. These are insulin and glucagon. Liver is the most important target organ for the action of these two hormones.

The basic unit of Insulin consists of two polypeptide chains held together by cross-linkages of two disulphide bonds belonging to the amino acid cystine.

Insulin

Surgical removal of pancreas in dogs has been found to elicit symptoms similar to those in diabetes mellitus. This disease is characterised by a pronounced increase in the blood sugar level (hyperglycemia), the appearance of sugar in the urine (glycosuria), an increase in the concentration of ketone bodies in the blood (ketonaemia) and in the urine (ketonuria) and the excretion of large volume of urine (polyuria). These symptoms can be corrected by the parenteral administration of a pancreatic extract, the active principle of which has been identified to be insulin, a protein secreted by the islets of langerhans in the pancreatic tissue. The molecular weight of insulin is about 6000. Excessive blood glucose levels damage the blood vessels and nerves of the body's extremities, increasing the risk for injury, infection, and tissue death.

Insulin is secreted by the beta cells of the islets of langerhans in the pancreas. Insulin is synthesized as a precursor of insulin called proinsulin, which is converted to active insulin by the selective removal of a portion of the molecule.

The secretory rate of insulin by the beta cells is dependent upon the blood glucose concentration. As the level of blood glucose rises, insulin secretion is augmented and when the blood glucose concentration falls, the insulin production by the pancreas declines. Insulin facilitates the transport of glucose into cells by increasing the affinity of membrane carrier molecules for glucose. In addition, insulin activates enzymes involved in the synthesis of glycogen from glucose, one of which is glycogen synthase.

Insulin, like all peptide hormones, binds to specific receptors in the cell membrane, but instead of being confined to activating membrane bound enzyme system, the insulin receptor complex is internalized to act at specific intracellular sites or in the nucleus.

Baseline Blood Glucose Level

42-80 mg/dl in cattle, sheep and goat

62-120 mg/dl in dog, cat, horse and pigs

- Blood glucose concentration in mature ruminants is substantially lower than those in new born ruminants.
- In ruminants 30-60 mg/dl of blood glucose is required for normal physiological processes.
- Below this amount ketosis and other clinical signs become evident.
- Starvation in ruminants often causes a drop in blood glucose concentration to 20-25 mg/dl.

Adiponectin and resistin are very vital adipokines which influence the energy homeostasis, insulin sensitivity and mobilization of body fat stores.

Glucagon

Glucagon is a polypeptide with 29 amino acids and has a molecular weight of about 3500 daltons. Glucagon is composed of a single chain of amino acids with no disulphide bridge.

Glucagon causes a rise in blood sugar upon intravenous injection into experimental animals. Glucagon is secreted by the alpha-cells of islets of Langerhans.

Glucagon acts by stimulating the glycogen breakdown in the liver. Glucagon increases the concentration of cyclic AMP in specific target cells. Glucagon is secreted whenever the blood glucose level drops below the normal value of about 80 mg/100 ml.

The glucagon so released causes the liver to break down glycogen to restore the blood glucose to its normal level. Glucagon thus counter balances the action of insulin, which is secreted into the blood when the blood glucose level is high and subsequently causes glucose to be removed from the blood by the peripheral tissues.

Glucagon when synthesized is an inactive precursor, proglucagon, which contains additional amino acid residues at the C - terminal end of the glucagon chain.

Glucagon acts by binding to specific glucagon binding sites on the liver cell membrane, resulting in the stimulation of adenylate cyclase. The resulting increase in cyclic AMP causes an increase in the concentration of phosphorylase in the liver.

Insulin : Glucagon Ratio

- 50-on carbohydrate rich diet
- 2-during fasting or low carbohydrate rich diet

Somatostatin

The delta cells of islets of langerhans secrete somatostatin, an inhibitory peptide, that is also found in the brain and gastrointestinal mucosa. Somatostatin originally received its name from the function with which it was first associated, that is, the inhibition of tissue growth, so it is also called growth hormone-release inhibiting hormone (GIH). Pancreatic somatostatin appears to inhibit the release of both insulin and glucagon.

- Somatostatin is a paracrine hormone
- It inhibits release of insulin and glucagon

Somatostatin first isolated from the hypothalamus.

There are 2 main form of somatostatin

- 14 amino acids form – Predominates in pancreas and hypothalamus
- 28 amino acids form – Predominates in GIT.

Both have similar biological activity.

Pancreatic Polypeptide

The PP cells of the islets of Langerhans secrete pancreatic polypeptide, a hormone that inhibits pancreatic secretion of digestive enzymes. It is thought to play a role in appetite, as well as in the regulation of pancreatic exocrine and endocrine secretions. Pancreatic polypeptide released following a meal may reduce further food consumption; however, it is also released in response to fasting.

Gastrin

The delta cells of the islets of Langerhans secrete gastrin, a peptide hormone that stimulates cells in the gastric mucosa to produce gastric juice.

Adrenal

Adrenal glands, also known as suprarenal glands, are small, triangular-shaped glands located on top of both kidneys. Adrenal glands produce hormones that help regulate your metabolism, immune system, blood pressure, response to stress and other essential functions. Adrenal importance is indicated by its extreme vascularity. Histologically the gland is composed of two distinct parts: a cortical (outer) layer and a medullary (inner) portion. These two parts differ in function and development. The medullary portion is derived from the embryonic tissue which also gives rise to the sympathetic nervous system. The cortex originates from tissues from which the reproductive glands (gonads) are developed. The adrenal cortex and adrenal medulla are enveloped in an adipose capsule that forms a protective layer around an adrenal gland.

There are two endocrine organs in the adrenal gland, one surrounding the other. The main secretions of the medullary portion are catecholamines namely epinephrine, norepinephrine and dopamine. The outer cortex secretes corticosteroids.

Adrenal glands produce hormones in response to signals from the pituitary gland in the brain, which reacts to signaling from the hypothalamus, also located in the brain. This is referred to as the hypothalamic pituitary adrenal axis. In response to stress, the hypothalamus produces corticotropin-releasing hormone (CRH) that stimulates the pituitary gland to secrete adrenocorticotropic hormone (ACTH). ACTH then stimulates the adrenal glands to make and release cortisol hormones into the blood.

Adrenal Cortex

The adrenal cortex is the outer region and also the largest part of an adrenal gland. It is divided into three separate zones: *zona glomerulosa(*named after the Latin word for 'ball of wool'*), zona fasciculata (named after the Latin for a 'bundle of sticks')* and *zona reticularis*. Each zone is responsible for producing specific hormones.The adrenal cortex is essential for the life of an individual.The hormones from the adrenal cortex are chemically steroids. They are derived from the esterified cholesterol by a series of enzymatic reactions. Over 30 different steroids have been isolated from the adrenal cortex which include aldosterone cortisol and corticosterone.

Cortisol is a glucocorticoid hormone produced by the zona fasciculata that plays several important roles in the body. It helps control the body's use of fats, proteins and carbohydrates; suppresses inflammation; regulates blood pressure; increases blood sugar; and can also decrease bone formation. This hormone also controls the sleep/ wake cycle. It is released during times of stress to help your body get an energy boost and better handle an emergency situation.

Aldosterone is a mineralocorticoid hormone produced by the zona glomerulosa plays a central role in regulating blood pressure and certain electrolytes (sodium and potassium). Aldosterone sends signals to the kidneys, resulting in the kidneys absorbing more sodium into the bloodstream and releasing potassium into the urine. This means that aldosterone also helps regulate the blood pH by controlling the levels of electrolytes in the blood. Aldosterone is required by the kidneys to promote normal reabsorption of sodium ions in the tubules. Aldosterone also increases the reabsorption of chloride ions from the tubules. At the same time that aldosterone causes increased tubular reabsorption of sodium, it also increases the loss of potassium in the urine. Aldosterone also acts on extracellular fluid volume, cardiac output and arterial pressure, sweat glands, salivary glands and intestinal glands. The effect on glands is similar to that on renal tubules.

The adrenal cortical steroids augment secretion of HCL and pepsinogen by the gastric mucosa and trypsinogen by the pancreas. Cortisol and certain synthetic steroids are anti-inflammatory substances (e.g. Betamethasone and Dexamethasone).

The adrenal cortical insufficient subject does not readily cope with challenge to homeostasis by noxious stimulus.

Adrenal Medulla

The adrenal medulla is located inside the adrenal cortex in the center of an adrenal gland. It produces "stress hormones," including adrenaline. The adrenal medulla is not essential for the life of an individual while adrenal cortex is essential for life. This portion is credited with the secretion of hormones known as adrenaline (epinephrine), noradrenaline (norepinephrine) and dopamines. The adrenal medulla is practically a sympathetic ganglion where the postganglionic neurons have lost their axons and became secretory cells. The adrenal medullary hormones are mostly emergency "Fight or flee" response of the body. The fight-or-flight response (also called hyperarousal, or the acute stress response) is a physiological reaction that occurs in response to a perceived harmful event, attack, or threat to survival.

Beta blockers block the action of endogenous catecholamines—epinephrine (adrenaline) and norepinephrine (noradrenaline) in particular—on β-adrenergic receptors, part of the sympathetic nervous system that mediates the fight-or-flight response. They are particularly used for the management of cardiac arrhythmias, cardiac protection after myocardial infarction (heart attack), and hypertension.

Adrenaline and noradrenaline are amino acids derivatives collectively known as catecholamines.

Norepinephrine is also released as a neurotransmitter at sympathetic nerve endings and then affects the immediate postsynaptic cells.

Epinephrine promotes glycogenolysis in muscle and liver, resulting in elevation of the blood glucose level and increased lactic acid formation in muscle. Norepinephrine has little effect on carbohydrate metabolism.

The catecholamines have a profound lipid mobilizing activity, increasing the blood level of non-esterified fatty acids.

Epinephrine administered intravenously produces a marked rise in blood pressure and an increase in heart and pulse rate and in cardiac output. Norepinephrine exerts much weaker inhibitory influence on smooth muscle then does epinephrine. Epinephrine does not relax bronchial musculature and augments both systolic and diastolic blood pressure due to increased total peripheral resistance with little effect on cardiac output.

Epinephrine and norepinephrine are often activated in physically and emotionally stressful situations when your body needs additional resources and energy to endure unusual strain. Adrenal cortical hormones are released during short term stress response whereas long term stress response is mediated by adrenal medulla hormones.

Adrenal Gland Disorders

Cushing syndrome results from excessive production of cortisol from the adrenal glands. Cushing disease, also referred to as hyperadrenocorticism, is a common endocrine disease in adult and aged dogs. The signs result primarily from chronic excess of the hormone cortisol. Increased cortisol levels in dogs may result from one of several mechanisms. The most common cause (85% to 90% of cases) is a tumor in the pituitary gland. The pituitary tumor produces a hormone that triggers excessive development of the adrenal gland. Less common (10% to 15% of cases) is a tumor in the adrenal glands themselves.

Prostaglandins

Prostaglandins were first discovered in 1933 in extracts of human seminal plasma and in the vesicular gland of sheep but since then they have been found in a wide variety of tissues. The term 'Prostaglandin' was coined by von Euler (1935) in the belief that the biologically active substance found in human semen was a secretion of the prostate gland.

Structure of Prostaglandins

Many different prostaglandins are now known all with structures similar to that of PGE, which is a C_{20} carboxylic acid with two hydroxyl groups, one trans double bond and one keto group in a five membered ring.

Prostaglandins of the E and F series are formed in the seminal vesicles by cyclization and oxidation of polyunsaturated fatty acids. They have diverse pharmacological effects including stimulation of myometrial contraction; PGE_2 has been used clinically to induce labour in pregnant women.

The nomenclature of prostaglandin is based on the parent saturated fatty acid prostanoic acid, in which a five membered ring is formed by ring closure between carbon atoms 8 and 12. For example PGE is designated 9-keto-11, 15-dihydroxyprost-13 enoic acid. All the prostaglandins have unsaturated carbon chains and the different series are characterised by variations in the 5 membered ring. For example prostaglandins of the E series have a keto group on position 9 while those of the F series have a hydroxyl group at this position. All the prostaglandins are formed in the animal body by ring closure and oxygenation of essential polyunsaturated fatty acids such as arachidonic acid.

Occurrence, Biosynthesis and Metabolism

Although originally isolated from human seminal plasma and sheep seminal vesicles, PGs occur naturally in the tissues of many organs such as the brain, heart, lung, kidney, stomach, gut and iris, as well as uterus, placenta and testis.

The fatty acid precursors seem to be stored as part of the phospholipids of all membranes. PGs are rapidly synthesized from these precursors and are released at their site of action. They are rapidly inactivated in tissue by 1, 5-hydroxyprostaglandin dehydrogenase (PGDH) and D^{13} prostaglandin reductase and also by oxidation in the liver. The concentration of plasma PG are, therefore, low. The synthesis of prostaglandin is inhibited by aspirin.

Actions

In the reproductive system PGE, and PGE_2 increase the contraction of the pregnant uterus, but inhibit the motility and tone of the nonpregnant uterus. PGE_1 and PGF_2 are given intravenously and intravaginally to induce therapeutic abortion. PGF_2 increases the motility of both sperm and uterine tubes.

Evidence is accumulating that PGs are mediators of inflammation and some anti-inflammatory drugs, such as aspirin, have been shown to inhibit the biosynthesis of PG *in vitro*.

It has recently been suggested that prostaglandins play a part in hypothalamic control of body temperature. In the gastrointestinal system PGs increase motility and diminish gastric acidity. They increase renal blood flow, inducing a sodium and water diuresis, but also redistribute blood from medulla to cortex, thus antagonizing renin production. They also antagonise the action of vasopressin, and increase the motility of bladder and ureters.

Prostaglandins of different groups exert opposing effects on the cardiovascular, respiratory and hematological systems. Thus, while they exert positive inotropic and chronotropic effects on the heart and increase capillary permeability, PGEs and PGAs reduce the blood pressure in systemic arteries and veins while PGFs increase it. PGEs and PGAs increase regional arterial blood flows, including the coronary flow, but PGFs diminish regional arterial flow. Bronchial dilatation is produced by PGE and PGE_2 but bronchial constriction by PGF_2. PGE_1 inhibits platelet aggregation, while PGE_2 stimulates it.

PGs even inhibit spinal reflexes and the release of noradrenaline after stimulation of sympathetic nerves. They can cause contraction of the iris and cutaneous hyperaemia. They seem to act as local regulators of hormonal activity in vitro. They increase the levels of cyclic AMP and the synthesis of hormones in many endocrine organs and in the target tissues they can modulate the activities of many hormones or drugs mediated by cyclic AMP.

Prostaglandins exhibit their actions by binding to G-protein coupled receptors which are in turn linked to various G-proteins namely Gi, Gs and Gq. The G-proteins further activates adenylyl cyclase which forms cAMP and which further activates protein kinase enzymes.

All of the prostanoid receptors are G protein-coupled receptors. Prostaglandin receptors or prostanoid receptors represent a subclass of cell surface membrane receptors that are regarded as the primary receptors for one or more of the classical, naturally occurring prostanoids viz., prostaglandin D2, (i.e. PGD2), PGE2, PGF2alpha, prostacyclin (PGI2), thromboxane A2 (TXA2), and PGH2.

Prostaglandin in Testicular Function

Testis is a dual endocrine organ producing androgens as well as prostaglandins. Prostaglandin are needed for testicular capsular contraction, for seminiferous tubule contractions, sperm transport and androgen biosynthesis or release. Prostaglandins are needed for normal male fertility. Excesses of PGs, however, may cause infertility.

Prostaglandins in Animal Reproduction

1. $PGF2\alpha$ is the uterine luteolytic factor.
2. Prostaglandins have been used successfully in the **synchronization of estrus** in several species.
3. Prostaglandins play a role in oviposition in birds.

Prostaglandins play a central role in the initiation of labour. Potent analogues of prostaglandin such as cloprostenol and Fluprostenol have found use as luteolytic preparations in synchronization of estrus and induction of parturition.

Hormones of calcium metabolism- disorders

Calcium metabolism, particularly the levels of Ca found in blood and tissues, is regulated mainly by three hormones: (1) parathyroid (PTH) from the parathyroid glands; (2) calcitonin (CT) from the C cells of thyroid and ultimobranchial bodies, and (3) dihydroxycholecalciferol (calciferol), formed from vitamin D in liver and kidney, which increases calcium absorption from the gut.

The Parathyroid Glands

In the man and horse, the parathyroid glands consists of one or two pairs of beanlike organs located at or within the thyroid gland. In ruminants and the pig, the external parathyroid glands lie cranial to the thyroid near the carotid bifurcation. Ruminant internal parathyroids are usually found embedded in the thyroid gland, while in the pig no internal parathyroid is present. Parathyroid glands secrete parathormone which is mainly responsible for regulating the calcium metabolism in the body.

Histology

Each parathyroid is surrounded by a connective tissue capsule from which septa extend into the substance of the gland and imperfectly divide it into lobules. The substance of the gland consists of densely packed masses and cords of epithelial cells between which are interspersed small blood vessels. There are two types of cells in the parathyroid, the chief or the principal cells and the oxyphil cells. Parathyroid hormone is secreted by the chief or the principal cells.

Structure of Parathormone

The parathormone is composed of a single polypeptide chain with a molecular weight of 8500. There are 84 amino acids with no disulphide bridge. In the secretory granules, the peptide is present as a 90 residue prohormone containing six extra residues at N-termini.

Functions

Parathormone causes the calcium ion concentration in the blood plasma to increase. In this respect, parathormone is antagonistic to calcitonin, which prevents the plasma calcium to increase to an abnormal level. This in turn results in an increased renal excretion of calcium and because of the excessive loss of calcium, the bones become decalcified. Removal of the parathyroids has the opposite effect, leading to a fall in blood calcium concentration, followed by tetanic muscle cramps by the low blood calcium level.

Parathormone also causes an increased phosphate excretion by the kidney. Parathormone causes increased absorption of calcium from the gastrointestinal tract.

Control

The normal secretion from the parathyroid is apparently controlled by a simple feedback mechanism, because a high plasma level of calcium inhibits release of hormones from the parathyroid and a low level stimulates release.

The actions of parathormone are explained by its ability to stimulate adenyl cyclase enzyme.

Disorders of Parathyroid

Parathyroid hormone deficiency causes tetany (Tetany is a symptom characterized by muscle cramps, spasms or tremors). caused by malfunction of the parathyroid glands and a consequent deficiency of calcium. This can be reduced by giving very high doses of vitamin D or by injection of parathormone. Hypocalcemia in cows is not definitely related to decreased parathyroid activity. In dogs, hyperparathyroidism leads to a condition called "rubber - Jaw syndrome".

Thyrocalcitonin or Calcitonin

Calcitonin, is a calcium lowering hormone secreted by the 'C' cells or parafollicular cells of the thyroid. These cells are rich in mitochondria. Calcitonin is composed of a single polypeptide chain of 22 amino acids and has a molecular weight of approximately 3,600 daltons.

Calcitonin acts directly on the bones and inhibits the release of calcium. The secretion of this hormone is regulated by negative feedback. A high concentration of calcium in the blood causes release of calcitonin while at the same time the secretion of parathormone is decreased. Conversely, a low serum concentration of calcium causes the suppression of secretion of calcitonin while increasing the secretion of parathormone. Thus, blood calcium level is maintained by the actions of two hormones parathormone and calcitonin.

The serum calcium level is important as calcium is required for nerve transmission, muscle function and for many other metabolic reactions of the body. Excessive secretion of calcitonin, may lead to lowering of serum calcium to such an extent, that result in muscle tetany.

Calcitonin inhibits osteoclast resorption of bone and in this manner prevents loss of calcium and phosphate to the blood.

The anorectic and gastrointestinal motor effects of calcitonin are centrally mediated by the release of prostaglandins.

Renin-angiotensin System

Angiotensin

Angiotensin is a polypeptide secreted by the kidney. It has a profound effect on blood pressure. Extracts of kidney tissue if injected can cause acute hypertension.

The key information molecule is renin, an enzyme produced by the juxtaglomerular cells of the kidney and released into the blood under certain conditions, including ischemia. This triggers a series of reactions, beginning with the conversion by renin of renin-substrate, a globular protein in blood that originates in the liver, to angiotensin I. Asp-Arg-Val-Tyr-Iso-His-Pro-Phe-His-Leu. (Angiotensin -1) Another blood protein, known as Angiotensin converting enzyme, cleaves histidine and leucine from this decapeptide produce the octapeptide, angiotensin II. It is this molecule which, by constricting arterioles, causes the hypertension of renal origin.

The principal action of Angiotensin II is to cause general constriction of smooth muscle, but it apparently also acts on the zona glomerulosa of the adrenal gland to cause aldosterone to be released. Aldosterone is the principal agent of the adrenal that enhances sodium and water absorption by the kidney.

Bradykinin

Like angiotensin, bradykinin is a linear polypeptide that is released from plasma globulins and acts on smooth muscle. It is released in the mammalian plasma from bradykinogen by the action of proteolytic enzymes such as trypsin and plasmin. When released it gives rise to a fall in blood pressure due to vasodilation, but produces a slow contraction of certain smooth muscles and can cause pain sensations.

Atrial Natriuretic Factors

Discovery of the endocrine heart provided a shift from the classical functional paradigm of the heart that regarded this organ solely as a blood pump to one that regards this organ as self-regulating its workload humorally and that also influences the function of several other organs that control cardiovascular function. The concept of the heart as an endocrine organ arises from the observation that the atrial cardiomyocytes in the mammalian heart display a phenotype that is partly that of endocrine cells. Investigations carried out between 1971 and 1983 characterised, by virtue of its natriuretic properties, a polypeptide referred to atrial natriuretic factor (ANF). Another polypeptide isolated from the brain in 1988, brain natriuretic peptide (BNP), was subsequently characterised as a second hormone produced by the mammalian heart atria. These peptides were associated with the maintenance of extracellular fluid volume and blood pressure. The natriuretic peptide (NP) family comprises three principal members which are released in response to hypervolemic and hypertensive states.

Hormones of Heart (Natriuretic peptides)

Natriuretic peptides play a fundamental role in cardiovascular homeostasis by modulation of fluid and electrolyte balance and vascular tone. There are three main types of natriuretic peptides.

ANP (Atrial natriuretic peptide)

BNP (Brain natriuretic peptide or B-type natriuretic peptide)

CNP (C-type natriuretic peptide)

Atrial natriuretic Peptide (ANP)

Atrial natriuretic factor (ANF) also called atrial natriuretic peptide (ANP), is a peptide hormone which is secreted by cardiac cells of the body. Heart cells of atrial walls release this hormone to regulate the blood volume and arterial blood pressure. The atrial natriuretic factor is a potential vasodilator viz. it dilates the blood vessels to reduce the pressure. In response to the high blood pressure, cardiac cells secrete Atrial natriuretic factor which leads to vasodilation (dilation of the blood vessels) and thus, decreases the blood pressure.Circulating form has 28 amino acids. Has characteristic 17 amino acids rings formed by disulfide bonds. Also isolated form the brain.

Brain Natriuretic Peptide (BNP)

Brain natriuretic peptide (BNP), also known as B-type natriuretic peptide, is a hormone secreted by cardiomyocytes in the heart ventricles in response to stretching caused by increased ventricular blood volume.Has 32 amino acids. It is also present in the human brain but more is present in the human heart, including the ventricles. Have similar ring of 17 amino acids as in ANP.

C-type Natriuretic Peptide (CNP)

C-type natriuretic peptide (CNP) represents the paracrine element of the natriuretic peptide axis which complements the endocrine actions of atrial natriuretic peptide (ANP) and brain natriuretic peptide (BNP). CNP is produced by the endothelium and the heart and appears to play a prominent role in vascular and cardiac function, both physiologically and pathologically. It is composed of 22 amino acids.

- Present in brain, pituitary gland, kidney and vascular endothelial cells.
- Very little present in the heart and the circulation.
- It appears to be primarily a paracrine mediator.

Actions

- ANP and BNP in circulation act on the kidney to increase Na^+ secretion.
- Dilate afferent arterioles and relax mesangial cells -Increases glomerular filtration.
- Inhibits Na^+ reabsorption from kidney tubules.
- They relax vascular smooth muscles in arterioles and venules.
- CNP has a greater dilator effect on veins than ANP and BNP.
- Elevated plasma CNP levels are found in patients with heart failure, septic shock and renal dysfunction.
- Cardioprotective roles of CNP have evolved the possibility of use of use of neutral endopeptidase inhibitors in cardiac medicine.

Erythropoietin

Erythropoietin is a hormone, which regulate the process of erythropoiesis. Erythropoietin (EPO), is a peptide hormone secreted by a non-endocrine tissue, kidney. It is also known as hemopoietin. Erythropoietin secreted by the juxtaglomerular cells of the kidney which functions by triggering the RBC production in the bone marrow, especially when the oxygen level in the blood reduces. The formation of RBC is called erythropoiesis.

Erythropoietin (EPO) is a 30,400 daltons glycoprotein, consisting of 165 amino acids produced mainly in the kidney and in the liver

GI hormones

Gastrin, secretin, cholecystokinin (CCK) and gastric inhibitory peptide (GIP) are four peptide hormones secreted by endocrine cells of the gastrointestinal tract (GIT). These hormones help in the digestion by stimulating the secretion of different enzymes and gastric juices.

Gastrin: This stimulates the release of HCl and pepsinogen for digestion by acting on the gastric glands.

Secretin: Secretin stimulates the exocrine portion of the pancreas for the secretion of water and bicarbonate ions.

Cholecystokinin: CCK stimulates the secretion of pancreatic enzymes and bile by the pancreas and gallbladder respectively.

Gastric inhibitory peptide: As the name suggests, it has an inhibitory action on gastric glands and thus inhibits the gastric secretion.

Growth factors which help in normal growth and repairing of tissues are also a non-endocrine tissue secretion.

Secretion and motility in the gastrointestinal tract are regulated by a combination of nervous and hormonal stimuli. The hormones involved are polypeptides produced by the mucosa of various parts of the tract and either act locally or are released into the blood, when they may act on the same or different parts of the digestive system.

Bayliss and Starling (1902) was the first to show that a substance released into the blood from the duodenal mucosa of the dog stimulated pancreatic secretion. They named this substance as secretin. Several of the gastrointestinal hormones have been isolated in pure form.

Hormones from Placenta

The placenta connects the developing fetus to the wall of the mother's uterus during pregnancy. It grows in the wall of the uterus and is attached to the fetus within the uterine cavity by the umbilical cord. Although placenta is mainly an organ for the support and nourishment of the developing embryo, it also functions as an endocrine gland during pregnancy. The placenta is a temporary endocrine organ formed during pregnancy, which produces hormones important in the maintenance of a healthy pregnancy and in preparation for labour. Placenta is known to secrete estrogen and progesterone in the later part of pregnancy in several species. It is evident from the fact that in these species (eg sheep) ovariectomy during later part of pregnancy does not lead to abortion. It has been assumed that the steroid hormones produced by placenta are sufficient to maintain pregnancy. The estrogen and progesterone secreted by the placenta are used for the continued maintenance of pregnancy. Progesterone suppresses the ability of the muscular layer of the uterine wall to contract, which is important in preventing labour from occurring before the end of pregnancy.

The placenta also releases several protein hormones, which include human chorionic gonadotropin, human placental lactogen, placental growth hormone, relaxin and kisspeptin. Human chorionic gonadotropin is the first hormone to be released from the developing placenta and is the hormone that is measured in a pregnancy test. It acts as a signal to the mother's body that pregnancy has occurred by maintaining progesterone production from the corpus luteum, a temporary endocrine gland found in the ovary. Kisspeptin is a recently identified hormone. Kisspeptin (KISS1), a recently discovered neuropeptide that acts upstream of gonadotropin-releasing hormone (GnRH) neurons, is critical for maturation and function of the reproductive axis.

Endorphins and Enkephalins

It has become increasingly evident that the central nervous system produces more chemical substances with specific physiological actions than any body imagined a few years ago. A series of remarkable discoveries has come from studies of the action of such well known opiate drugs as morphine and heroin. These are used to suppress pain, but they also cause euphoria and, as everybody knows, are addictive. Because opiates do not occur naturally in animals, it was reasonable to assume that the opiate receptors must have some other normal physiological role and that there might be endogenous materials that normally act at these sites. The hypothesis has led to the tracking down of a whole series of endogenous substances that participate in the normal functioning of the nervous system-substances that may be involved not only in the suppression of pain, but also in change in mood and emotions and possibly also in certain types of mental disease.

The naturally occurring substances that interact with the opiate receptors are called endorphins. Among them are two pentapeptides, known as enkephalins. Several active polypeptides with somewhat longer chains are also known, and new active substances are constantly being found.

Some of them have the exact same amino acid sequence as certain fragments from longer peptide hormones, such as B lipotropin, which serves to mobilize fat from adipose tissue and is a chain of 91 amino acids. Because of the demonstrated action of smaller and larger chains, it is difficult at the present time to say which specific compounds are normally active in the nervous system and which are precursors or breakdown products.

Pheromones

A chemical substance produced and released into the environment by an animal, especially a mammal, affecting the behavior or physiology of others of its species. Pheromones are ectohormones meaning they act outside the body of the individual that is secreting them. Pheromones are usually produced by glands located on the skin, or by ducts within the body that have ducts leading to the body's exterior; the second variety of glands are known as exocrine glands.

Male effect in sheep and goats : In sheep and goats, the seasonally anestrous endocrine state of females is changed to the estrous state upon exposure to male scents . This so-called "male effect" is one of the most conspicuous primer pheromone effects. An olfactory molecule (4-ethyloctanal) has been shown to activate the central reproductive axis.

Summary

- Hormone is a molecule that is produced by an endocrine gland, secreted to the blood circulation and transported to other parts of the body, and recognized there by a specific receptor protein. Hormones are very much like neurotransmitters in that only cells that have receptors to the hormone can respond.
- Hormones are secreted from the endocrine glands in the body. Some of the major endocrine glands in the body include: Pituitary gland, Pineal gland, Thymus ,Thyroid, Adrenal glands,Pancreas,Testes,Ovaries.
- While hormones are essential to reproduction, they are fundamental to all the systems of your body.
- Growth hormone (GH) is essential for postnatal somatic growth, maintenance of lean tissue at maturity in domestic animals and milk production in cows.
- The hormonal substances used for growth promotion in cattle are the naturally occurring steroids: estradiol-17β,progesterone, and testosterone, as well as synthetic compounds such as zeranol, which has high affinity for estrogen receptors, trenbolone acetate, which has affinity to androgen receptors, and melengestrol.

14

Female Reproduction

Reproduction is essential for the survival of the species but not for the survival of the individual. The female reproductive system is entrusted with the responsibility to produce female gametes ie ova and hormones that regulate and integrate the functional activity of the female reproduction.The reproductive system of female domestic animals consists of (1) A pair of ovaries attached with ligaments to the uterus and (2) A pair of fallopian tubes the distal ends of which (infundibulum) serve to receive ova expelled from the ovary and the proximal ends enter the uterus (3) The uterus proper with its outer smooth myometrium and inner mucous endometrium which either sloughs off periodically or develops in part into a placenta, depending on whether pregnancy occurs , (4) cervix and (5)Vagina which serves to receive sperm. The female reproduction is slightly different from the male in that the reproductive processes are cyclic and substantially fewer gametes or ova are released at each ovulation. For successful reproduction, the reproductive processes of male and female must be in synchrony.

Genetic & Endocrine Control of Gonadal Development

Genetic Regulation of Fetal Sex Development involves a complex genetic cascade in which several factors either promote or repress each other in order to allow an initial bipotential gonad to differentiate into a testis or ovary .

The ovary is the primary female reproductive organ and has two important functions: Producing the female reproductive cell (the egg or ovum) and Producing the hormones estrogen and progesterone. This dual role is complementary, interdependent and necessary for successful reproduction.The two ovaries are connected to the back of the female with ligaments inside the main body cavity. Gonad development, sex determination, and reproductive success of offspring are highly dependent on sex hormone systems. The developing organism is exquisitely sensitive to alterations in hormone function. In the early embryonic state, the gonads of males and females are morphologically identical. Sex determination is the process by which the bipotential gonads develop as either testes or ovaries.

The first appearance of the gonad is essentially the same in the two sexes, and consists in a thickening of the mesothelial layer of the peritoneum. The thick plate of epithelium extends deeply, pushing before it the mesoderm and forming a distinct projection. This is termed the gonadal ridge. The gonadal ridge, in turn, develops into a gonad. This is a testis in the male and an ovary in the female.

At first, the mesonephros and gonadal ridge are continuous, but as the embryo grows the gonadal ridge gradually becomes separated off from the mesonephros. However, some cells of mesonephric origin join the gonadal ridge. Furthermore, the gonadal ridge still remains connected to the remnant of that body by a fold of peritoneum, namely the mesorchium or mesovarium. About the seventh week the distinction of sex in the gonadal ridge begins to be perceptible.

Sexual differentiation begins under hormonal influence during the prenatal period of fetal development, and thus, alterations in hormones during this highly sensitive period can have profound consequences. The balance of estrogens and androgens is critical for normal development, growth, and functioning of the reproductive system. Normal gonadal differentiation and sex development depend on the meticulous choreography and synchrony of a network of endocrine, paracrine, and autocrine signaling pathways reflecting the actions and interactions of specific genes, transcription factors, and hormones. Knowledge of the many genes, proteins, and hormones involved in gonadal sex determination and sexual differentiation is rapidly increasing. The expression of the male determining gene Sry is regulated by histone modification and DNA methylation. It is increasingly evident that epigenetic mechanisms contribute to establish the male fate.

Sexual differentiation and gonadal development are directed by the balance between gonadal oestrogen and androgen production. In the female fetus, there is no secretion of antimüllerian hormone (AMH), which is synthesized by the Sertoli cells of the fetal testis, Müllerian duct development in the female proceeds normally into the uterus and fallopian tubes.

Modification of Gonadotropin Release

GnRH agonists (e.g., goserelin, triptorelin, buserelin and leuprolide) are decapeptides, with similar structure to native GnRH and a great affinity to the GnRH receptors. After their binding to the receptors on gonadotropes, they initially cause gonadotropin release (flare-up effect) GnRH-agonists (GnRH-A) are generally used to down-regulate the secretion of pituitary gonadotropins and to inhibit ovarian steroid secretion. Gonadotropin-releasing hormone (GnRH) agonists (e.g., triptorelin) are used for androgen suppression therapy e.g. for the treatment of hormone-resistant prostate cancer.

Gonadotropin-releasing hormone (GnRH) and its analogs have been extensively used in clinical medicine since they were identified and synthesized in 1971. Native GnRH stimulates gonadotrophs of the anterior pituitary and has been used for induction of ovulation.

Ovarian Functions

When puberty, or sexual maturity is reached, the ovaries begin to function with a rhythm or cycle of activity, the most evident manifestation of which is estrus or heat. The production of oocytes causes the reduction of chromosome number to the haploid number by meiosis under the influence of meiosis-initiating factor. During meiosis, specific genes are more highly transcribed. Both transcriptional and translational controls determine the broad restructuring of meiotic cells needed to carry out meiosis.

Meiosis is divided into meiosis I and meiosis II which are further divided into Karyokinesis I and Cytokinesis I and Karyokinesis II and Cytokinesis II respectively. Meiosis I and II are each divided into prophase, metaphase, anaphase, and telophase stages.

The ovary performs two major functions.

1. The cyclic production of fertilizable ova
2. The production of balanced ratios of steroid hormones that maintain the development of the genital tract, facilitate the migration of the early embryo and secure its successful implantation and development in the uterus.

The shape of the ovary varies according to the species and stage of the estrous cycle. The epithelium covering the mammalian ovary is a single layer of cuboidal cells called the germinal epithelium.

Ovarian functions are regulated by the endocrine hormones of the hypothalamus, the anterior pituitary, the ovary itself and the uterus. The estrus period or heat is the period when the female is receptive to the male. The duration of heat in cattle is around 19 hours. The estrous cycle has a duration of about 21 days and it is composed of two main phases, the follicular and the luteal phase. The follicular phase precedes ovulation and is marked by fast follicular growth while the luteal phase is characterized by the presence of a corpus luteum.The duration of estrus and cycle is variable in different individuals and in different seasons of the year.

The ovarian parenchyma contains a large number of potential egg forming cells. There are many more of these than are required for the breeding life of females. New follicles begin to grow each estrus cycle one of which finally ovulates. The initiation of meiosis, the formation of the follicles and differentiation of steroidogenic cells are three major developments or events in the development of the ovary.

The ovary can be visualized and evaluated by transrectal ultrasonography technique. A 5-MHz or 7.5-MHz linear array or sector transducer allows imaging of ovaries, uterine horns, uterine body, and cervix. The technique is particularly useful for evaluation of the morphological and functional status of ovarian follicles and corpora lutea in the cycling animal.

The ovary in addition to producing germ cells or ova, acts as an endocrine gland. The ovarian hormones are chemically Steroids. There are two major types of ovaries steroids namely estrogens and progesterone.

Both Estrogens and progesterone have a cyclopentanoperhydrophenanthrene nucleus (three benzene rings and one pentane ring) in their structure.

The ovaries and placentas of cattle, pig and horses are known to secrete two estrogens namely-estradiol and estrone. In human beings only, a third estriol is also secreted. All the three steroids are c18 steroids. They are secreted primarily by the granulosa cells of the ovarian follicles, the corpus luteum and the placenta. Their biosynthesis depends on the enzyme aromatase, which converts testosterone into estradiol and androstenedione to estrone.

Estradiol 17 beta has been isolated from cattle placentas and appears to be the only identifiable estrogen in sheep and goat placentas.Pregnant mares excrete estrogens with additional unsaturation in ring B equilen and equilenin. Hydroxyestradiol - 6 has been found in the follicular fluid of pregnant mares.

LH Surge

LH release from anterior pituitary increases 7-10 times during 24 hrs prior to ovulation.

It promotes final development of primary oocytes.

The process of luteinization begins prior to ovulation so estrogen level decreases and level of progesterone increases prior to ovulation.

Following LH surge granulosa cells produces

Prostaglandin

Thromboxane Induces Local Response Similar to Inflammation

Leukotrienes

Weakens the follicular wall and promotes its rupture

Oxytocin ⟶ Promotes muscular activity ⟶ Assists spermatozoal transport in the female reproductive tract.

Progesterone has negative feedback effect on LH secretion so during diestrus secretion of LH decreases

Follicular Development Dynamics

The ovary is covered by the peritoneum except the attached border where the vessels and nerves enter. In most animals the ovary is somewhat divided into a cortex, in which the follicles with the developing ova are located and a medulla which is rich in blood vessels, lymphaticis and nerves.

The ovary contains several thousand tiny structures called primary follicles. Each follicle consists of a germ cell surrounded by a layer of cells. This germ cell has the potential to mature into an egg if the follicle completes development. However, most of the primary follicles never develop. Rather, they die, are absorbed by the ovary, and are replaced by newly formed primary follicles.

The relatively few primary follicles that develop completely do so through a series of phases. Many layers of cells are added to the single layer of cells surrounding the egg in the primary follicle, forming a central cavity. As the follicle and cavity grow larger, the egg becomes attached to the back of the follicle (opposite the ovulation site) by a stalk of cells. As the follicle continues to grow rapidly, the side opposite the egg bulges from the surface of the ovary and becomes very thin. Once the follicle reaches this mature state it is called a Graafian follicle. At ovulation, the thin portion ruptures to release the contents of the follicle, including the egg.

The follicle is the basic functional unit of the ovary containing the oocyte which is surrounded by specialized epithelial cells (granulosa and theca cells) which perform endocrine function.The bovine estrous cycle is characterized by two or three waves of follicular growth. These waves involve synchronous development of a group of follicles. Follicle development is controlled primarily by a feedback system involving gonadotropin releasing hormone (GnRH), follicle stimulating hormone (FSH), luteinizing hormone (LH), estrogens, androgens, progestin and other proteins. Follicular stimulating hormone is the main hormone responsible for the growth and development of follicles in the ovary. The dominant follicle of a follicular wave becomes larger than the other follicles and through the production of steroidal and non-steroidal substances cause atresia of the subordinate follicles of the wave and the static dominant follicle of the previous wave.

After two or three follicular waves, when the dominant follicle reaches a diameter of around 13mm., a surge of luteinizing hormone will cause ovulation. The LH surge is caused by the increasing amounts of estrogens produced by the granulosa cells of the dominant follicle. Once the follicle has released the oocyte, it will undergo luteinization. During the next phase of the estrous cycle, the dominant reproductive hormone is progesterone, produced by the corpus luteum. This hormone inhibits hypothalamic function via a negative feedback signal and consequently impedes any further follicular maturation during the life span of the corpus luteum.

Graffian follicles are follicles in which an antrum is clearly visible. Each Graafian follicle normally contains only one developing ovum. The follicles vary in size according to their stage of development, the more advanced one's project the surface of the ovary slightly.Ovulation is the release of mature ovum from the ovarian follicle. At maturity the follicle ruptures, thus allowing the egg / oocyte and follicular fluid to escape. The egg cell, or ovum (plural ova), is the female reproductive cell, or gamete. The key event in the process of ovulation is the preovulatory surge in luteinizing hormone (LH). LH Surge-LH release from anterior pituitary increases 7-10 times during 24 hrs prior to ovulation. Following ovulation, the cells that developed within the follicle differentiate to form the corpus luteum, which has the important function of producing progesterone.

Ovulation or the rupture of follicle is followed by haemorrhage, a blood clot which fills the old follicular cavity. After this process, the cells lining the walls of the follicle (stratum granulosum cells) take on renewed activity. They finally got converted to become the corpus luteum. The corpus luteum (CL) is a dynamic endocrine gland within the ovary secreting progesterone that plays an integral role in regulation of the estrous in domestic animals and menstrual cycle in human beings and maintenance of pregnancy. Progesterone is necessary for implantation of the blastocyst. Following implantation, the continued secretion of progesterone is essential to maintain a quiescent uterus and an intrauterine environment that is conductive to continued development of embryos. If implantation occurs, then the embryo signals the corpus luteum either directly or indirectly to continue to secrete progesterone and to prevent the corpus luteum from regressing. If fertilization or implantation does not occur, the corpus luteum regresses, and the consequent withdrawal of progesterone secretion leads to increased frequency of luteinizing hormone secretion, increased follicular estrogen synthesis and a new follicular phase.

The fimbriae of the oviduct picks up the ovum till fertilization takes place in the ampulla of the oviduct. Ovulation is either spontaneous (in response to gonadotropins and ovarian steroids) after endogenous surge of LH or induced (in which ovulation occurs in response to LH surge induced after coitus). The domestic animals cattle, buffalo, sheep, goat, mare, sow and bitch are spontaneous ovulator species. Animals like cat, camel, rabbit are induced ovulator species.

Endocrine and Receptor Profiles

Amongst different steroid hormones, estrogens are the most important hormones of reproduction and plays a vital role in development of anatomical, functional and behavioral characteristics that are necessary for reproduction of the species. Estrogens are the products of androgen metabolism catalyzed by the enzyme complex known as cytochrome P450 aromatase, encoded by CYP19 gene. The bovine CYP19 is mapped on chromosomes 10.

The corpus luteum is an important endocrine gland secreting progesterone required for the maintenance of pregnancy. The removal of corpus luteum during early stages of pregnancy is followed by abortion.

Thus ovulation encompasses the following events.

1. Cytoplasmic and nuclear maturation of the oocyte.
2. Disruption of cumulus cell cohesiveness among the cells of the granulosa layer.
3. Thinning and rupture of the external follicular wall.

Follicle-stimulating hormone (FSH) and Luteinizing hormone (LH) is a glycoprotein hormone of pituitary origin that regulates gonadal function, including steroidogenesis and gametogenesis. In cattle, two major specific hormones Follicle-stimulating hormone (F.S.H) and Luteinizing hormone (L.H.), their action mediated by receptor gene viz. Follicle-stimulating hormone receptor (FSHR) and Luteinizing hormone receptor (LHR) play important role in reproductive traits. The FSH receptor gene is expressed in gonads and the actions of FSH are mediated to ovarian and testicular somatic cells through these receptors. The Follicle-stimulating Hormone (FSH) starts and maintains follicular development by binding to its specific receptor (FSHR) in the surface of the granulosa cells in the ovary. This binding allows the activation of the FSHR coding gene. These changes in the molecular structure of the FSHR gene cause desensitization of the FSH receptors in the cell membrane, which results in a less afficient hormone signal transmission. The changes in the DNA sequence can affect the activation of the FSHR gene and indicate that the genotype plays an important role in ovarian physiology. The bovine FSHR is mapped on chromosome 11.

LH in females plays a role in the stimulation of the ovarian follicle to secrete estrogen, female sex hormone; also a surge of LH is responsible for ovulation. LH also has a role in the development of corpus luteum (CL), which is responsible for secretion of progesterone hormone associated with the pregnancy maintenance. The luteinizing hormone receptor (LHR) is a member of the subfamily of glycoprotein hormone receptors within the superfamily of G-protein coupled receptor (GPCR)/seven transmembrane domain receptors. The size of the mature receptor is 80-90 KDa. LHR has been localized in the target or classical, gonadal tissues as well as in the non-classical or non-target, extragonadal tissues.

Ovulation rate and litter size are important reproduction traits and are of high economic value. Prolificacy is defined as the number of live offspring per parturition. Some animals like Merino sheep , Garole sheep and Black Bengal goats have multiple ovulation and high prolificacy probably due to a single gene (Booroola). Average litter size of Garole has been reported as 2.27. There are evidence for the presence of naturally occurred beneficial gene (FecB) in these prolific sheep. The production of transgenic animals provides methods to rapidly introduce 'new' or modified genes and DNA sequences into livestock without crossbreeding or hybridizing. Efforts are on to produce prolific animals through transgenesis. Introduction of a mutated or engineered estrogen receptor (ESR) gene could increase litter size in a number of diverse breeds of pigs. The manipulation of reproductive processes using transgenic methodologies is only beginning and should be a rich area for investigation in the future.

Oviduct

The oviducts are a pair of tubes which carry the ova from the ovary to the uterus. The oviducts are suspended in the mesosalpinx, a peritoneal fold that is derived from the lateral layer of the broad ligament. The length and degree of coiling of the oviduct vary in farm animals. The oviduct is composed of fringe like fimbriae, funnel shaped infundibulum, the distal ampulla and proximal isthmus. The isthmus connects the ovary with the uterine lumen.

Functions of the Oviduct

The oviduct has a unique position in reproduction. It is in the oviduct that the ova are first exposed to conditions outside of the ovary. It is here where the sperm cells await the arrival of ova. Within the oviduct fertilization takes place, syngamy occurs, and the initial stages of clearance and development begin. The oviduct combines the essential components, environment, hormonal balances and biochemical constituents-which make it possible for all of these functions to take place normally and in orderly fashion, thus making the process of reproduction possible.

Uterus

The uterus is a fluid filled organ which is responsible for the development and nourishment of the embryo till its final expulsion as a calf or kid. The uterine fluid is the medium which provides a proper environment for embryonic development. In short, the uterine fluid is isotonic, having buffering capacity, provides nutrients for the embryonic development.

The uterus is a hollow muscular organ which is capable of expanding greatly, as it does during pregnancy. It consists of two horns, the body and the cervix. The horns are continuous with the oviducts but they are much larger. In most species, the line of demarcation is quite sharp, but in others one blends into the other gradually. The horns are about 10 inches long in mare, about 15 inches in the cow, 6 inches in the ewe and 4 or 5 feet in the sow. Implantation of fertilized egg and development of the embryo occurs in the uterus. The two layers of the uterus are endometrium and the myometrium.

Functions of the Uterus

The uterus serves the following functions

1. Transports sperm from the site of ejaculation to the site of fertilization in the oviduct.
2. Initiation of implantation, pregnancy and parturition.
3. Secretes substances responsible for the proper functioning of corpus luteum.

Cervix

Cervix is a sphincter like structure that projects caudally into the vagina. The cervix is characterized by a thick wall and constricted lumen. The cervix secretes cervical mucus, the consistency of which varies with the stage of estrous cycle. The cervical mucus during estrus shows a fern pattern of crystallization upon drying on a glass slide.

1. It facilitates sperm transport through the cervical mucus to the uterine lumen.
2. It acts as a sperm reservoir
3. During pregnancy, a highly viscid, thick and turbid mucus occludes the cervical canal, which prevents the invasion of bacteria in the uterine lumen and the fetus from coming out.

Vagina

Vagina is the copulatory organ in which semen is deposited and coagulated until spermatozoa are able to pass through the cervical mucus.

Vulva

The vulva is the terminal organ of both the urinary and the genital systems. It is a continuation of the vagina and the urethra and leads to its floor. The diameter of the vulva is considerably larger than that of the vagina. The walls of the vulva are well supplied with glands which are especially active during sexual excitement.

The clitoris lies partially embedded in the posterior floor of the vulva. It is a homologue of the penis and excepting the urethra, consists of the same parts.

Sperm Transport in the Female Reproductive Tract

During coitus the sperms are deposited either in the vagina (dog, ewe, cow) or in the uterus (cow, mare etc.). Sperms are carried from the site of insemination to the site of fertilization by muscular contraction of the duct system.

Efficient transport of a number of viable spermatozoa from the site of insemination or deposition in natural service to the site of fertilization is essential to successful fertilization.The spermatozoa gets transported to the oviduct by uterine contractions and spermatozoal motility.Other factors which influence sperm transport include ciliary movement in the oviduct and negative intrauterine pressure. The sperms are usually deposited during natural service at the cervix, the uterotubal junction and sometimes in the uterine lumen also during artificial insemination. Peristaltic contractions occur in the wall of the oviduct. During follicular phase these contractions occur from uterine to the ovarian end and during the luteal phase towards the uterine end of the oviduct.

Although quite a large number of sperms are deposited in the female genital tract, only a few reach the fertilization site. The fertilizing capacity of sperms is of much shorter duration than the duration of their motility. In the cow the duration of fertilizing capacity of the sperm is 28-50 hours while the maximum duration of motility is 96 hours.

Role of Seminal Plasma

Seminal plasma acts as a vehicle for transport of spermatozoa in the female genital tract. Besides, the seminal plasma is a source of metabolic substrates for the spermatozoa and supplies requisite enzymes effective in fertility.

Sexual Receptivity and Ovarian Sycle

Adult non pregnant animals undergo a cycle of sexual receptivity and a period during which the female will not accept the male. When the female is not pregnant, estrous occurs at regular intervals. The length of oestrous cycle varies from 16-24 days in domestic animals i.e. in ewe 16-17 days, cow, water buffalo (river type), sow, goat; 20-21 days; water buffalo (swamp type) 30-33 days; mare 20-24 days. However the dog has only one or two estrous cycles in the year, when ovulation and receptivity coincides with the males sexual interest in the female. The duration of estrus varies greatly with different individuals and species. The estrus is generally accompanied by ovulation which generally occurs 24 to 30 hours after the onset of estrus in most ewes, does and cows, 35-45 hours in sows and 4 to 6 days in mares.

The estrous cycle is composed of two distinct phases. The follicular phase is characterised by high estrogen content secreted by the Graafian follicles. The luteal phase is characterised by high progesterone content which is secreted from the corpus luteum. The corpus luteum is formed as a result of ovulation from the Graafian follicles. The estrogen and progesterone are steroid hormones which bring about distinct changes in the body. The progesterone secretion regresses abruptly some days before the next estrous. The decrease is brought about by the regression of corpus luteum function by several luteolytic factors , like prostaglandin from the uterus. The secretion of luteolytic factors is controlled by the hypothalamus. The duration of the luteal phase lasts from 14-15 days in ewes, and 16-17 days in cows and sows. The oestrus behaviour is of paramount importance to improve reproductive efficiency of dairy animals and is influenced by season. In buffaloes, the oestrus behaviour during summer is much depressed. The LH peaks are depressed in summer which has been suggested to be the reason for the decreased reproductive efficiency during summer in cattle and probably buffaloes, too.

Fertilization

If the cow is inseminated by a bull during estrus, it may get pregnant. The insemination can be either natural or artificial using fresh or frozen semen. The process of fertilization can be defined as the fusion of the male and female gametes to form one single cell, the zygote. The first important step of fertilization involves the passage of spermatozoa through the zona pellucida with the aid of acrosomal enzymes such as hyaluronidase and acrosin. The motility of the sperm is also an important aid for the penetration of the zona pellucida. The sperm genome has to be intact to participate in embryo development.

Zona Reaction

When the spermatozoa penetrates the zona pellucida, the zona reaction occurs. This reaction is a protective mechanism preventing penetration of the vitelline membrane by other spermatozoa. This is important since polyspermy is deleterious to the development of a normal zygote.

Once the spermatozoa penetrates the ovum, its head enlarges and converts into male pronucleus. Both male and female pronuclei enlarge before they move towards each other through the cytoplasm. The gamete pronuclei membranes come in contact and eventually fuse, incorporating the sperm and egg nuclei into a single cell. This process, known as syngamy, signals the completion of fertilization and the formation of the zygote. In most domestic animals, ova remains viable for about 12 to 18 hours after ovulation. If no spermatozoa is able to penetrate the ova during this period, the ova degenerates.

Postpartum Ovarian Activity

After calving, cows go through a period of temporary infertility known as postpartum anestrus. Cows will not experience estrous cycles during this time. Postpartum interval, is the time from calving to the subsequent conception.

The biggest impact of postpartum anestrus is the extension of the interval from calving to conception, which consequently impacts the calving interval. During gestation, circulating progesterone and estrogen concentrations remain high, exerting a suppressive effect on the hypothalamic–pituitary axis. The causes of postpartum anestrus in cattle are often multifactorial, but can be broadly categorized into physiological, nutritional, managerial, environmental, and pathological.

Cows or buffaloes must complete uterine involution and may experience short estrous cycles during their postpartum anestrus period. Uterine involution can be defined as the structural and functional regression of the uterus to a status that is capable of supporting another pregnancy. This process is completed in approximately 20–40 days following calving.

Suckling and presence of the calf has an important effect on resumption of normal reproductive activity postpartum. Suckling triggers a complex system of neural responses and hormonal feedback loops that result in reduced LH pulse frequency and amplitude by altering GnRH release. This results in decreased or hindered follicular development and a lack of follicles eligible for ovulation.

Nutrition plays an important role in postpartum anestrus.Demand of fetus during pregnancy puts the animal in negative energy balance at the time of parturition and postpartum period. Low negative energy balance decreases LH pulse frequency, growth rate and diameter of dominant follicle (DF), IGF-I, glucose, insulin concentrations and increases GH and certain blood metabolites. Females with restricted intake of energy have decreased levels of LH secretion, which is the hormone that signals ovulation.

Ovum transport

Since the survival time of ova and sperm is relatively short (20 to 48 hours), fertilizations depend primarily on the synchronous transport of the gametes in the female reproductive tract. The fimbriated end of the infundibulum picks up the ovum and the ovum is transported down the uterine tubes into the uterus by the combined actions of the cilia on the mucosal surface of the epithelial cells and contractions of the uterine tubes. The sperm-egg complex undergoes various maturational changes in preparation for fertilization. The transport time of ova in the oviduct varies with the species. In cattle, sheep, and swine, the transport time ranges from 72 to 90 hours. The fertilizable life of the egg is the maximal period during which it remains capable of fertilization and normal development. In most species, the egg is capable of being fertilized for some 12 to 24 hours. The attachment of sperm head to the zona pellucida is regulated by receptor sites on the zona surface. The mature oocyte synthesis a glycoprotein ZP3, which functions as the sperm receptor to which the sperm with intact acrosome can bind. The presence of glycosyl transferases, proteinases and glycosidases on the plasma membrane covering help the sperm head to bind with ZP3.

Transuterine migration of the egg through the common body of the uterus is common in ungulates.

Capacitation

Spermatozoa must undergo some change after they are deposited in the female reproductive tract in order to acquire the ability to penetrate the zona pellucida and fertilize the ova. This process, referred to as capacitation. Release of the acrosomal contents, which consist of the enzyme acrosin, a trypsin-like protease, and of hyaluronidase, plays a role in the spermatozoon's passage through the cumulus oophorus and the zona pellucida, allowing contact with the oolemma, the egg plasma membrane.Capacitation comprises at least three events.

1. There is removal or neutralization of the decapitation factor in those species having such an agent. Decapacitation factor is defined as that factor in seminal plasma which will inhibit capacitated sperm from fertilizing eggs.
2. Sperm of all species appear to acquire an acrosome reaction. This involves fusion and vesiculation of the plasma and outer acrosome membranes to form ports through which the acrosomal enzymes escape.
3. There is release and/or activation of lytic substances that allow the sperm to pass through the outer investments of the egg. Activation is defined as the removal of seminal plasma enzyme inhibitors from the sperm in the female reproductive tract.

The following enzymes seem to be activated in the capacitation process.

Acrosomal proteinase or Acrosin.

Hyaluronidase

Corona penetrating enzyme

Arylsulphatase

Acid phosphatase

B-N-Acetylglucosaminidase.

The role of acrosomal proteinase in fertilization can be inferred from the zona pellucida dissolving action of acrosomal extracts.

Estrogen facilitates capacitation in the rabbit uterus and oviduct. Progesterone may inhibit capacitation in the uterus or have other deleterious effects on the sperm. These results correlate well with natural events i.e. in most species sexual intercourse occurs only with defined periodic time limits (estrus) when the female tract is under estrogenic influence. So it is well for the continuation of these species that estrogen facilitates capacitation.

Fertilization

The oviduct has the unique function of conveying the eggs and spermatozoa in opposite directions, almost simultaneously. The fertilization of ova takes place in the ampulla. The embryos remain in the oviduct for three days before they are transported to the uterus. The oviductal fluid provides a suitable environment for fertilization and cleavage of fertilized eggs.

Fertilization is the union of the haploid sperm and the haploid ovum to form a diploid individual; the actual beginning of pregnancy. Fertilization is the union of viable ovum and sperm. It takes place in the ampullary isthmus junction of the oviduct.

At the time of fertilization, the ovum consists of a nucleus surrounded by a plasma (vitelline) membrane. The ovum is covered with a mucoprotein coat called the zona pellucida. The special granulosa cells (cumulus oophorus) that surround the zona pellucida are usually lost after ovulation.

Following capacitation and contact with the ovum, when the spermatozoa penetrates the zona pellucida, zona reaction occurs. This protective reaction prevents the penetration of the vitelline membrane by other sperms. This penetration is accomplished by the acrosomal enzymes, hyaluronidase and acrosin and trypsin like enzyme break down the hyaluronic acid – protein matrix of zona pellucida.

The spermatozoa upon penetrating the zona attaches to the vitelline membrane and stimulates the second meiosis in the ovum to form the second polar body and the ovum forms the female pronucleus. Once the spermatozoa penetrates the ovum its head enlarges and converts into the male pronucleus.

Both male and female pronuclei enlarge many times before they move towards each other.

The gamete membrane comes in contact with each other and fuse incorporating sperm and egg nuclei into a single cell. This process is known as syngamy.

Estrogen and progesterone hormones affect immune cells in the endometrium to prevent sperm rejection and to prepare the endometrium for implantation of the embryo. Abnormal inflammation which can be related to infection or an exaggerated immune response contributes to common reproductive disorders including endometriosis, infertility and pregnancy complications.

Reproductive Cycles in Farm Animals

The reproductive cycle relates to various phenomena: puberty and sexual maturity, the breeding season, the estrous cycle, postpartum sexual activity, and aging. These components are regulated by nutritional, environmental, genetic, physiologic, hormonal, behavioral, and psychosocial factors.

The level of fertility initiated at the time of puberty is maintained for a few years before it begins to gradually decline due to aging. The age at puberty is influenced by genotype, nutrition, management and climate. At the onset of the pubertal period, gonadotropin secretion rises.

Estrus or "heat" is a period during the reproductive cycle when female animals become sexually receptive. The oestrus cycle in the domestic animals like cow, buffalo etc can be divided into four phases: Proestrus; Oestrus; Metoestrus; Dioestrus. The mean length of the oestrous cycle in buffaloes is 21 days.

Recently nanomaterials based biosensors have been developed for monitoring the livestock reproductive cycles.

Hormones Present in the Biological Fluids During Pregnancy and Their Uses for the Diagnosis of Pregnancy

If the ovum becomes fertilized, a completely new sequence of events called gestation or pregnancy takes place and the fertilized ovum eventually develops into a full term fetus. The establishment of pregnancy in the cow involves a complex series of interrelationship between embryo, its uterine environment and the corpus luteum. The embryo is known to produce proteins, steroids and prostaglandins and also regulatory effect on the uterine blood flow, nutrient transfer, embryo migration and other events associated with the establishment and maintenance of pregnancy.

Implantation: Implantation is the most critical stage in the establishment of pregnancy. In cows, the conceptus remains detached from the uterus till it is getting implanted and it occurs by day 19 after fertilization. The first signal for maternal recognition of the pregnancy is interferon-tau (IFNt). The various key steps that are involved in the establishment of pregnancy include granulocyte involvement in follicle differentiation and gamete transfer, monocyte invasion of the peri-ovulatory follicle and their subsequent role in corpus luteum formation and the pivotal roles of maternal macrophage and dendritic cells. Different immune cells are involved during the critical period of implantation, but the information on the contribution of the maternal immune system to reproductive function in cattle is less as compared to humans. Neutrophils are the first immune cells to sense the implantation of the embryo in the uterus.

Although development before birth is a continuous process, gestation is sometimes considered in three stages.

- The period of ovum
- The period of the embryo
- The period of the foetus

The period of ovum: The interval from fertilization until about the twelfth day of pregnancy in the cow, is so named because during this time, the zygote retains its original shape. At first, it travels slowly down the oviduct, cell division has started and zygote changes from one cell to two, two to four and so on. At about the sixteen cell stage (fourth day) the zygote reaches the uterus, which has been prepared for it by hormone action. About the eight day the zona pellucida begins to break up and cells push outward. Layers of cells form and from these layers membranes grow that will nourish the developing embryo.

During this time the zygote is nourished by the stored materials that were in the ovum and by the nutrients absorbed from the oviduct and uterus. It changes from a single cell to several cells, which gradually form a hollow sphere, the blastula. During this stage a mass of cells accumulates at one side of the hollow sphere. This inner cell mass is destined to become the body of the embryo. The thin layer of cells around the outside of the blastula function primarily to nourish the embryo, it is called the trophoblast (germ nourishers). Usually the blastula remains in the same side of the uterus from which the ovum was released and only rarely does migration to the opposite side occur. At about 12 or 13 days the blastula ceases to float freely and remains in one place, held to the uterine wall by a weak surface attachment. Its elongation also tends to stop free movement. Firm attachment must await the development of extra embryonic membranes.

Period of the embryo: The period of the embryo, arbitrarily set in cattle as the interval from 13th day to the 45 day is characterised largely by the first formation of most organs and body parts. During this period the digestive tract, the lungs, the liver and the pancreas develop from the primitive gut. During this period the extra embryonic membranes are also formed and by means of them the embryo becomes attached to the uterine wall. By the end of the embryonic period the **placenta** is the sole source of nutrients for the developing calf.

Period of the Foetus : The period of the foetus is considered to extend from the 46th day after conception to birth of the calf at about 280 days. During this period the main changes are in the size of the fetus and in the differential growth of the various parts that were laid down during the period of the embryo. Early in the period of the fetus the eyelids are formed, the ossification of bone starts and rapid changes occur in the relative appearance and size of the limbs.

Hormones of Pregnancy

Progesterone is the key hormone of pregnancy which is secreted from the corpus luteum. The value for cattle are 6 to 7 ng/ml (nanogram/ml) for the first 14 days of pregnancy. The values increase somewhat with the onset of pregnancy and are maintained for most of pregnancy. Blood progesterone falls to 1 ng/ml on the day of calving and still lower during lactational anestrus. The estrogen levels remain low but a rise after day 250 is observed. The values reach maximum between the fifth and second prepartum days. In other animals also a rise and fall is observed in progesterone content during pregnancy and just prior to parturition. In some of the species, corpus luteum is not the only source of progesterone during the later part of gestation. Instead placenta replaces the function of the corpus luteum to secrete progesterone to maintain pregnancy. Ovariectomy in such animals during late gestation do not end up in an abortion (e.g sheep).

The corpus luteum is a transient endocrine gland that develops from a Graafian follicle following ovulation. The corpus luteum secretes progesterone and has an important regulatory role. Length of estrous cycle and menstrual cycle are determined by the duration of progesterone secretion.

The control of progesterone secretion by the corpus luteum is under the control of secretion from anterior pituitary gland, ovary, embryo and placenta. Luteinizing hormone from the anterior pituitary stimulates progesterone synthesis and is considered an important luteotropin. Administration of LH in cattle increases the luteal life span, whereas anti bovine LH causes luteolysis.

FSH has also been implicated in the control of progesterone secretion by the corpus luteum and FSH receptors have been located in the bovine corpora lutea.

The LH induced progesterone synthesis by luteal tissue occurs through a receptor mediated action. Luteinising hormone binds to a specific membrane receptor and activates adenylate cyclase resulting in cAMP synthesis. The hormone receptor complex is internalized subsequently by endocytosis and degraded within a lysosome. Increased intracellular cAMP concentrations stimulate protein kinase activity which may phosphorylate steroidogenesis enzymes (i.e. cholesterol esterase etc.) and thus increasing progesterone synthesis.

Prostaglandin F2 alpha and oxytocin have been regarded as the luteolytic agents which bring about cessation of progesterone secretion. The former is secreted by the uterus at the end of gestation and the latter is secreted from the posterior pituitary. It has been reported that prostaglandin F_2 alpha can increase oxytocin concentration.

The blood flow through the uterus is increased upto 20 fold during pregnancy. In this way the oxygen supply made available for the growing fetus is correspondingly increased. Just before parturition there is a sudden fall in the uterine blood flow which may represent a preparatory protective closing down of the placental circulation.

The placenta functions as an endocrine and paracrine organ by secreting a wide range of chemical messengers comprising proteins and growth factors into the maternal circulation. Pregnancy-associated glycoproteins (PAGs), a placental-derived family of inactive aspartic proteinases, are abundantly produced and released by the trophoblastic placental layer during pregnancy in ruminants .

Parturition

A normal pregnancy ends with the birth of the offspring. At parturition (the process of giving birth), the fetus is expelled from the uterus, passing through the cervix. The membranes that had formed around the fetus are also expelled and, collectively, are called afterbirth.

Successful parturition depends on Myometrial contraction and Capacity of cervix to dilate. Parturition is triggered by the fetus and completed by complex interaction of endocrine, neural and mechanical factors.

After parturition, the corpus luteum on the ovary begins to degenerate, a developing follicle on the ovary begins to release estrogen, estrus occurs, and the estrous cycle begins again.

The induction of parturition at or near term in domestic animals may be required for physiological and pathological reasons. Parturition can be induced by the injection of corticosteroids in cattle, sheep, horses and swine. PGF2α and its analogues (cloprostenol or fluprostenol) have luteolytic properties and the end of the progesterone inhibition on the uterine motility results in abortion or calving with a high rate of success. Oxytocin is also supplemented alongwith corticosteroids or prostaglandins. However, induction of parturition is accompanied by higher incidence of placenta retention.

An early and precise pregnancy diagnosis is an important criterion for better reproductive management in livestock like cows and buffaloes.

The pregnant human female secretes a hormone –human chorionic gondatropin estimation of which in the urine forms the basis of most pregnancy tests. The immunological tests are based on double antigen antibody reactions.

But no equivalent hormone is secreted by domestic ruminants so an equivalent test is not feasible in ruminants. Early pregnancy diagnosis is crucial to shortening the calving interval through enabling the farmer to identify open animals so as to treat and/ or rebreed them at the earliest opportunity.

In animals like cattle, buffaloes and mare's recto genital palpation and trans-rectal ultrasonography are the methods of choice for an accurate and early pregnancy diagnosis. Compared to cattle, rectal palpation in buffaloes must be gentle as the rectal mucosa is more fragile and bleeds easily. In sheep, goat, sow, bitch and cat ultrasonography is the only reliable method of pregnancy diagnosis. A 5-MHz or 7.5-MHz linear array or sector transducer allows imaging of ovaries, uterine horns, uterine body, and cervix. In the camel cocking of the tail is an effective method of pregnancy diagnosis and recto genital and ultrasonography are also useful.

As an alternative to USG, laboratory methods based on detection of progesterone hormones or specific antigens,such as Pregnancy Associated Glycoproteins (PAGs) have been developed/refined for farm animals. If progesterone is low 21 days after breeding, the cow cannot be pregnant. However, if the progesterone is high, the test is only 80% accurate at diagnosing pregnancy. This test is based on the assumption that cow have a normal cycle of 21 days and cows with short and long cycles can cause misinterpretation of the test.

The Early Pregnancy Factor (EPF) or Early Conception Factor (ECF) test was reported accurate on day 2 but the test was later shown to be inaccurate at any time. Other tests measure the biological response to interferon-t (day 16 to 18), progesterone in blood or milk (day 18 to 23), or pregnancy associated glycoproteins (PAG; after day 25). The three most studied bovine PAGs PSPB, PAG 67 kDa or bPAG-1.These molecules appear in the maternal circulation and can be determined with accuracy from 29 to 30 days post breeding.ELISA system developed to measure PAGs is a useful technique for early pregnancy detection.

Proteomics provides an opportunity to analyse proteins from a complex mixture of proteins in various body fluids. Future pregnancy diagnosis methods will involve proteomic methods to identify PAGs for pregnancy diagnosis.

Maternal Foetal Placental Participation in Pregnancy & Parturition

Maternal adaptations to pregnancy are largely mediated by the placenta; the functional interface between the mother and fetus that secretes hormones and growth factors into the mother with physiological effects. The important placental hormones secreted during pregnancy and parturition include prolactin-growth hormone family (e.g., prolactin, placental lactogen and growth hormone), steroids (estrogens and progesterone) and neuropeptides (serotonin, melatonin and oxytocin).

Immunology of Gestation

Reproductive Immunology is a very important yet poorly understood field which affects fertility and pregnancy outcomes. Healthy endocrine and immune systems work closely together to enable reproduction while providing immune protection against infections. Pregnant state has long been considered a state of relative immunosuppression to protect the allogeneic fetus. Pregnancy is not a state of total systemic immunosuppression but rather a state of dramatic immune modulation.The immunology of pregnancy has been considered as a host–graft response characterized by immune suppression and consequently a period of increased risk of bacterial and viral infection. Pregnancy is a more complex immunological condition. A successful pregnancy requires a robust, dynamic and responsive immune system. Embryo implantation and trophoblast invasion require a local inflammatory environment that promotes cell clearance, angiogenesis, cell growth and tolerance.

The immune system of the mother during pregnancy is tightly regulated to prevent an unwanted immune response against the paternal antigens present in the developing conceptus . Pregnancy is an immunological balancing act in which the mother's immune system has to remain tolerant of paternal major histocompatibility (MHC) antigens and yet maintain normal immune competence for defense against microorganisms. Interferon-β is a crucial immune modulator during pregnancy; it protects the fetus against viral infections and contributes to the process of immune regulation at the maternal–fetal interface.

Maternal inflammation due to viral or bacterial infections has detrimental consequences for fetal development. Uterine decidual and placental cells produce a huge array of cytokines which also help in modulation of immune function during pregnancy. Trophoblast - d NK (Natural Killer)cell interaction is essential for the success of pregnancy. The most common cells responsible for innate immunity are decidual natural killer cells, macrophages, dendritic cells and T-lymphocytes. It has recently been recognized that natural killer cells (NK) are very important in promoting fetal development because they secrete growth promoting factors. The immunological relationship between the mother and the fetus is a bi-directional communication determined on the one hand by fetal antigen presentation and on the other hand by recognition of and reaction to these antigens by the maternal immune system. During normal pregnancy, the implanting fetus is usually recognized by the maternal immune system and immune responses, including proinflammatory/proangiogenic responses to fetal antigens have been demonstrated. Impaired activation of Immune cells lead to pregnancy complications, including abortion and congenital infections. Several autoimmune factors have been investigated as possible influences on reproductive success and failure.

Priparturient Endocrine Events

Parturition encompasses the various physiological processes involved in the birth of the young. The young one is expelled from the uterine lumen, after the completion of the period of prenatal growth (gestation period). The gestation period is defined as the period from the time an animal conceives until she gives birth to the young. The gestation period varies considerably between different species and among animals of the same breed as well as between different breeds. The gestation period of various domestic animals is given below.

Primiparous heifers will average approximately two days less than pluriparous cows of the same breed. The gestation period of buffaloes is longer than that of cows and is approx. 310 to 330 days. Murrah tend to have a shorter gestation period (315 days) than swamp buffaloes (330 days). In some cows, mares and pigs, the gestation period may get unduly prolonged (Delayed parturition) which may result in complication at the time of birth and the delivery of considerable large fetuses. The variation in gestation length of different cattle and buffaloes breeds is shown in table below.

When the period of embryonic growth ends, the fetuses are expelled from the uterine lumen. For delivery of the fetus it is necessary that the uterine myometrium be converted from a quiescent organ to an actively contracting one. This change in the uterine myometrium is brought about by a complex interplay of neuroendocrine mechanism at the time of parturition.

Parturition is the physiologic process by which a fetus is expelled from the uterus. Parturition is a complex physiologic process involving fetal, placental, and maternal signals. A variety of endocrine systems play a role in the maintenance of uterine quiescence and the onset of parturition, with its attendant increase in uterine contractility and cervical ripening. It requires the presence of regular painful uterine contractions, which increase in frequency, intensity and duration leading to progressive cervical effacement and dilatation.

The major hormones during pregnancy is *progesterone* which is secreted in high amounts from the corpora lutea as well as from placenta.

Progesterone prevents the uterine myometrium from contracting or expelling the fetus prematurely.

The other hormone present in the plasma is estrogen. The levels of estrogens rise just prior to parturition. The estrogens are important for the production of uterine contractile proteins during the last stage of pregnancy.

Another change which occurs at the time of parturition is the decrease in the level of progesterone, thus removing the progesterone block on the contraction of the uterine myometrium. This decrease in progesterone concentration is brought about by a complex interplay involving fetal pituitary and adrenal cortex. It is thought that the fetal hypophyseal-adrenal system causes the secretion of fetal cortisol which in turn causes the synthesis of estrogens instead of progesterone by the placenta. The increased estrogens cause the release of PGF 2 alpha which acts as a luteolytic factor and causes the regression of the corpus luteum of pregnancy. Prepartum luteolysis passively allows the myometrium to become contractile.

Further progress in the parturition is brought about the release of oxytocin from the posterior pituitary. The release of oxytocin is initiated via impulses through the spinal cord to the hypothalamus, once the fetus becomes engaged in the pelvic canal. It enhances the rhythmic contraction of the uterine musculature during the delivery process.

Another important hormone in the parturition process is relaxin which brings about the softening of the cervix. Relaxin is produced by the placenta as well as by the corpus luteum.

The biochemical connective tissue changes in the cervix usually precede uterine contractions that, in turn, lead to cervical dilatation. Fetus hormones are important in control of timing of parturition. Activated fetal hypothalamic-pituitary-adrenal (HPA) axis leads to a surge in adrenal cortisol production. Fetal cortisol stimulates activity of placental 17 α hydroxylase/17, 20 lyase (CYP 17) enzyme, which catalyzes the conversion of pregnenolone to estradiol. The altered ratio of progesterone: estrogen in favor of later, up regulates the synthesis of uterine prostaglandins (PG). Prostaglandins or inflammatory cytokines, may directly affect the contractile mechanisms. Oxytocin, CRH, or relaxin supplement the effects of other hormones on the contractile mechanisms. Estrogens promote a series of myometrial changes including increased receptor expression of oxytocin. The control of the softening of the cervix involves rearrangement and realignment of collagen, elastin, and glycosaminoglycans such as decorin.

Assisted Reproductive Biotechniques

Farm animals, an important component of agriculture in Asia and other countries of the world, plays a pivotal role in the agricultural economy in the form of meat, milk and drought power. This important animal resource needs to be genetically improved owing to considerable dependence of the state economy, food chain as well as the farmer's security upon them. The limitation to genetic improvement imposed by inherent biological factors can be overcome by the use of reproductive bio-techniques which aim to manipulate reproduction - related events and/or structures to achieve pregnancy with the final aim of producing healthy offspring in the females. Assisted Reproductive Techniques (ART) manipulate structures and/or events related to ovulation, fertilization and embryo transfer. It corners around manipulation of female/ male reproductive tract physiology, biochemistry, health and thereby longevity. Recently developed bio-techniques used for improving reproductive efficiency of farm animals include

- Artificial insemination,
- Cryopreservation of Embryos and Ova
- Multiple ovulation and embryo transfer technologies,
- In vitro embryo production, ovum pick-up, cloning by nuclear transfer (NT) of embryonic and somatic cells,
- Stem cell biology and transgenics.

The expanding field of embryo transfer (ET) can be viewed as the female counterpart of artificial insemination.

Use of these techniques could enable scientists and researchers to understand and overcome the key issues responsible for limiting full utilization of domestic animals like cattle, buffalo, sheep and goat to improve the economy.

Multiple Ovulation and Embryo Transfer Technologies

The normal development of mammalian eggs transferred from one animal to another was first demonstrated by Heape in 1890. Using rabbits in his experiment he showed that the offspring were not influenced by the genetic characters of foster parents. The first report of a calf having developed to term from a transplanted bovine embryo appeared in 1951 by Willet and colleagues. Embryo transfer is an important method of genetic improvement as much as the embryos from genetically superior animals can be transferred to genetically inferior animals.

Females of superior genetic merit are superovulated with gonadotropic hormones, their eggs fertilized in vivo or oocytes fertilized in vitro, then the resultant embryos are transferred to recipients, genetically less distinguished surrogate mothers. Remarkable progress has been made during the past decade in the refinement of procedures for induction of ovulation, synchronization of estrus, in vivo and in vitro embryo production and cryopreservation of embryos. The non-invasive techniques of ultrasonography for oocyte aspiration from adult and prepuberal animals, and the non-surgical techniques and laparoscopy for routine ET have accelerated the growth of embryo transfer technology in farm animals.

Essentially there are three stages involved in the procedure for egg transfer to recipients Eggs may be successfully recovered from the donor tract by surgical and non surgical method. The surgical method involves mid ventral laparotomy immediately anterior to the mammary gland. The exteriorized uterus may be flushed with a physiological medium which passes to the exterior via a cannula inserted into its lumen. Alternatively the fluid may be passed into the uterus and out through a cannula inserted into the oviduct. Nowadays, non surgical flushing of embryos using Folley's catheter is a common practice. Surgical methods are still used in small ruminants where non-surgical methods are not so successful.

A genetically superior high milk yielding cow is selected as a donor. The donor cow is treated with super ovulating hormones such as PMSG or Follicle Stimulating Hormone. Semen from top pedigree bull is introduced in this cow for fertilization. Seven days after such insemination, the fertilized eggs or embryos are flushed out from the uterus of the donor cow, and kept in a nutrient media for a few hours under controlled temperature. On an average 4 to 6 embryos are recovered from a donor cow and such embryos recovered from a donor cow are transferred into the uterus of a separate genetically inferior local cow. Thus the local cow who receive these embryos act as recipients (foster or surrogate mother).

Assuming an average success of 50%, it is possible to get 2-3 calves from one donor cow as against only one calf by natural breeding/ artificial insemination. Again the same donor cow can be used for obtaining further embryos say about 4 times in a year. Thus, instead of one donor cow delivering only one calf by natural breeding/artificial insemination, it can donate at least 16-24 embryos which when transferred to local cows can result in 8-12 superior calves. The foster mother works as an incubator for the young one and does not impart any of the genetic characters of her own.

Cryopreservation of Embryos and Ova

In 1949, the first human cells, sperm cells, were successfully cryopreserved (Polge *et al.,* 1949). Since then a number of other cells and tissues have been added to the list. Whittingham, Leibo and Mazur first reported successful freezing and thawing of mouse embryos in 1972. The procedure for cryopreservation includes initial exposure to and equilibration with the cryoprotectants, cooling to sub zero temperatures, storage, thawing and finally dilution and removal of the cryoprotectant with return to physiological environment that will allow further development. Cells must maintain structural integrity throughout the cryopreservation procedure. Storage is usually at -196ºC, the temperature of liquid nitrogen. Above a temperature of -80ºC, cells gradually lose viability, but below -130ºC, there is insufficient energy for most reactions. Several cryoprotectants such as glycerol, dimethylsulfoxide, propylene glycol etc ensure protection from cryo-injury during freezing. The exact mechanism by which each of the various cryoprotectants exerts their protective action remains to be determined but partly due to the ability of cryoprotectants to prevent ice crystal formation.

Two problems that occur during thawing can reduce the survival of frozen cells : recrystallization with intracellular ice formation and osmotic shock. Ice formation may be avoided by thawing rapidly past the melting point of ice. Plastic ministraws of 0.25ml capacity are widely used for cryopreservation of cow embryos.

Cryopreservation of mammalian embryos was developed during the late 1970s. Since then, the cryopreservation techniques have been diversified and improved to try to cryopreserve embryos from most species, at different developmental stages, and more sensitive embryos such as in vitro produced, cloned or biopsied embryos. Slow freezing (or equilibrium freezing) and vitrification are the main cryopreservation techniques commonly used. Slow freezing attempts to maintain a delicate balance between cryoprotectants and the aqueous embryo compartment, whereas the strategy of the vitrification method is a rapid solidification of liquid without ice crystal formation.

In vitro Embryo Production

In vitro embryo production is normally designated IVF, even though in domestic animals it consists of three distinct in vitro phases: maturation of oocytes (IVM), fertilisation of oocytes with capacitated spermatozoa (IVF), and finally culture of the presumptive zygotes (IVC). Chang (1959) published the first report of the birth of rabbits after IVF. Brackett et al. (1982) were the first to report the live birth of a calf after IVF, using in vivo matured oocytes aspirated from follicles at laparotomy, with surgical transfer of the presumptive zygotes to the oviduct of synchronised heifers after 24 to 48 hours of in vitro culture.

Different steps of in vitro production of bovine embryos up to the blastocyst stage include: (1) oocyte maturation, (2) in vitro fertilization, and (3) in vitro development.

Cumulus oocyte complexes (COC) from slaughterhouse-derived ovaries are generally aspirated from follicles more than 2 mm in diameter, as they have proved to contain developmentally competent oocytes. Oocytes obtained from slaughtered animals by aspiration, slicing, puncture or ovum pick by use of a transvaginal ultrasound-guided needle up in live animals are graded as follows.

Grade A: Compact cumulus-oocyte-complexes (COCs) with an unexpanded cumulus mass having ≥4 layers of cumulus cells, and with homogenous evenly granular ooplasm

Grade B: COCs with 2-3 layers of cumulus cells and a homogenous evenly granular ooplasm

Grade C: Oocytes partially or wholly denuded or with expanded or scattered cumulus cells or with an irregular and dark ooplasm

Irrespective of species, oocytes without a cumulus investment (denuded oocytes) and oocytes with signs of degeneration are normally discarded before IVM. Once harvested, these oocytes are brought to the lab and placed in solutions that mimic the uterine environment. The oocytes undergo the process of maturation (IVM). The processes encompassing oocyte maturation are essential for the transition from a gamete to an embryo competent to give rise to a healthy new individual. Aspects of oocyte maturation include (1) nuclear maturation, (2) cytoplasmic molecular maturation, (3) cytoplasmic organelle maturation, and (4) epigenetic maturation. Cytoplasmic oocyte maturation involves the synthesis of proteins from nuclear and mitochondrial transcripts used by the oocyte during early embryonic development. Nuclear maturation is judged by the appearance of the first polar body under a microscope. Epigenetic maturation involves de novo DNA methylation that silences maternal imprinted genes, exchanges of histone variants, and histone modification that support genome remodeling and gene transcription during oogenesis and preimplantation development.

In vitro fertilization includes the preparation of sperm and matured oocytes for in vitro fertilization and the culture of the obtained embryos up to expanded blastocyst stage of development.

Stem cell biology and transgenics

Stem cells (SC) are biological cells found in almost all multicellular organisms that can divide and differentiate into diverse specialized cell types and can self-renew to produce more stem cells. Stem cells have the remarkable potential to develop into many different cell types in the body during early life and growth. In many tissues they serve as a sort of internal repair system, dividing essentially without limit to replenish other cells. Stem cells are unspecialized cells from which other more specialized cells can be derived. Stem cells may be obtained from

- Blood in the umbilical cord of a baby after it is born (donated by the mother)
- Bone marrow (bone marrow transplantation)

Stem cells are undifferentiated cells that have the potential to become one of 200 types of cells in the body, including blood, nerve, muscle, heart, glandular, and skin cells. Stem cells divide, producing more stem cells, until they are triggered to specialize. Stem cells are of two types: 1. Embryonic stem cells derived from embryo 2. Adult stem cells derived from adults. Typically, stem cell division produces one cell that remains a stem cell while the other daughter cell differentiates into a specialized cell with the usual life span. The cell that continues being a stem cell does not lose any developmental capacity and can divide indefinitely, continuing to produce additional stem cells and additional differentiated cells.

By triggering certain genes, researchers may be able to cause the stem cells to specialize and become the cells that need to be replaced. Stem cell transplantation is the removal of stem cells (undifferentiated cells) from a healthy person and their injection into someone who has a serious blood disorder. Stem cells are most commonly used in clinical veterinary medicine in therapeutic applications for the treatment of musculoskeletal injuries in horses and dogs. Spermatogonial stem cell culture has been used for conservation of endangered species. One such project is use of spermatogonial stem cells for conservation of doom pig breed of Assam. Stem cell therapies in veterinary patients are still in an experimental stage but likely to play an important role in future.Stem cells improve tissue repair through secretion of immunomodulatory and bioactive trophic factors but the exact mechanisms are still a matter of investigations.

Mesenchymal and spermatogonial stem cells on transplantation into the recipient animals provide a powerful tool for enhancing reproductive performance of female and male animals, respectively. High genetic merit semen of exotic male could be produced from indigenous animals in harsh tropical climates. Moreover, sperm could be harvested from prepubertal animals via its germ cell transplantation to less valuable animals thus reducing the time of sire evaluation markedly and helping in utilizing the less valuable males in the breeding program. Production of sperm / ova from male / female animals of desired genetics can be ensured even after its death. The technique includes spermatogonial stem cell isolation, characterization and their long term preservation.

Sex Selection

Manipulation of sex of offspring has great potential for the livestock industy. The ability to determine the sex of the embryos prior to transfer to the recipients has commercial application in the embryo transfer and artificial insemination programme.

Many methods have been proposed for separating X- and Y-chromosome bearing spermatozoa, , e.g.

Cytological method

X-linked enzymes

Differential development rates

Detection of male specific antigen

Y-specific DNA probes

PCR amplification of Y-chromosome specific gene

However, the only method which has been shown to work reliably is that of selection and separation of spermatozoa whose DNA is stained with a bis benzimidazole dye, H33342, using the sorting capacity of a flow cytometer. This method functions because the X chromosome is larger than the Y, therefore taking up more of the DNA-specific stain and showing a higher fluorescence when the spermatozoa are passed through a laser beam. In bulls, for example, the difference in DNA content between the X and Y- chromosome is approximately 4.2%. However, the process of sorting sufficient numbers for an insemination dose in the flow cytometer takes too long, since the stained spermatozoa must pass one at a time through a laser beam for detection of their DNA content. Moreover, the pregnancy rate after insemination of sexed bull spermatozoa is lower than with unsexed spermatozoa, making the procedure inefficient and expensive.

Generally, the procedures are costly, clumsy, time consuming, damaging to embryos and costly but research is likely to overcome these limitations in near future.

Fertility genes

Fertility is a complex phenotype, which depends on both genetic and Environmental factors. CYP19A1 gene is a strong candidate gene for fertility. One important fertility factor is the Aromatase cytochrome P450 which is encoded by the CYP19 A1 gene which is directly involved in estradiol production.

Summary

- The female gonads have a dual function: Production of female germ cells and the secretion of sex hormones.
- The ovaries secrete a large amount of estrogen and progesterone and a small amount of androgens.
- Progesterone, a steroid hormone secreted by the corpus luteum in the ovary, prepares the uterus for pregnancy.
- The three estrogenic steroids produced by the ovaries are 17beta estradiol, estrone and estriol. They are secreted primarily by the granulosa cells of the ovarian follicles, the corpus luteum and the placenta.
- The biosynthesis of estrogenic steroids is dependent upon the enzyme aromatase , which converts testosterone to estradiol, and androstenedione to estrone.
- The fertilization of ova takes place in the ampulla. The embryos remain in the oviduct for three days before they are transported to the uterus. The oviductal fluid provides a suitable environment for fertilization and cleavage of fertilized eggs.
- Spermatozoa must undergo some change after they are deposited in the female reproductive tract in order to acquire the ability to penetrate the zona pellucida and fertilize the ova. This process, referred to as capacitation.
- Pregnancy is not a state of total systemic immunosuppression but rather a state of dramatic immune modulation.The immunology of pregnancy has been considered as a host–graft response characterized by immune suppression and consequently a period of increased risk of bacterial and viral infection.

15

Male Reproduction

The male reproductive system consists of a pair of testes that produce sperm (or spermatozoa), ducts that transport the sperm to the penis and glands that add secretions to the sperm to make semen. The adult mammalian testis performs two important functions, spermatogenesis and male sex hormone production. It is an organ structurally designed to produce the haploid male gametes from diploid postnatal germ-line stem cells, i.e. type A spermatogonia. The process of morphological and functional differentiation of type A spermatogonia into the haploid male gamete, the spermatozoon, is termed spermatogenesis. In addition, the testis elaborates a steroid hormone, testosterone, that is responsible for maintaining the spermatogenic process as well as the secondary male sexual characteristics. Reproduction in the males culminates in the production of semen containing fertile spermatozoa and deposition of these in the female reproductive tract at an opportune time.

The male gonads, the testes, lie outside the abdomen within the scrotum, which is a purse-like structure derived from the skin and fascia of the abdominal wall.The testes produce the spermatozoa and the male sex hormones (androgens) . The spermatozoa pass from the testis into the epididymis where they acquire motility and attributes essential for fertilization and are then stored there. At ejaculation they are squeezed along the vas deferens into the urethra and mixed with the secretions of the accessory glands to constitute the ejaculated semen. The assessory sex glands include the Bulbo-urethral gland also known as Cowper's gland, ampullae and prostate. The seminal vesicles and prostate are absent in chicken. Boar seminal vesicles are very large. In the case of a dog, the prostate is almost absent.

The scrotum is absent in birds and testes remain within the abdominal cavity.

Largest testes in proportion to body weight

- Among common domestic animals – Boar
- Among all mammals – Golden hamster

Each testis is covered with a thick fibrous capsule, the **tunica albuginea**. Functionally testes have 3 compartments

1. **Interstitial tissue** : Have leydig cells
2. **Basal compartment** : Contains spermatozoa
3. **Ad-luminal compartment** : Here spermatozoa undergoes meiosis.

Basal compartment and adluminal compartment is present within the seminiferous tubule.

Mechanism of Penile Erection

The process of penile erection is caused by increased blood flow into the penis as well as mechanical compression of the venous drainage. The corpus cavernosum penis pressure is several times higher than arterial pressure during erection. The abolition of peak corpus cavernosum penis pressure observed during peak erection by anesthetizing the ischiocavernosus muscle supports the hypothesis that muscles are the source of energy for the pressure of CCP greater than arterial pressure. During erection there is mechanical compression of the internal pudendal arteries; deep arteries of the penis external to or within the tunica albuginea of the crus and veins against the ischium by contraction of the ischiocavernosus muscles.

Thus, general erection of penis is considered to be produced by a combination of elevated arterial pressure, dilation of the arteries to the penis, relaxation of the walls of the cavernous spaces and contraction of the external penile muscles.

Erection is produced by physical and psychic stimuli. Physical stimuli, such as touch and massage of the penis, relay the afferent impulses to the pudendal nerve, to the spinal cord reflex center and to higher brain centres. Erection is caused by parasympathetic impulses that pass from the sacral portion of the spinal cord and to the penis. These parasympathetic impulses dilate the arteries of the penis.

Ejaculation during coitus or intercourse deposits spermatozoa into the vagina or cervix uteri. Through the combined action of sperm motility and the muscular contractions of the female reproductive tract spermatozoa are transported through the uterus and into the oviducts where fertilization occurs.

Frequency of copulation among domestic animals varies with the species and a number of factors such as breed, health, ratio of males to females and dimensions of the breeding area.

Seminal plasma plays a major role in the transport and physiology of sperm in the female reproductive tract.

Ejaculation depends on the normal integrity and function of the autonomic nervous system, which coordinates seminal emission, closure of the urinary bladder sphincters and ejaculatory displacement of the seminal components through the penile urethra. The contractile activity of the urethral musculature is under the control of catecholamines and adrenergic receptors in the urethra.

Spermatogenic Cycle and Wave

The testis are composed of long tubes called seminiferous tubules and interstitial tissue. The spermatozoa are produced within the seminiferous tubules. Spermatogenesis is a highly organized and complex sequence of differentiation events that yields genetically distinct male gametes for fertilization.This process is known as spermatogenesis. Spermatogenesis is the process by which haploid spermatozoa develop from germ cells in the seminiferous tubules of the testis. This process starts with the mitotic division of the stem cells located close to the basement membrane of the tubules. Sperm production is a continuous process, initiated at puberty and continuing throughout life.

The interstitial compartment consists of Leydig cells, immune cells (macrophages and lymphocytes), and fibroblasts. In addition, it also contains blood and lymph vessels, nerves, and loose connective tissue. The tubular and interstitial compartments of the testis perfonn the defined functions of spermatogenesis and steroidogenesis, respectively.

A spermatogenic cycle is defined as the time it takes for the reappearance of the same stage within a given segment of the tubule. Each stage of the cycle follows in an orderly sequence along the length of the tubule. The distance between the same stage is called the spermatogenic wave. One tubule can contain numerous complete waves. The number of stages within a spermatogenic cycle and the number of cycles required for the completion of spermatogenesis varies between species.

Spermatogenesis can be divided into three distinct phases: mitosis, meiosis, and spermiogenesis.

The first phase is referred to as spermatogonial proliferation and renewal. During this period, relatively undifferentiated diploid spermatogonia, the immature germ cells, undergo several mitotic divisions to generate a large population of cells called primary spermatocytes.

In the second phase the spermatocytes go through the process of two meiotic divisions leading to the formation of haploid germ cells, spermatids.

In the third phase, the spermatids go through a complex series of cytological transformations and dedifferentiate to form stem cells that cyclically develop into highly specialized spermatozoa.

Spermatogenesis is the process of sperm cell development. Rounded immature sperm cells undergo successive mitotic and meiotic divisions (spermatocytogenesis) and a metamorphic change (spermiogenesis) to produce spermatozoa. Spermatogenesis is the process by which haploid spermatozoa develop from germ cells in the seminiferous tubules of the testis. This process starts with the mitotic division of the stem cells located close to the basement membrane of the tubules. Spermatogenesis is the process by which stem cells develop into mature spermatozoa. There are three phases:

(1) **Spermatocytogenesis** (Mitosis)- Spermatocytogenesis (also called Mitosis): Stem cells (Type A spermatogonia; singular = spermatogonium) divide mitotically to replace themselves and to produce cells that begin differentiation (Type B spermatogonia). Spermatogonia have spherical or oval nuclei, and rest on the basement membrane.

(2) **Meiosis**- Meiosis is the process by which the diploid number of chromosomes present in spermatogonia (the stem cells) is reduced to the haploid number present in mature spermatozoa. Cells in prophase of the first meiotic division are primary spermatocytes. They are characterized by highly condensed chromosomes giving the nucleus a coarse chromatin pattern and an intermediate position in the seminiferous epithelium. This is a long stage, so many primary spermatocytes can be seen. Primary spermatocytes go through the first meiotic division and become secondary

spermatocytes. The cells quickly proceed through this stage and complete the second meiotic division. This stage is very short.

The products of the second meiotic division are called spermatids. They are spherical cells with interphase nuclei, positioned high in the epithelium. Since spermatids go through a metamorphosis into spermatozoa, they occur in early through late stages. All of these progeny cells remain attached to each other by cytoplasmic bridges. The bridges remain until sperm are fully differentiated.

(3) **Spermiogenesis-** This is the metamorphosis of spherical spermatids into elongated spermatozoa. No further mitosis or meiosis occurs. During spermiogenesis, the acrosome forms, the flagellar apparatus forms, and most excess cytoplasm (the residual body) is separated and left in the Sertoli cell. Spermatozoa are released into the lumen of the seminiferous tubule. A small amount of excess cytoplasm (the cytoplasmic droplet) is shed later in the epididymis.

Hormonal regulation. Spermatogonia continue to divide, but in reduced numbers, after hypophysectomy. Spermatocytogenesis is completely arrested at the primary spermatocyte stage in hypophysectomized animals; this step is restored by testosterone. Androgen-binding protein (the testicular counterpart of SHBG) sequesters testosterone within the seminiferous tubule (and caput epididymis). Meiosis II is hormonally-independent. Follicle-stimulating hormone participates in spermiogenesis.

Protamines and Transition nuclear proteins (TPs) are the major proteins important for histone displacement and chromatin condensation during mammalian spermatogenesis.

Seminiferous Tubules has 5 types of Germ Cells

1. Spermatogonia
2. Primary spermatocytes
3. Secondary spermatocytes
4. Spermatid (round and elongated)
5. Spermatozoa

Within seminiferous tubules, sertoli cells and various stages of sperm forming cells form seminiferous epithelium.

Blood-Testis Barrier and Seminiferous Tubules

The seminiferous tubules are not penetrated by blood or lymph vessels.

Two principal components of blood – testis barrier are

1. Incomplete or partial barrier of myoid cells that surrounds the tubules.
2. Unique junctions between sertoli cells.
   - It is formed by sertoli cells and myoid cells.
   - Sertoli cells are joined by specialized tight junctions that separate seminiferous epithelium in to adluminal and basal compartments and thereby, preventing formidable B-T-B

- Sertoli cells are essential for the maintenance of spermatogenic cell glutathione (GSH).

i.e. The junctions divide the seminiferous tubule into 2 distinct compartments:

1. Basal compartment containing spermatogonia and preleptotene spermatocyte.
2. An adluminal compartment containing a more advanced stage of spermatocytes and spermatids, this freely communicates with the lumen of the tubule.

Functions of Blood Testis Barrier

There are two main functions of blood testis barrier

1. It provides isolation of the luminal environment in which the metabolism of the developing sperm cells is controlled e.g. K^+ is secreted in this space and they serve to maintain spermatozoa in quiescent state.
2. It prevents developing spermatozoa from moving into interstitial tissue and thus immune reactions against spermatozoa can be prevented.

Testosterone is required for spermatogenesis, especially for the process of meiosis.

Function of Sertoli cell-leydig cell

Two types of somatic cells are present in the seminiferous tubules.

1. Myoid cells (like smooth muscles cells)
2. Sertoli or sustentacular or nurse cells

Sertoli cells multiply during fetal and prepubertal life but after puberty mitotic events are infrequent, although there is apparently an annual loss and regeneration in seasonal breeding species.

At all stages of differentiation, the spermatogenic cells are in close contact with Sertoli cells which are thought to provide structural and metabolic support to the developing sperm cells. The Sertoli cell extends from the basement membrane to the lumen of the seminiferous tubule.

They are characterized by the presence of a vesicular, oval, basally positioned nucleus which contains a prominent nucleolus. Sertoli cells are endocrine cells - they secrete the polypeptide hormone, inhibin, a dimeric 32-kD glycoprotein. Inhibin acts at the level of the pituitary to reduce the secretion of follicle stimulating hormone. Inhibins are gonadal messengers that exert a physiological negative feedback control on FSH release at the pituitary gland. There are at least two active molecular forms in circulation, inhibin A and inhibin B.

The interstitial tissue contains Leydig cells or interstitial cells of Leydig which are responsible for the production of the male hormone called androgens. The process of testosterone formation from its precursor, cholesterol, is termed steroidogenesis.The androgens are produced under the influence of hormones from the anterior pituitary namely ICSH (LH) and FSH.

The testes are suspended from the body in the loose sacs called scrotum, present in the inguinal region. The scrotum in addition to its container function, also acts as a regulator of temperature required for spermatogenesis. The testes develop in the abdominal cavity and normally migrate to the scrotum during fetal development.

It must be pointed out that there is a narrow temperature range suitable for male gametogenesis. This temperature range is lower than the body temperature. Tying the testes close to the body wall in rams causes temporary sterility by preventing them from cooling off when the environmental temperature rises.Hence the scrotum functions in the maintenance of lower temperature than the body. Scrotal temperature is regulated by two distinct mechanisms. First, it accomplishes this by a double muscle system that draws the testes close to the body wall for warmth or lets them fall away from the body wall for cooling. The two muscles involved are the external cremaster and the tunica dartos. Exposure to cold makes the dartos contract, thus causing the scrotal skin to pucker and forcing the testes closer to the body wall. The second mechanism involved is the countercurrent mechanism in the pampiniform plexus. The pampiniform plexus is the intricately and prodigiously (prodigiously meaning extremely great in ability, amount, or strength) looped system of veins and arteries that lies on the surface of the epididymis.The arterial branch to this plexus is supplied by the spermatic artery and the venous part empties into the spermatic vein.

Epididymis

The sperms are carried from the seminiferous tubules into the epididymis. Epididymis is a compact fibrous organ closely attached to the superior or posterior border of testis longitudinally. Epididymis can be differentiated into three parts, the proximal caput, the middle thin corpus and distal sac like cauda. The epididymis is a single long convoluted tube, passage through which confers the immotile and infertile spermatozoa the properties or the ability to move and to fertilize. This process is called the maturation of spermatozoa. During the process of maturation , the spermatozoa are altered morphologically, physiologically, biochemically and immunologically. The membrane changes are important in the maturation. The epididymis also acts as a storehouse for the spermatozoa. For this most of the fluid secreted by the rete testes is absorbed in the caput and corpus parts of the epididymis so as to concentrate the spermatozoa and also to bring the maturation factors to critical concentrations.

During the process of maturation, the cytoplasmic droplet migrates distally along the tail of the spermatozoon and falls off; this event is correlated with an increase in cellular motility (Jindal and Panda, 1980).The passage of spermatozoa through the epididymis takes several days. The spermatozoa from the cauda epididymis are drained into the thick walled muscular vas deferens.

Accessory Glands

These accessory glands secrete substances and fluid which forms a major part of the seminal plasma in which sperms are suspended. There are three major accessory glands of the male reproductive tract viz - Seminal vesicles, prostate and bulbo-urethral glands.

Seminal Vesicles

Each vesicle is a muscular convoluted tube lined by an epithelium which secretes an alkaline yellow viscid fluid which forms much of the volume of the ejaculated semen. The vesicular fluid contains an abundance of fructose, and smaller amounts of ascorbic acid, inositol, ergothioneine, amino acids, phosphorylcholine, prostaglandin and fibrinogen. The fructose and other substances in the seminal fluid are of considerable nutritive value for the ejaculated sperm until one of them fertilizes the ovum.

Prostate

The prostate secretes the seminal fluid that helps to nourish and transport the sperm that comes from the testicles. The fluid is then stored in the seminal vesicles. The gland itself surrounds the urethra, which is the tube that carries urine from the bladder out through the tip of the penis

The prostate is a small organ about the size of a walnut. It lies below the bladder (where urine is stored) and surrounds the urethra (the tube that carries urine from the bladder). The prostate makes a fluid that helps to nourish sperm as part of the semen (ejaculatory fluid).

The prostate gland consists of many follicle-like spaces leading into ducts. The epithelium of the follicles secretes the prostatic fluid, which is thin and opalescent and gives the semen the characteristic odour. Between the follicles there is a good deal of muscular tissue. The prostatic fluid contains citric acid, calcium and several other substances and is slightly alkaline in nature. The prostatic fluid neutralizes the acidity of the fluid in the female reproductive tract and thus greatly enhances the motility and fertility of the sperms. The secretions of the prostate gland are under androgenic control.

As the prostate grows larger, it may press on the urethra. This narrowing of the urethra can cause some men with prostate enlargement to have trouble with urination. Prostate enlargement may be the most common health problem in men older than 60 years of age.

Prostate Specific Antigen (PSA) is an androgen dependent glycoprotein secreted by glands of the prostate, released in serum by disruption of normal prostatic tissue—cancer, inflammation, BPH, or trauma. An elevated PSA occurs in prostatic cancer and is widely used as a screening test for this disease. PSA is a single-chain glycoprotein containing 237 amino acids and four carbohydrate side chains (molecular weight: 28,430). The Canine Prostatic Specific Esterase (CPSE) has been identified as a suitable biomarker to be included in a prostate health screening program in dogs, following the model of prostate-specific antigen (PSA) in human medicine. A higher CPSE in dogs suffering from several prostatic diseases, such as benign prostatic hyperplasia, bacterial prostatitis, or prostatic carcinoma, has been reported.

Castration is the destruction or removal of the testicles of the male. It is carried out on animals which are not wanted for breeding. Male sheep, cattle, goats and pigs are routinely castrated in order to reduce aggression and subsequent injury. Methods of castration are either by blade or rubber ring. Castration is generally done to prevent the development of secondary sexual characteristics. In order to prevent development of boar taint, it is customary to castrate male pigs intended for meat production.

Semen-composition

Semen is a mixture of various fluids that carry live spermatozoa to the female genital tract for fertilization. Semen is composed of spermatozoa suspended in seminal plasma. The mammalian spermatozoa, the male gamete, is a microscopic motile cell whose essential function is to serve as the nuclear bridge between generations. It is composed of three parts, the head, midpiece and tail.

Head

The apical portion of the spermatozoa is called head and contains the genome in the form of nucleus. The head is oval in shape in most domestic animas and it is elongated in chicken. Its haploid nucleus is surrounded anteriorly by a double-walled membranous cap, the acrosome. The acrosome as well as the other parts of the sperm which include the neck, the middle piece and the tail are contained by an outer limiting plasma membrane.

Anomalies of the spermatozoal head are defined by changes in the shape of the spermatozoal head and usually involve both the nucleus and acrosome.

Middle Piece

The middle piece, more commonly referred to as the mid piece, is that region of the gamete containing mitochondria that supplies the energy for the sperm's activity.

Tail

The tail is made of protein fibers that contract on alternative sides, giving a characteristic wavelike movement that drives the sperm through the seminal fluid. The tail of the spermatozoon consists of a thick middle piece, a long thin principal piece and a short terminal piece. The bovine sperm tail consists of 20 fibres arranged concentrically in a 9+9+2 pattern. This arrangement of fibrils is in all mammalian sperm and the 9+2 pattern is in fact characteristic of many flagella and cilia.

These cells are produced by the process of spermatogenesis, which occurs within the seminiferous tubules of the testis. In a human life span possibly a trillion or more such sexual cells are generated. Once formed, spermatozoa pass from the testis into and through the tubule of the epididymis to the cauda or tail of this organ. Therein these cells are stored until removal. At ejaculation the spermatozoa are intermixed with secretions from the accessory glands producing semen.

Seminal plasma is contributed by the accessory sex glands eg epidymis, prostate and seminal vesicles etc. The seminal vesicles produce a yellowish viscous fluid rich in fructose and other substances. The prostatic secretion is a whitish (sometimes clear), thin fluid containing proteolytic enzymes, citric acid, acid phosphatase and lipids. A small amount of fluid is secreted by the bulbourethral and urethral glands; this is a thick, clear, lubricating protein commonly known as mucus. Seminal plasma normally contain fructose, amino acids, citric acid, phosphorus, potassium, and hormones known as prostaglandins.

Though sperm can live for many weeks in the male genital tract, once they are ejaculated in the semen, their maximal life span is only 24 to 72 hours at body temperature. At lowered temperatures, however, semen may be stored for extended periods, say at liquid nitrogen temperatures, sperms after being suspended in suitable diluter containing cryoprotectants can be stored for several years.

Capacitation

Freshly ejaculated spermatozoa are not able to penetrate oocytes; they must undergo a series of calcium-dependent biochemical and structural changes before they become capable of fusing with the egg plasma membrane.Spermatozoa must undergo plasma membrane modifications termed capacitation, which render them able to undergo the acrosome reaction. This process consists of loss of the plasma membrane of the rostral portion of the spermatozoon head, shedding of the acrosomal cap (a modified secretory granule situated over this region of the sperm head), and exposure of the inner acrosomal membrane.

Semen can be collected by electroejaculation or by use of artificial vagina in most domestic animals. The massage method is the most common approach for semen collection in birds.

Semen Evaluation

The standard method of evaluating the fertility of breeding males of farm animals, other than directly evaluating their ability to produce a pregnancy, is by examination of semen. No single test accurately predicts fertility of a sperm sample, however examining various physical characteristics of semen can determine greater fertility potential. Semen should have a relatively uniform, opaque appearance indicative of high sperm cell concentration. The sample should be free from hair, dirt, and other contaminants; frequent ejaculation results in lower average volume.

The quality and preservability of semen varies between individual breed and season. The semen of crossbred bulls in India was found to be superior during winter, spring and autumn season but was most affected during summer. Low ambient temperature does not interfere with testicular development, sperm production or semen quality of boars. Age and frequency of semen collection account for much of the variability in semen characteristics of different species of livestock. Plane of nutrition can also be an important determinant.

Evaluation of semen quality parameters is very important before selection of breeding cocks used for fertility and hatchability of eggs. In birds, the semen quality parameters normally evaluated include color, volume, sperm concentration, semen pH, sperm motility, sperm viability, HOST and acrosome integrity.

Colour *:* The semen of most domestic animals is white (milky). The semen of healthy buffaloes is milk white. It becomes thin and watery when collections are repeated too frequently and during the hot season. The natural colour of poultry semen is white or pearly white.

Volume: The volume of semen varies considerably in different domestic animal species. It may vary from less than 1 ml. in the buck and ram to more than 500 ml, in case of boar and stallion.An average human ejaculates a spoonful i.e. 5 ml of semen.

Concentration : Sperm concentration measures the concentration of sperm in bulls semen ejaculate.A lower sperm count is considered oligozoospermia. Counting chambers have been used to do microscopic evaluation of semen. The concentration of sperm in semen samples varies widely. Say for example in water buffalo, reports from India, give figures from 630 to 1034 millions/ml; in Egypt, 210 to 2000 million/ml and in the USSR 980 million/ml.

Motility: Sperm function requires progressive motility. Sperm motility (expressed as %) is evaluated by counting moving and nonmoving sperm in several microscopic fields.

Semen fertility assessment is on the basis of quality of semen. The quality is generally assessed on the basis of volume, mass activity, progressive motility, sperm concentration, sperm viability or dead and live count, sperm morphology and abnormalities count as well as several biochemical tests such as acrosomal integrity, HOST and tunnel test for DNA damage.

DNA damage in sperm cells that can be probed by analysis of DNA susceptibility to denaturation. DNA damage can be assessed by Terminal deoxynucleotidyl transferase dUTP nick end labeling (TUNEL) assay. DNA damage is related to fertility.

The methods of evaluating sperm quality from frozen semen are associated with motility and intact acrosomes. Motility assessment involves subjective estimation of the viability of spermatozoa and the quality of the motility. Evaluation of sperm motility is conducted with raw and extended semen. Morphologic abnormalities of sperm have the greatest relationship to fertility of livestock. Heat stress causes high numbers of damaged sperm.

Some of the tests for measuring metabolic activity of semen are Methylene Blue reduction time, Resazurin reduction time, fructolysis, oxygen uptake etc.

The hypo-osmotic swelling test (HOST) is widely used as a valuable test for determining sperm quality by evaluating the membrane integrity of spermatozoa of various domestic animals including cattle, horses and swine. The HOST has also been used as an indicator of the fertilising capacity of spermatozoa. The HOS test predicts membrane integrity by determining the ability of the sperm membrane to maintain equilibrium between the sperm cell and its environment. Influx of the fluid due to hypo-osmotic stress causes the sperm tail to coil and balloon or "swell." A higher percentage of swollen sperm indicates the presence of sperm having a functional and intact plasma membrane.

Zona binding assays are sometimes used for in vitro assessment of the fertilizing ability and quality of semen in the laboratory. Such assays require skilled technicians and sophisticated equipment.

Computer Assisted Semen Evaluation

Seminological assessment constitutes the basic examination in the early diagnosis of male infertility. Bull semen analysis commonly depends on a manual microscopy method in semen freezing laboratories worldwide. However, some of the major disadvantages of this technique are that it is labour-intensive, subjective, laboratory-based and time-consuming. Computer-assisted semen analysers (CASAs) have enabled partial automation of routine semen analysis. Most CASA systems are based on image analysis. Computer-assisted techniques are most-often used for the assessment of sperm concentration and mobility characteristics, such as velocity and linear velocity. Computer-aided sperm analysis (CASA) system has been accepted and used ín some of the semen laboratories as a routine semen analysis instrument. Sperm concentration, motility and morphology can be assessed more objectively with the use of CASA.

CASA-is a computer system which requires a high-resolution camera connected to a phase-contrast microscope.

Semen of Birds

The **semen of birds** is highly concentrated and as a result total volume per ejaculate is very small. The average ejaculate volume is 0.5 ml. Semen from cockerels contains between 3-7 billion sperm cells/ml. Cocks start producing semen from the age of 16 weeks. At the time of ejaculation a lymph-like fluid (also known as transparent fluid) of cloacal origin may be added to the semen in varying amounts. The addition of transparent fluid to semen at the time of ejaculation act as an activating medium for the previously non-motile spermatozoa, thus ensuring their transport from the site of deposition to the sites of sperm storage tubules in the utero-vaginal junction of the hen's oviduct.

Testosterone-function and Regulation

Androgens (testosterone, androstenedione and dihydrotestosterone (DHT)) are the male sex hormones required for development of the male reproductive system and secondary sexual characteristics.The principal androgens produced by the testis are testosterone, androstenedione and dihydrotestosterone. Testosterone , the principal hormone of the testes, is a C_{19} steroid with an –OH group in the 17position.

Adrenal cortex also secretes androgens, normally testosterone, androstenedione and dehydroepiandrosterone (of these last one is more important). The actions of adrenal androgens are unimportant under normal physiological conditions because their quantity is insignificant.

Major functions of androgens include regulation of gonadotropic secretion by the hypothalamic pituitary system, initiation and maintenance of spermatogenesis, formation of male phenotype during sexual differentiation and promotion of sexual maturation at puberty. The testes developed in the abdominal cavity is pushed into the scrotum through the inguinal canal just before birth. Testosterone is necessary for this descent of testes.

Testosterone's effects are generally broken into two classes: anabolic and androgenic. Both appear to result from the same signalling pathway as there are no proteins with anabolic effects independent of androgenic effects. Testosterone causes nitrogen retention in the body (positive nitrogen balance) and causes accelerated growth of the body and skeletal muscles in particular. Androgens increase the rate of linear growth of the bones causing a rapid increase in stature in human male at puberty (pubertal growth spurt). Bone loss and osteoporosis are prevented by the androgens in adult males.

Mechanism of Androgen Action

Steroids work by binding with the cytoplasmic (free within the cell) androgen receptor. Like all steroids, the steroid-receptor complex has a strong affinity for the nucleus. The complex is translocated into the nucleus and binds to DNA. It is also possible that the steroid and receptor dissociate in the nucleus and act on DNA separately. The rate limiting factor in this process appears to be the cytoplasmic concentration of the receptor, rather than the concentration of the steroid or translocation of the complex.

Once in the nucleus, the steroid appears to enhance transcription of specific genes. The resulting mRNA is processed and sent out of the nucleus, resulting in increased protein synthesis.

Testosterone circulates in plasma primarily bound to two proteins, testosterone binding globulin and albumin. More than 98% of secreted testosterone is bound to plasma proteins, 68% is bound to albumin and 30% is bound to testosterone-binding globulin. The protein bound steroid is in dynamic equilibrium with unbound or free hormone comprising 1 to 3% of the total. The free fraction alone is physiologically active in the target tissues as only the free hormone can enter cells and there exists a specific mechanism for the entry.

Inside the cell, testosterone can be converted to dihydrotestosterone by 5 alpha reductase. The two hormones then bind to the same high affinity androgen receptor protein in the cytosol. The hormone receptor complexes then diffuse into the nuclei and interact with acceptor sites before effecting a biologic response. This interaction results in increased transcription of specific structural genes and subsequent appearance of a new messenger RNAs and proteins in the cytoplasm.

Hormonal Control of Spermatogenesis

Several pituitary and sex steroid hormones are involved in the hormonal regulation of spermatogenesis. Androgenic hormones such as testosterone provide the major stimulus for spermatogenesis. Production of testosterone by the Leydig cells is regulated by FSH & LH (ICSH) from the anterior pituitary. Evidence has accumulated that high intratesticular testosterone concentrations are essential for the completion of the meiotic division of the spermatocytes. The Sertoli cell is the primary site of action of FSH on the testis and that the production of a specific androgen binding protein (ABP) by the Sertoli cell is stimulated by FSH. It has been suggested that the effect of FSH on spermiogenesis is mediated by creation of high androgen concentrations in the vicinity of germ cells.

The actions of androgens such as testosterone and dihydrotestosterone are mediated via the androgen receptor (AR), a ligand-dependent nuclear transcription factor and member of the steroid hormone nuclear receptor family.Androgen regulated genes are critical for the development and maintenance of the male sexual phenotype. The androgen receptor (AR), also known as NR3C4 (nuclear receptor subfamily 3, group C, member 4), is a type of nuclear receptor that is activated by binding any of the androgenic hormones, including testosterone and dihydrotestosterone in the cytoplasm and then translocating into the nucleus. The main function of the androgen receptor is as a DNA-binding transcription factor that regulates gene expression. AR signalling may also be involved in the development of tumours in the prostate, bladder, liver, kidney and lung.

Cryptorchidism

Cryptorchidism refers to a condition in which the descent of the testes may fail to occur or may be incomplete. Cryptorchid animals whose testes remain inside the body cavity instead of descending into the scrotum are sterile. Generally, unilateral cryptorchids are usually fertile, while bilateral cryptorchids are generally sterile. Failure of one or both testes to descend into the scrotum may be due to genetic predisposition, insufficient androgen (i.e. testosterone) stimulation, and other factors.

Horses are one of domestic animal species with the highest prevalence rate of cryptorchidism. Cryptorchid testes may be located under the skin outside of the inguinal canal, within the inguinal canal or inside of the abdominal cavity. A single cause of equine cryptorchidism has not been established and contributing causes remain obscure. The condition is likely the result of a complex combination of genetic, hormonal, and mechanical factors. All breeds of horses may exhibit cryptorchidism, but there is a higher frequency in Quarter Horses, Saddlebreds, Percherons, and ponies. The condition is considered heritable.

The incidence of cryptorchidism is higher in dogs or pigs than in cattle or sheep. In dogs, it is believed to be an autosomal sex-linked recessive gene. Cryptorchidism is a common congenital anomaly in pigs, and a genome-wide association study of Large White and Landrace pigs localizes the associated gene or genes to candidate genes to SSC8 (Sus scrofa chromosome) between 65 and 73 Mb.

Puberty -photoperiod

Puberty, the transition from an immature to a reproductively mature state, is a neuroendocrine process with broad ramifications for anatomy and physiology. Puberty is defined in both the male and female as the ability to accomplish reproduction successfully (acquiring reproductive competence). Onset of puberty in the male domestic animals occurs at approximately the same time after birth as puberty in females of the same species.The age at onset of puberty is dependent on neuro-endocrine mechanism, nutrition of the animal, season, photoperiod and presence of the female in the vicinity.

Definition of Puberty in Male

a. Age at first sexual behavioral activities

- Mounting and erection
- Not sperm production

b. Age at first ejaculation

- Development of muscles, nerves, accessory glands

c. Age at first ejaculation with spermatozoa

d. Age when the ejaculate contains enough sperm cells to accomplish fertilization

Puberty is a consequence of the reactivation of pulsatile gonadotropin-releasing hormone (GnRH) secretion by the hypothalamus. GnRH-secreting neurons are regulated by peptides and neuromodulators, including kisspeptin, neuropeptide Y, glutamate, gamma-aminobutyrate and neurokinin B. The age of puberty onset is characteristic for each species, as each species has its own time-course for hypothalamo-pituitary–gonadal development. Increased release of the gonadotropin-releasing hormone (GnRH, a synonymous term for LHRH, luteinizing hormone-releasing hormone) from the hypothalamus triggers the onset of puberty. Several genes are involved in regulating the GnRH release from hypothalamus which include G-protein coupled receptor 54 and neurokinin B receptor.

Photoperiod is defined as day length or the period of daily illumination received by an organism and remains constant between years at any given geographic location. Photoperiod has been shown to influence a variety of physiologic rhythms, including thermoregulation and reproduction. The pineal gland, and its hormone melatonin, mediates photoperiodic time measurement in mammals.

Uses of Androgens, Progestogens, Estrogens

Steroid hormones have been used in animal production for various applications like increase in growth rate, induction of lactation etc. In the earlier years of last century, Diethylstilbestrol was extensively used for increasing the growth rate of veal calves until the use of steroids was restricted. Poultry generally do not appear to respond to oestrogens by increased gain but by changes in lipid deposition.

Mammary duct growth is stimulated by estrogen, while estrogen and progesterone in combination stimulate lobule-alveolar development of the mammary gland . Artificial induction of lactation can be induced in infertile animals by the combination of steroid hormones estrogen and progesterone. Success rates can be increased by using Reserpine, a tranquilizer that increases blood prolactin, and dexamethasone, a synthetic glucocorticoid. Selected animals should have good genetic merit for milk production, healthy and with good body condition. For good results, a thorough and frequent massage of udder is essential.

Summary

- The male reproductive system includes the penis, scrotum, testes, epididymis, vas deferens, prostate, and seminal vesicles.
- The purpose of the organs of the male reproductive system is to perform the following functions: To produce, maintain, and transport sperm (the male reproductive cells) and protective fluid (semen). To discharge sperm within the female reproductive tract during sex. To produce and secrete male sex hormones responsible for maintaining the male reproductive system.
- The above reproductive functions of the male is assisted by hormones and the autonomic nervous system
- Semen is ejaculated into a female's vagina, millions of sperm "swim" up from the vagina through the cervix and uterus to meet the egg in the fallopian tube. It takes only one sperm to fertilize the egg.
- The prostate and bulbourethral glands pour their secretions into the urethra, where at the time of ejaculation, they are mixed with the fluid suspension of sperm and ampullary secretions from the ductus deferens.
- Male reproduction in the bird is different from mammals in that the testis is located within the body cavity in the bird and Internal structure of the testis is similar to mammals. There is no pampiniform plexus in the male bird, instead, of an epididymis as found in mammals, the sperm are stored in the vas deferens

16

Mammary Gland Function

Lactation is the process of milk secretion by the mammary gland. Lactation is the final phase of the complete reproductive cycle of mammals. Newborns of most species are dependent on maternal milk during the neonatal period. Lactation is therefore essential for survival of the species.

Milk is one of the most fascinating biological fluids whose role as a nearly complete food in sustaining life processes is well known. Milk provides an essential and highly digestible form of nutrients for the mammalian young during the critical period after birth. Milk also forms the first meal of the mammalian young.

Most mammals produce milk according to the requirements for their young ones. However, man for centuries have selectively bred several animals, so that they produce milk, far in excess of the requirements of their young. The excess milk is harvested by man for his own and his children's nurture. The physiology of the mammary gland or the mechanism of milk secretion forms an important part of the man's strategy to manipulate it to its own advantage. Milk forms the raw material for the multi million dollar dairy industry all over the world. In India, dairying is the second largest agriculture based industry.

The most important animal domesticated by man for production of milk is undoubtedly the cow. Buffalo as a milk producer is important only in Asia & parts of Africa. In India its importance is as much or even more as compared to the cow in milk production ability. The other important milk producing animals are goat, sheep, camel, yak, and mithun.

The ability to produce milk is dependent on several factors including breed, season, feed etc. Majority of our animals in India do not conform to any descript type, some 20 percent of them belong to 50 cattle breeds and 17 buffalo breeds. The major milk producing breeds of buffaloes are Murrah and Nili Ravi. The season affects the milk producing ability of domestic animals. Goat milk has a composition similar to cow milk.

Animal productivity of milk has significantly increased in the last 75 years, with annual milk yield per cow increasing over 4-fold.

Functional and Metabolic Organization of Mammary Glands -Structure and Development

Milk is a complex mixture of solutes that are secreted by specialized epithelial cells within anatomically distinct glandular units found in the mammary glands of mammals.

Milk is a record of the exquisite functioning of a cell, a fascinating cell that might be described as a factory, but a factory with the unusual property of becoming, to a certain extent a product. Indeed the lactating mammary cell ranks second in importance only to the photosynthesizing cell as a factory in sustaining life. Lactation is a physiological event that is exclusive to mammals. Lactation evolved as a strategy to improve the survival of the young by providing them with the complete nutrition that is required for survival upon birth.

Milk is produced and secreted by most mammals in specialized skin glands called mammary glands. Mammary glands are present in both sexes but in males they remain rudimentary but in females they are well developed after puberty. Mammary gland development commences embryonically and continues post natal even during lactation.

External Morphology of the Mammary Gland

The mammary glands of most dairy animals are located in the inguinal region i.e. cattle, buffalo, sheep, goat, horses, camel and donkey. The number of teats is normally four in case of cattle and buffaloes whereas sheep, goat, camel and horse have two. Udder of the camel cow have four quarters with its own teat.

The mammary gland of man, other primates such as monkey, langoor, chimpanzee & elephants are two in number and are located in the pectoral region. The fully developed breast in human females is a soft, rounded, elevated structure present over the pectoral region having central dark pigmented area (areola). The central part of areola, projected above the surface, is called nipple.

In the case of dog, cat, pig, rabbit, rat and mouse, multiple paired teats (4 to 6) are distributed along the thoracic and abdominal wall.

The pig has got several teats. The glands and teat are collectively known as udder in domestic animals. Udder is not found in Pig, rabbit and Humans. Udder is found in Horse, Cattle, Buffalo, Sheep and goats. In cow, buffalo and mare, four mammary gland form an udder but in sheep and goats 2 mammary glands form an udder.The teat functions as the only exit for milk and through which the neonate receives milk. Usually one teat drains one gland.The teat size is greater in case of buffaloes as compared to exotic cows, which make them less suitable for machine milking. The size of udder determines milk yield. Teat size and shape determine milk flow rate rather than milk yield.

Supernumerary, or extra teats in ruminants are defined as any teat that is in excess of the normal number of teats. Supernumerary teats are the most common congenital abnormality and the condition is likely heritable in dairy cattle. Most of the extra teats in cattle are blind, and do not have a streak canal or attachment to mammary tissue. Each supernumerary teat may or may not be connected to a functional gland. These extra treats sometimes render the cows unsuitable for machine milking. The presence of a patent streak canal in the supernumerary teat serves as a source of infection to the mammary gland. The occurrence of supernumerary teats in exotic cows is quite common as compared to the Indian or Zebu cows. Buffaloes have a very small number of animals having supernumerary teats (4%). Supernumerary teats may also cause nipple confusion; occasionally, a newborn can get so focused on a bogus teat that he inadvertently ignores the real milk supply and ends up with hypoglycemia or failure of passive transfer (FPT).

Structure of the Mammary Gland

The mammary gland is a skin gland and is covered with hair except for the teats. The udder is separated into two halves by a longitudinal groove, the intermammary groove, externally.

One of the important anatomical adaptations of the udder that allows dairy cows to carry large amounts of milk is the development of a suspension system for the udder. Internally the right and left halves are separated by the medial suspensory ligament, which is made up of two layers of dense connective tissue. The medial and lateral suspensory ligaments support the bovine udder. Although no specific membrane separates the fore and rear quarters of each udder half, the duct system is independent of each other.

The mammary gland mainly consists of (1) Glandular epithelium (2) Blood and lymphatic vessels and (3) connective tissue.

The mammary tissue is made up of a group of alveoli which are surrounded by connective tissue capsules called stroma. A group of alveoli surrounded by a thin layer of connective tissue is called a lobule and a group of lobules surrounded by thick layer of connective tissue form a lobe. Each alveoli is a group of mammary cells which are arranged in a single layer around a central duct. The ducts of several alveoli are joined together to form a large duct and so on which ultimately drain into the gland cistern. Each gland cistern is supplied by 12-20 larger ducts and open into the teat cistern. The teat cistern is the cavity within the teat. The junction between the teat cistern and gland cistern is surrounded by a constriction called annular fold. The teat cistern opens to the outside of the teat through a small opening called streak canal or teat meatus.

Furstenburge's Rosette : The Furstenberg's rosette is located in the internal streak canal of the teat. It radiates upward into the teat cistern. It often is considered a barrier for pathogens, yet it offers little resistance to milk leaving the teat. It is composed of about 7 or 8 loose folds of double layered epithelium and underlying connective tissue. Each fold have number of secondary folds. The teat canal serves as the first line of defence protecting the mammary gland against new infections manifesting as mastitis.

Galactophore : The opening of the teat canal to the exterior is known as galactophore. Number of galactophores represents the number of primary sprouts. Number of galactophores per teat varies among the animals. In mare there are two galactophores and two teat canals. In bitch and cat there are multiple galactophores on each teat.

The interior anatomy of mammary tissue is divided into:

I Connective tissues

II. Secretory tissues

Connective tissue consists of fibrous tissues made of collagen and fatty tissue made of adipose cells. The essence of these tissues is to provide support to the mammary gland in order to exhibit optimal performance (milk production).

Secretory Tissues

These are tissues made up of cells, which produce milk. The milk is synthesized by the alveolar cells and from there it is secreted into the alveolar ducts. The milk from ducts is finally carried via the gland cistern, teat cistern, to the young calf. The alveolar tissue of the mammary gland is highly vascularized to facilitate the synthesis of large amounts of milk.

Alveolus : The basic unit of milk synthesis in the mammary gland is an alveolus. Alveoli are sac-like structures where milk is synthesized and secreted. An alveolus is the discrete milk-producing unit. It is comprised of a single layer of secretory epithelial cells that surround a cavity called lumen. Each alveolus is roughly spherical and is surrounded on the outer side by a basement membrane called membrana propria. Myo-epithelial cells are located between the basement membrane and epithelial cells. When activated by oxytocin (a hormone secreted from the posterior pituitary), the myo- epithelial cells contract so as to squeeze the alveolus and to cause milk ejection from the lumen of the alveoli.

The milk is stored after secretion into gland cistern and teat cistern. The size and shape of the cistern varies with species, stage of lactation and physiological status of the animal.

Effect of Estrogens and Progesterone-Mammary Development

The development of mammary function is divided into several distinct stages. (1) Mammogenesis, the growth and differentiation of mammary alveolar tissue (2) Lactogenesis, the onset of copious milk secretion around parturition (3) Lactation, the continuing production of milk and (4) involution, the return of the mammary gland to a less differentiated state at cessation of lactation.

Mammogenesis is the process of development of the mammary gland and starts as soon as the embryo develops (30 days). Mammary gland growth in the female takes place during five distinct phases of the development. 1. Prenatal, 2. Prepuberal, 3. Post pubertal (during estrus cycle), 4. Pregnancy and 5. Early lactation.

1. Prenatal development or fetal development of the mammary gland : During fetal development, hormonal influences are not necessary for the development of the gland. The first mammary growth in the fetus occurs as a raised area of ectoderm on both sides of the midline in either the inguinal region or on the entire abdominal surface. This mammary band is further converted to mammary line and gives rise to mammary buds equal to the number of teats in the adult. Internally the duct system is developed at birth but the alveolar system has not developed yet.

2. Mammary gland growth from birth to puberty : Most of the development in mammary gland from birth to puberty is due to an increase in connective tissue and deposition of fat in the mammary gland. However, a small amount of secretory tissue growth also takes place.

Initially the growth of the mammary gland is parallel to increase in metabolic body weight (weight of the body raised to the power 0.72, $W^{0.72}$). This type of growth is called **isometric growth** (iso- similar). At about 3 months of age the growth of the mammary gland becomes faster than the body growth. Such type of growth is called **allometric growth** (allo-dissimilar).

3. Mammary gland development during recurring estrous cycles : During estrous cycle, the ovary is active and produces two hormones, namely estrogen and progesterone. In addition the pituitary also secretes two hormones during this period namely prolactin and somatotropin (STH, Growth Hormone) which are concerned with mammary gland growth. Estrogen and progesterone are concerned with the lobulo-alveolar development of the mammary gland.

Thus two points stand out clearly; that the development of the mammary gland during the estrous cycle is not as much as during pregnancy and also that this growth is under hormonal control.

4. Mammary gland growth during pregnancy : The majority of the mammary growth occurs during pregnancy. This growth is dependent on the presence of pregnancy hormones. The great increase in the size of udder during the last part of pregnancy is due to the accumulation of secretory material within the mammary gland. The major hormone prominent during pregnancy is progesterone secreted by the corpus luteum of pregnancy as well as by the placenta. In addition estrogen, prolactin, thyroxine, insulin, corticosteroids are also involved. Specific placental lactogens have been found in several species.

5. Mammary gland growth during lactation : Although a large proportion of secretory tissue has developed by the end of pregnancy, some additional growth also takes place during the early part of lactation.

Puberty brings about an increase in the level of sex hormones. These hormones in the females are estrogen and progesterone, required for the proper functioning of the estrous cycle & pregnancy. These two hormones are also important for the proper development of the mammary gland. In general estrogen alone causes duct development and progesterone is required for the alveolar development. Estrogen and progesterone together bring about the lobulo-alveolar growth but the ratio of the two hormones required for optimum mammary development varies with the species. The two hormones act in unison with one hormone mimicking the effect of other to a limited extent and it is not entirely possible to separate out the role of these two.

The role of ovarian hormones, viz. estrogen and progesterone was demonstrated by experiments in which the reintroduction of ovarian tissue into ovariectomised animals permitted continued growth of mammary glands. Similarly, mixture of estrogen and progesterone stimulated mammary proliferation equivalent to late pregnancy in female rabbits, but progesterone alone was ineffective. The ratio of estrogen and progesterone as also the source of their origin varies with the species. These hormones are in addition assisted by a number of other hormones from the anterior pituitary. Somatotropin (STH), Adrenocorticotropin (ACTH) and prolactin are such hormones.

The extrapituitary hormones known to help in the mammogenesis process are insulin and thyroxine.

The mammogenic effect of prolactin manifests itself as increased alveolar development, and the presence of mitotic activity and thymidine incorporation. Insulin increases the mitotic activity of mammary gland explants of pregnant rats. Adrenocorticotropic hormone(ACTH) and thyroid stimulating hormone(TSH) acting on the adrenal gland and thyroid gland also play a minor role in growth of the mammary gland

Hormonal Control of Mammary Growth

Estrogens (estradiol 17β; E2), progesterone (P4), prolactin (PRL) and growth hormone (GH) are essential for physiological mammary growth and development, which not only take place during pregnancy but also occur with every reproductive cycle. While estrogens induce ductal growth, P4 is essential together with PRL for lengthening and tertiary branching of the ductal system and stimulation of lobulo-alveolar development

Lactogenesis (Initiation of Lactation)

The sudden surge in secretion of milk at parturition is called lactogenesis. Lactogenesis is caused by an interaction among several hormones. Major among these hormones are prolactin and adrenal corticoids. Several nonspecific stresses, drugs and neural stimuli can initiate lactation by actions mediated through the hypothalamus and pituitary. Adrenal corticoids aid prolactin in the initiation of lactation, which alone is ineffective. ACTH also has the same effect as that of injecting adrenal corticoids.

The high levels of estrogens and progesterone during pregnancy act synergistically to inhibit lactation. At parturition, the levels of estrogen and progesterone declines removing the block for initiation of lactation & prepares the ground for full potential of prolactin and corticoids to initiate lactation. Progesterone is the key negative regulator of lactogenesis. Progesterone suppresses onset of synthesis of lactose, alpha-lactalbumin, and casein. Progesterone in fact competes for glucocorticoid receptors and suppresses prolactin secretion from the pituitary.

Insulin and/or IGF-I seems to be necessary for lactogenesis and causes alveolar cells to undergo cell division. Insulin and /or IGF-1 also stimulates glucose uptake by mammary cells by stimulating glucose transporters in the mammary cell. This action is essential for lactogenesis as glucose is a needed precursor for lactose synthesis.

Glucocorticoids also help in lactogenesis as they are involved in transcription of casein and alpha-lactalbumin genes and in other changes needed for protein synthesis. Mammary Glucocorticoid receptors increase late in pregnancy.

Prolactin controls Prolactin release from pituitary and increases Prolactin receptors peripartum.

Galactogenesis (The production of milk by the mammary gland).

Galactopoiesis (Maintenance of Lactation)

Once the lactation starts, the milk yield rises gradually until it reaches its peak and then starts declining. The lactation length varies considerably among different genetic groups and species. Lactation is stopped when the young are weaned or milking is stopped abruptly or gradually.

Hormones required for the maintenance of milk secretion are similar to those required for the initiation of lactation. Hypophysectomy of the animals, stops the milk production. Thus involvement of prolactin, along with Adrenal corticotropic Hormone, Thyroid and Growth Hormone is indicated. Suckling stimulus is important in the continued release of galactopoietic hormones from the pituitary gland (i.e. ACTH, TSH & STH).

Ablation of the neural lobe of the hypophysis abolishes the milk ejection reflex and the young die from starvation unless injections of oxytocin are given to the mother.

In addition to prolactin and somatotropin, placental lactogens are galactopoietic hormones in cattle. Placental lactogens are Type I cytokines produced by the placenta during pregnancy that share structural homology with PRL and GH and can also influence pregnancy-related mammary development. Human Placental Lactogen is a single-chain, nonglycosylated polypeptide composed of 191 amino acid residues and two disulfide bridges, with a molecular mass of 21,600 Da.

Milk production is a function of mammary gland size and activity, these components increase during recurring lactations. It is to be mentioned that the nutritional demands of a cow or human mother during pregnancy are considerable, but those during lactation are far greater. The enormous output of nutrients, of carbohydrate, protein, fat and calcium, necessitate a large food intake by the lactating cow.

Growth Hormone (GH1) gene has been reported to be a candidate gene for milk production in cattle. The genetic markers related to GH1 gene could be used for early selection of young males for improving milk production and milk composition in dairy cattle. bGH gene is approximately 2800bp long, having five exons and four introns. Identified genetic markers in the intron 3 and exon 5 region of the GH1 gene can be used for selection for improvement of milk production.

Milk Ejection Reflex

Milk ejection is the discharge of milk from the mammary gland. Milk ejection is a reflex phenomenon. It is called milk ejection reflex or milk let-down reflex. It is a neuroendocrine reflex.The rate and extent to which milk is ejected from the mammary gland during suckling or milking depend upon the relative functioning of a complex array of facilitatory and inhibitory factors which are entwined and capable of adapting. Some of these operate to regulate the release of oxytocin from the neurohypophysis; others function peripherally to regulate the contractile effectiveness of oxytocin sensitive moyo-epithelial cells within the mammary gland.

When the calf suckles, the sensory impulses are transmitted to the hypothalamus through somatic nerves to the hypothalamus. The activation of hypothalamus causes release of oxytocin and prolactin from the pituitary gland. The oxytocin is carried to the teats through blood, where it causes contraction of myoepithelial cells that surround the outer wall of the alveoli. This process is called milk ejection or milk expulsion or milk let down.

Even stimuli such as sight or sound of calf also cause milk ejection, indicating the psychological component in the neuroendocrine reflex.

Milk Removal

To extract milk, a calf presses its tongue around the teat and against the palate of its mouth and creates a vacuum by separating its jaw and retracting its tongue. More than 100 suck and swallow cycles may be observed per minute. Milk removal during nourishing is also dependent on the differential pressure across the teat canal.

Milk removal is dependent on the reflex release of oxytocin from the posterior pituitary. Oxytocin is transported via blood and causes milk ejaculation by contracting the moyo-epithelial cells that surround the mammary alveoli. The act of suckling or milking reflexly stimulates both milk secretion and milk ejection. The time taken by the hormones to reach the site of moyo-epithelial cells surrounding the alveoli & exert its action is the time required for milk let down.

The afferent component of the reflex arc is nervous, whereas the efferent limb is hormonal. The sensory stimuli associated with suckling excite receptors in the mammary glands and impulses are conveyed over spinal and brainstem tracts to the diencephalon and supra-optic nuclei of the hypothalamus. Through the mediation of the supra-optic-hypophyseal tracts, the neural cells of the hypothalamus discharges oxytocin which is transported to the hypophysis. Oxytocin in the blood forms the effector component of the arc and the moyo-epithelial basket cells around the mammary alveoli constitute the effector tissue. The milk ejection reflex may be excited by various kinds of conditioned stimuli, and it is also subject to inhibition by emotionally stressful situations.

Milking Rate

It determines the speed with which animals can be milked. The milking rate of cattle is inherited characteristic. Maximum and average rate of milk flow increases with lactation after the first lactation.

Size of Teat Orifice

The most important physiological factor determining the rate of milk flow is the teat opening. This involves both the diameter of the teat meatus and the tautness of the sphincter muscle surrounding the meatus. Significant positive correlation between the size of the teat orifice and the maximum milking rate has been reported. The tautness of the sphincter muscles was more closely related to the maximum rate of milk flow than was the size of the orifice. The size of orifice determines the rate of passage of a liquid through it and the tonus of sphincter muscle affects the size of the opening.

Internal Udder Pressure

Internal udder pressure develops due to the accumulation of milk within the mammary gland. It may be equivalent to 2-3 inch of Hg. It has a relatively small influence in the milking rate.

Machine Factors

The machine factor that causes the greatest change in milk flow rate is the *level of vacuum*. Increase in vacuum level, increases maximum and average rate of milk flow. Fluctuation in vacuum decreases the rate of milk flow. The milking rate can be increased slightly by increasing the *number of pulsations per minute*.

Physiology of Mammary Gland During Dry Period- Involution of Mammary Gland

Once lactation is induced at parturition, it is maintained through continued ejection of milk from mammary glands. If milk ejection is curtailed, the production of milk ceases and the mammary gland involutes. After the peak secretion of milk, the milk yield gradually decreases until it is finally stopped. This is due to the involution of the mammary tissue. The exact mechanism which causes involution is not known though the mammary cell fatigue and decrease in the number of milk secreting cells may be the factors responsible for it. The involution of lactation is important as it gives the body the necessary time to replenish the body stores, for the mammary gland to function again at next parturition. During involution, the alveoli become distended, their walls stretched and the alveolar cells flattened, the capillaries become compressed and the blood supply is greatly reduced. Within 3 to 4 days, the alveolar cells break up, lysosomal enzymes are released and there is digestion of the cellular components and resorption of the secretary products, which diffuse into the interstitial spaces and are carried away in the lymph. Macrophages play an important role in the removal of fat from the regressing gland.

Artificial Induction of Lactation

Estrogen, progesterone, prolactin and glucocorticoids work synergistically at the onset of lactogenesis. Estrogen stimulates mammary ductal growth, and the combination of estrogen and progesterone regulates lobular-alveolar development of the mammary gland. This development does not occur in infertile animal or animals suffering from reproductive disorders due to relative absence of sex steroid hormones. Artificial induction of lactation can be induced in such animals by the combination of steroid hormones estrogen and progesterone. Additionally reserpine (tranquilizer-increases prolactin level) and dexamethasone (a synthetic glucocorticoid) can be used in induction protocols to increase the success rate. Artificial induction reduces the involuntary culling rate as well as the genetic losses. To save such genetically superior bovines, induction of lactation is the most appropriate technology used under Indian conditions. The treatment is more effective in well-fed animals with good body condition scores and having normal teats and udders. Hormonal induction of lactation should be practiced only in infertile animals; it should not be followed as a routine practice, as an alternative to normal lactation. Estrogen and progesterone in 1:2.5 ratios is effective in exotic and cross bred while 1:1 ratio is effective in indigenous cows and buffaloes for artificial induction because of short luteal phase. These methods of artificial induction of lactation yield 60 to 70% milk of previous lactation.

Colostrum

Colostrum is the first biological fluid from the mammary gland of mammals following parturition. Calves are highly susceptible to disease immediately after birth because of inadequate nutritional reserves. The colostrum specifically provides elements that enhance the calf's disease defences and accomplishes many nutritional demands. Colostrum is high in fat, protein and immunoglobulins, but low in lactose. It takes several days for the composition of milk to become normal.

Among non immunoglobulin important nutraceutical found in milk is lactoferrin is an iron-binding glycoprotein. Lactoferrin's main function is non-immune protection.It has the following activities

- antimicrobial activity, which has been presumed due to iron deprivation, but more recently attributed also to a specific interaction with the bacterial cell wall and extended to viruses and parasites;
- immunomodulatory activity, with a direct effect on the development of the immune system in the newborn, together with a specific anti inflammatory effects;
- a more recently discovered anticancer activity.

The colostrum though best suited for the feeding of the newborn, is not normally considered suitable for human consumption. The young of most and perhaps all mammalian species do not develop an effective immune system until after birth. Humoral immune protection (immunoglobulins) is supplied to the neonate by a process of transfer of passive immunity from the dam to the neonate. This generally occurs by transfer of maternal serum IgG from the dam to the offspring either in utero or, after birth, by ingestion of immunoglobulin-rich colostrum by the neonate. These maternal immunoglobulins offer immune protection until development of a competent immune system in the neonate and may even be involved in modulating the neonate's developing immune system. Therefore, lack of colostrum intake shortly after birth can lead to high neonatal mortality rates .

Colostrum, besides being a concentrated source of energy to the newborn, provides immuno-globulins (especially IgA antibodies) which helps in protecting the newborn calf against several diseases and also helps in the development of immunity. The immunoglobulins in the case of domestic animals are impermeable to the placenta, thus colostrum serves as the sole source of immunoglobulins in early life. In several other mammals, the placenta is permeable to these immunoglobulins and then the importance of immunoglobulins in these species is a minor one.

Immunoglobulin isotype G1 (IgG1) is the major immunoglobulin transported by the cow mammary gland during colostrum formation. The IgG1 and IgG2 make up the majority of immunoglobulin in cow colostrum and primarily come from the blood (that is they are preformed). Most of the IgA and IgM that are transported into colostrum are synthesized by the plasma cells (B lymphocytes) that reside in the mammary tissue. Transport of the IgGs and the IgA/IgM occurs through the epithelial cells by a process involving small transport vesicles. However, the receptors for the IgGs and the IgA/

IgM are different receptors. The receptor for IgA/IgM is called secretory component and is proteolytically cleaved off the membrane during transport of the IgA. The secretory component remains bound to the IgA and the SC-IgA complex is called secretory IgA.

The transformation from colostrum to normal milk takes 3 days in goat's milk and about a week in the case of camel's milk. Colostrum, the first secretion after parturition, is emerging as the most potent natural immune booster for human beings. Evidence suggests the beneficial effects of supplementation of bovine colostrum in improving health, athletic performance, diarrhea in persons with immune-deficiency syndromes, NSAID(Non steroidal anti inflammatory drug)-induced gastrointestinal disturbances, and aspects of the acute phase response that occurs secondary to surgery.

Milk Yield and Composition : The milk yield varies considerably with the breed, level of nutrition, stage of lactation, climate & various other factors. The yield of zebu cattle is much less than the exotic cattle. Part of the differences in milk yield are genetic. The capacity for milk yield is inherited. The amount of milk produced by an animal is important from the economic point of view. The whole dairy industry is dependent on the abundant and uninterrupted supply of milk.

Milk is mainly composed of carbohydrates (i.e. lactose), fat (triglycerides) and proteins (casein, L-lactalbumin, lactoglobulin etc.) though water comprises the largest component of milk of all domestic species. Minerals and vitamins constitute the minor components of milk though not so minor in importance. Normally milk is deficient in Vitamin C and Iron.

Cow and goat milk most nearly resembles human milk except for higher amount of protein and lower amount of lactose in them. Cow, sheep, goat and buffalo are the major producers of milk required for human consumption. Many ingenious processes are used to make cow's milk resemble human milk more closely for infant nutrition. The content of lactoferrin, wellknown antimicrobial and antiviral substance is higher in desi cow milk as compared to crossbred and buffalo milk.

Milk of Different Species of Domestic Animals

Cow milk : Cow milk contains approximately 3 to 4 percent fat, protein about 3.5 percent and lactose 5 percent, but the gross chemical composition of cow milk varies depending on the breed. The health effects of milk may depend on the breed of cow it came from. Currently, A2 milk is marketed as a healthier choice than regular A1 milk. Proponents assert that A2 has several health benefits and is easier for people with milk intolerance to digest. A2 milk generally refers to a variety of cow's milk that mostly lacks a form of β-casein proteins called A1, and instead has mostly the A2 form. There are 13 genetic variants of bovine beta casein; out of these A1 and A2 are the most common in dairy cattle breeds. The A1 and A2 variants differ only at position 67, which is histidine in A1 or proline in A2 milk. A1 and A2 beta-casein are genetic variants of the beta-casein milk protein that differ by one amino acid. A1 β casein could be responsible for several health disorders like diabetes, coronary heart disease etc, while A2 β-casein is generally considered safe for human consumption.

Indian native breeds of cows and buffaloes are of A2 milk type and hence are a source for safe milk.

Buffalo milk: Buffalo milk is rich in fat as compared to cattle. The buffalo fat does not contain carotene which is very much present in cow milk fat. That is why the butter or ghee prepared from buffalo milk is white while it is yellowish in case of cow milk.

Camel milk: Camel's milk composition approaches nearest to goat's milk. As compared to buffalo milk, the milk of camel is decidedly poorer in total solids. Camel milk seems to contain larger amount of total proteins, such as lactoferrin and immunoglobulins as compared to cow milk, which may be responsible for the better antimicrobial properties. The casein fraction of milk proteins consists of four caseins, namely αs1-casein, αs2-casein, β-casein and κ-casein. Casein genetic polymorphisms are important due to their effects on quantitative traits and technological properties of milk.

Goat milk: The average composition of goats milk resembles most nearly the human and cow's milk. Goats milk contains more protein and less carbohydrates as compared to human milk. Goats milk contains less sodium but more potassium and chlorine than cow's milk.

Equine milk : Equine milk contained low fat as compared to sheep, HF cows, camel and buffalo milk but lactose content was at par in milk of all the species. Protein content in equine milk was lower than sheep and buffalo milk.

Biosynthesis of Milk Constituents

Biosynthesis of Milk Proteins

Milk contains approximately 3.5% protein of which 80% are casein and 20% whey proteins. Caseins have been classified as α-, β- and k-caseins. Whey contains β-lactoglobulin, α-lactalbumin and several minor proteins with different biological activities such as enzymes, mineral-binding properties and immunoglobulins. Kappa-casein, an important protein component in mammalian milk, plays a pivotal role in formation and stabilization of milk micelles and preventing them from aggregating and therefore, helping to keep calcium phosphate in solution.

The lactating mammary gland is a prodigious protein-producing factory. Therefore, with the advent of genetic engineering of mammals it has the possibility of making use of the mammary gland to produce large quantities of proteins not normally found in milk. Use of transgenic animals for this purpose has been advocated and tried.

Arising from several origins including the blood stream and various cellular sources, many of the proteins found in milk are products of the secretory cells directly involved in the synthesis and secretion processes of various milk components. Blood proteins (Proteins derived from milk) are higher in colostrum and in the milk of early lactation, followed by a drop and tending to rise again in late lactation. Blood proteins amount to only a few percent of the normal mid lactation milk, which contains mostly lactation specific proteins synthesized de novo in the mammary gland. The lactation-specific proteins present in major amounts are synthesized in the rough endoplasmic reticulum

(RER) under genetic control and undergo further post-translational modifications in their secretory route from the RER through the Golgi apparatus and secretory vesicles before ejection into the lumen with other milk components.The molecular mechanism of milk synthesis is the same as in other cells. The endoplasmic reticulum, m RNA etc. are involved.

Milk secretory cells derive their requirements of all the essential and a few of the nonessential amino acids from the blood plasma but probably synthesize themselves the other ones. The major milk proteins casein and β-lactoglobulin are synthesized in the mammary gland itself from its nitrogen pool which is in equilibrium with free circulating amino acids.

Biosynthesis of Lactose

The lactose produced in the mammary gland is the main carbohydrate in the newborns' diet and an important source of energy. Lactose is the main carbohydrate in the milk of most species.The substance responsible for the sweet taste of milk is lactose, a carbohydrate with about a fifth of the sweetness of ordinary sugar. Chemically, lactose is a disaccharide consisting of glucose and galactose joined together by a beta linkage between C-1 carbon atom of galactose and C-4 carbon atom of glucose. Lactose is found exclusively in the milk and mammary gland is the only tissue having the unique capacity of its synthesis. The presence of lactose has a strong effect on ingredient processing and stability.

Lactose favours calcium and phosphorus absorption from the intestine and promotes the growth of favourable types of bacteria in the intestine and inhibits the multiplication of undesirable putrefactive ones.

In the mammary gland, lactose is synthesized from glucose. The first step of lactose biosynthesis is common with the first step of glycolysis in which glucose is phosphorylated in the C-6 position by the enzymes glucokinase or hexokinase.

Among the lactose synthesizing enzymes, lactose synthetase has a unique function. Its activity in the rat mammary gland increases markedly during lactation from an almost zero value on the last day of pregnancy. A comparison of the activity of lactose synthetase with other enzymes in the pathway indicates that the activity of lactose synthetase is a limiting step in milk production. Furthermore, the study of lactose synthetase delineated for the first time a metabolic function for one of the major milk protein components. The enzyme lactose synthetase is composed of two proteins. One of them, the b-protein has been identified as alpha-lactalbumin, a principal protein of milk whey. The A-protein is an enzyme that normally incorporates galactose into glycoproteins. In the presence of alpha-lactalbumin the enzyme has its specificity changed to the promotion of the reaction of glucose to form lactose. This seems to be the only case known where such a protein modified the specificity of an enzyme.

The galactosyl transferase is located in the Golgi apparatus of the lactating cell.

Digestion of lactose into usable monosaccharides, glucose, and galactose needs the activity of the genetically controlled, intestinal enzyme lactase.The enzyme Lactase is a transmembrane protein in intestinal epithelial cells, or enterocytes. Its function is to break lactose into its two constituent sugars: glucose and galactose. These constituent sugars can then be used in ATP manufacturing and other cellular processes.

The transcriptional regulation of lactose synthesis indicates that glucose transporters play an important role.

Milk and dairy food consumption can lead to adverse clinical symptoms probably due to lactose intolerance. Lactose intolerance is defined as experiencing gastrointestinal symptoms following the ingestion of lactose which is often caused by a genetically determined reduction of lactase production in adulthood.

Biosynthesis of Milk Fat

Milk fat is the most important constituent of milk because of its obvious economic implications. Milk fat has a great nutritional significance although recently milk fat importance has been mitigated because of association of saturated fat and cholesterol with coronary heart disease. Milk fat contains potential anticancer agents such as sphingomyelin and other sphingolipids, butyric acid, 13 methyltetradecanoic acid and vitamin A. There are other antimicrobial activities associated with milk fat . Milk fat as an energy source has obvious implications in body metabolism.

Milk fat invariably consists of triglycerides (i.e. glycerol combined with three fatty acids). The fatty acids of different species vary in their length of carbon chain and in the degree of saturation.

Milk fat is composed of fatty acids of varying chain length and degree of saturation. The fatty acids having a long carbon chain are either taken up from the circulating lipids in the blood or by synthesis de novo within the cells of the mammary gland. The medium chain fatty acids are invariably synthesized de novo in the cells of the mammary gland. Acetate and butyric acids absorbed from the rumen are used in the mammary glands to synthesize fatty acids. Butyric acid gets converted to beta hydroxybutyrate in the liver and released into the blood circulation where it gets taken up by mammary tissue for further synthesis of fatty acids in the milk.

3-hydroxybutyrate taken up from the blood which is used in some short chain fatty acid synthesis. Butyryl-coA is synthesized de novo from acetyl CoA and malonyl-CoA by fatty acid synthetase, thus serves as a primer for the de novo synthesis of most medium & long chain fatty acids. Acetyl-coenzyme A carboxylase is the major regulatory enzyme of fatty acid biosynthesis, catalyzes the conversion of acetyl-CoA to malonyl-CoA. Sequencing of the ACACA cDNA has indicated a silent single nucleotide polymorphism identified at exon 45 (C5493T). C5493T mutation was suggestively associated with fat yield, lactose content, and somatic cell count.

The synthesis of milk fat involves intracellular assembly of milk-lipid droplets and the nature and formation of the milk-fat globule membrane (MFGM). Triacylglycerols are synthesized in the rough endoplasmic reticulum by membrane-bound fatty acyl transferases. Microlipid droplets (less than 0.5 μm in diameter) so formed, are released into the cytoplasm and coated with protein and polar lipids from the reticular membrane. Expulsion of lipid droplets from the cell is completed by a budding process, during which the droplets acquire an outer membrane of proteins and phospholipids from the apical plasma membrane by a process known as exocytosis.

The synthesis of fatty acids is under hormonal control with insulin, cortisol, growth hormone & prolactin being important among others. Growth hormone-releasing factor is the main endogenous stimulator of somatotropin secretion has a role in milk fatty acid synthesis through growth hormone and does not have a galactopoietic role per se independent of growth hormone. Studies have shown a relationship between milk fat depression (MFD) and alterations caused in lipogenic gene expression by dietary nutrients.

Nutrition is the predominant factor affecting milk fat.

Production diseases such as milk fever or hypocalcemia, ketosis, fatty liver, metritis, retained placenta, displaced abomasum, and mastitis have all been shown to have a negative effect on potential production and to increase the risk of involuntary culling.

Bioactive Components of Milk

Milk contains specific proteins, peptides, and fatty acids that are bioactive components. The bioactive properties of a number of these components in milk have been examined with regard to a range of health-related variables eg Lactoferrin, a bioactive glycoprotein is a member of transferrin family and plays an important role in immune defense, iron homeostasis, antioxidant and regulation of cell growth.

The lactating mammary gland is a prodigious protein-producing factory. Therefore, it is little wonder that with the advent of genetic engineering of mammals someone would propose making use of the mammary gland to produce large quantities of proteins not normally found in milk. Application of the concept of genetic engineering and the use of the mammary gland as a bioreactor is being explored aggressively to produce novel proteins, biopeptides and pharmaceuticals is an area called gene pharming.

Immunoglobulin Transport in the Mammary Gland

The young of most mammalian species do not develop an effective immune system until after birth. Humoral immune protection (immunoglobulins) is supplied to the neonate by a process of transfer of passive immunity from the dam to the neonate. This generally occurs by transfer of maternal serum IgG from the dam to the offspring either in utero or, after birth, by ingestion of immunoglobulin-rich colostrum by the neonate. These maternal immunoglobulins offer immune protection until development of a competent immune system in the neonate. In most domestic animal species immunoglobulins are not transported across the placenta, therefore the colostral immunoglobulins are critically important to neonate survival. Lack of colostrum intake shortly after birth can lead to high neonatal mortality rates.

Mammary Cell & Secretion of Milk

The cells lining the alveolus which synthesize milk are similar in structure as any other cells in the body. As any other cell, they are composed of a nucleus and cytoplasm. They differ from other cells in that they have the enzymes responsible for milk synthesis in their cytoplasm and also have higher number, volume or surface of organelles which are required for synthetic activity of the mammary cell.

Most of the milk is stored in the alveoli. In ruminants a considerable amount of milk is stored in the gland cistern and teat cistern also.

The secretion of milk by the mammary cells involves both transcellular and paracellular pathways. The transcellular pathway involves the precursors for the synthesis of milk components are taken up by mammary which synthesizes the final secretory product for final secretion into the ducts by the process of exocytosis. The paracellular pathway for secretion of substances into milk involves passage between the epithelial cells rather than through them.

Among the major milk components, proteins, lactose, calcium, phosphate and citrate are packaged into secretory vesicles and secreted by exocytosis. Triglycerides (fat) synthesized in the cytoplasm and smooth endoplasmic reticulum of the mammary alveolar cells coalesce (unite) into large droplets which gradually make their way to the apex of the cell. The lipid droplets bulge against and gradually become entirely enveloped by apical plasma membrane, and finally separate from the cell as milk fat globule. The immunoglobulins secretion by the mammary cells from the blood is through the mediation of specific receptor protein.

The solid components of milk like proteins, fats and lactose are all formed in the alveolar cell. During peak lactation, the mammary gland synthesizes and secretes a prodigious complement of products into milk including proteins, carbohydrates, membrane-coated lipid droplets, water, and ions. The overall process of milk formation involves the biosynthesis and secretion of its components. Milk synthesis has been defined as synthesis within the cells and passage of the formed products into the alveolar lumen. Independent pathways have been advocated for synthesizing various components of milk. The efficiency of milk synthesis can be improved by taking advantage of the accumulated knowledge of the transcriptional and post-transcriptional regulation of genes coding for proteins involved in the synthesis of fat, protein, and lactose in the mammary gland. Recently it has been possible to direct nutrigenomic interventions to increase milk fat synthesis by feeding long-chain fatty acids and milk protein synthesis by feeding amino acids.

Mastitis

Mastitis is an infection of the mammary gland resulting in significant economic losses and an important threat affecting the world's dairy industry . High milk production is usually associated with higher incidence of mastitis. The most significant abnormality in milk due to subclinical mastitis is the increase in somatic cell count (SCC). Since cell numbers in milk are closely associated with inflammation and udder health, SCC constitutes an important criterion for the measurement of milk quality as an international standard. Milk somatic cells are primarily leukocytes or white blood cells. High SCC levels in the milk cause deterioration of milk quality.

Mastitis is caused by udder inflammation. Mastitis is the result of a bacterial invasion of the mammary gland where the immune system is either weakened or overwhelmed. The term, inflammation describes the response of a tissue or organ to injury. The purpose of inflammation is to destroy or neutralize infectious agents and associated toxins, thus allowing the gland to return to normal function. Bacterial invasion of the mammary gland occurs by bacteria entering the teat sphincter and moving into the teat cistern and beyond. The disease is multi-etiological complex in which Staphylococcus aureus has been found to be the most important pathogen worldwide for clinical as well as subclinical forms. Capsular polysaccharides produced by S. aureus isolates are considered important virulence factors in the pathogenesis of Staphylococcal infections. Bacterial presence within the udder results in the movement of white blood cells into the gland to help fight the disease. Once gland tissue becomes infected, numerous neutrophils will be drawn to the mammary gland, resulting in increased somatic cell counts. During mastitis condition, there is an increase in the somatic cell count which is directly related to proteolysis of milk protein due to the increase in plasmin activity. The milk somatic cells have a wide range of proteolytic and lipolytic enzymes, which are released during the intracellular mechanism, killing microorganisms in subclinical mastitis, and may significantly contribute to proteolysis and lipolysis of the milk constituents. Proteolysis associated with increased somatic cell count in milk promotes the breakdown of casein micelles. Increase of proteolysis has a negative impact on the quality and technological properties in milk and milk products. There are a range of adverse effects from the use of high (Somatic cell count)SCC milk in the production of cheese, such as reduced curd firmness, decreased cheese yield, increased fat and casein loss in whey, and compromised sensory quality.

In general goat milk contains higher SCC than cow milk due to the apocrine secretory process of goats. According to the National Mastitis council, to differentiate between healthy and infected udder secretion the limit of SCC has been decided as 10,00,000 cells/ml.

The reductions in milk production during mastitis is largely due to physical damage to the epithelial cells of the affected mammary gland, and a consequent reduction in the synthetic and secretory capacity of the gland as a whole. Effects of mastitis on milk composition are determined by severity of infection, extent of infection, secondary physiological changes which alter metabolism of mammary cells and/or the cow, and whether the epithelial cells are disrupted or milk components are destroyed by enzymatic action. The bacterial contamination could lead to alterations in milk composition through the action of hydrolytic enzymes released by the bacteria.

Lactoferrin is one of the important candidate genes for mastitis resistance. The gene is located on Bos taurus autosome (BTA) 22 and consists of 17 exons spanning over 34.5 kb.

Prolactin

Prolactin is a polypeptide hormone synthesized in and secreted by anterior pituitary lactotroph cells. The biological actions of prolactin are not limited to its essential role in reproduction, but also involve regulation of the immune system, osmotic balance, angiogenesis and behavior. Prolactin is a natural hormone in the body. It plays a role in breast growth and the production of milk . Prolactin is associated with the development of mammary tumors in rats and dogs. Estrogens and ionizing radiation can act synergistically in the development of malignant mammary tumors in female rats.

An increase in the concentrations of free estrogen and prolactin in the plasma following estrogen administration will result in an increase in the rate of DNA synthesis in the mammary gland and a concomitant increase in the susceptibility to tumorigenesis. In addition, prolactin and estrogens could act as promoters of tumor growth. The effects of prolactin are mediated by its receptor, and alterations in receptor expression are likely to play a role in tumor development.

Neoplasms of the mammary gland are among the most common diseases in female domestic dogs (Canis familiaris) and has been correlated with prolactin hormone. Mammary cancer has been found to have decreased expression of estrogen receptor-alpha (ERα, ESR1), progesterone (P4) receptor (PGR), prolactin (PRL) receptor (PRLR) and growth hormone receptor (GHR) associated with neoplastic differentiation of mammary tissues.

The contribution of prolactin (PRL) to the pathogenesis and progression of human breast cancer at the cellular, transgenic, and epidemiological levels is increasingly appreciated. Women with higher blood levels of prolactin have a slightly higher risk of breast cancer than women with lower levels. Acting at the endocrine and autocrine/paracrine levels, PRL functions to stimulate the growth and motility of human breast cancer cells. The actions of this ligand are mediated by at least six recognized PRL receptor isoforms found on, or secreted by, human breast epithelium. The PRL/PRL receptor complex associates with and activates several signaling networks that are shared with other members of the cytokine receptor superfamily. Coupled with the recently identified intranuclear function of PRL, these networks are integrated into the in vitro and in vivo actions induced by ligands. Antagonists of PRL/PRL receptor interaction or PRL receptor-associated signal transduction may be of considerable utility in the treatment of human breast cancer.

Mammary tumors represent the most common neoplastic disease in female dogs. Breast cancer has the strongest association with increased prolactin and prolactin receptor levels. Bromocriptine and cabergoline are also used to treat hyperprolactinemia with no known cause.

Lactation Cycle

Cows and buffaloes must calve to produce milk and the lactation cycle is the period between one calving and the next. Milk production changes during lactation characterized by an ascending phase from parturition to peak production (the maximum production) and a downward phase, from this peak to the dry period. The slope of this phase represents the persistency of lactation. The cycle comprises the early, mid and late lactation and the dry period. In an ideal world, cows calve every 12 months. A number of changes occur in cows as they progress through different stages of lactation.

The two major factors determining total lactation yield are peak lactation and the rate of decline from this peak (Persistency of lactation).

Lactation Curve

Milk production commences at relatively high rate after parturition. Amount secreted increases for 3 to 6 weeks. Higher producers peak later than lower producers. After peak, milk production gradually declines

Rate of decline = persistency

Milk Composition Changes

The concentration of milk fat and protein is highest in early and late lactation and lowest during peak milk production through mid lactation. Normally, an increase in milk yield is followed by a decrease in the percentages of milk fat and protein, while the yields of these constituents remain unchanged or increase. Late-lactation milk has higher levels of fat, protein, casein, whey proteins, non casein nitrogen, bovine serum albumin, sodium, and casein hydrolysis products than other stages of lactation. This change in milk composition could be due partly to reduced milk volume at late lactation resulting in the concentration of milk constituents within the udder.

Questions on Lactation Physiology

Write short note on following

1. Induction of lactation
2. Milk proteins
3. Endocrine control of lactogenesis
4. Lactose synthesis in mammary tissue
5. Synthesis of milk fat
6. Hormones involved in mammogenesis
7. Galactopoiesis
8. Write the hormonal control of mammary gland development and lactogenesis.

Summary

- Lactation is the process of milk secretion by the mammary gland of mammals.
- Milk is produced and secreted by most mammals in specialized skin glands called mammary glands. Mammary glands produce milk by which the young are nourished through the critical period from birth to weaning.
- Milk is a complex mixture of solutes that are secreted by specialized epithelial cells within glandular units found in the mammary glands.
- The initiation of milk secretion (lactogenesis) and the maintenance of milk secretion-galactopoiesis is under hormonal control.
- Prolactin, somatotropin and placental lactogens are galactopoietic hormones in cattle.
- The lactating mammary gland is a prodigious protein-producing factory. The major milk proteins casein and β-lactoglobulin are synthesized in the mammary

gland itself from its nitrogen pool which is in equilibrium with free circulating amino acids.

- Lactose, the main milk sugar, is found exclusively in the milk and mammary gland is the only tissue having the unique capacity of its synthesis. Lactose synthetase is a unique enzyme for the synthesis of lactose in the mammary gland.
- The synthesis of milk fat involves intracellular assembly of milk-lipid droplets and the nature and formation of the milk-fat globule membrane (MFGM). Triacylglycerols are synthesized in the rough endoplasmic reticulum by membrane-bound fatty acyl transferases.
- The secretion of milk by the mammary cells involves both transcellular and paracellular pathways. The transcellular pathway involves the precursors for the synthesis of milk components are taken up by mammary which synthesizes the final secretory product for final secretion into the ducts by the process of exocytosis. The paracellular pathway for secretion of substances into milk involves passage between the epithelial cells rather than through them.
- Mastitis is an infection of the mammary gland resulting in significant economic losses. Mastitis is the result of a bacterial invasion of the mammary gland where the immune system is either weakened or overwhelmed.

17

Growth and its Regulation

Growth is a correlated increase in the mass of the body in definite intervals of time, in a way characteristic of the species i.e. increase in size and weight. This means growth includes the protein, fat and mineral deposition in the body. Growth is an irreversible increase in the metabolically active protoplasm. There is a characteristic rate of growth for each species and a characteristic adult size and development. Maximum size and development are fixed by heredity and nutrition is an essential factor determining whether this maximum will be reached. An optimum nutritional regime is the one which enables the organism to take full advantage of its heredity.

Growth process involves both an increase in the size of cells called as hypertrophy and an increase in the number of the body cells called as hyperplasia.

Two fundamental components of growth are hyperplasia (increase in number of cells) and hypertrophy (increase in cell size). These processes cause change in body weight and body size (daily fluctuations like feed and water intake and disease conditions are not considered as growth). Monitoring of growth is essential to provide proper quality and quantity of feed economically for a viable animal industry.In early embryonic life both processes occur in the case of all cells. Ability of adult organisms to hypertrophy becomes less with age.

Growth and development have important implications for domestic animal production because they significantly influence the value of the animal being produced. By understanding the physiology of growth there lies a huge potential for improving the efficiency of animal production.

Growth rate and feed conversion ratio decrease with age and follow a curvilinear pattern in most domestic animals. This may be because of the fact that maintenance energy increases with increase in metabolic body weight. Therefore, it seems economical if livestock are produced and slaughtered at an earlier age. Lot of research has gone into the determination of the optimum age of slaughter of domestic animals like sheep, goat, cow, pig and poultry. Law of diminishing returns has been most applied in determination of optimum age for slaughter.

Growth in animals can be measured quantitatively by plotting a growth curve which indicates the rate of increase of mass or length over a period of time.

Absolute growth rate is measured as absolute weight gain per unit time. Relative growth rate is measured as weight gain in a given time in relation to initial weight and expressed in percentage.

Cells and Principles of Cell Growth

Cells are building blocks of all tissues. Cells are of various types and specialize in performing certain functions in the tissues.

Growth is achieved by increase in the mass and /or number of cells comprising specific tissues and organs of the body in a dynamic way which involves not only new cell or material additions but also the degradation of older dying cells and removal of cell constituents. Cells consist of proteins, lipids, nucleic acids, carbohydrates, water and mineral components, all of which are in a dynamic state of turnover (synthesis, accumulation, degradation and elimination). In order for there to be an increase in size or mass the rate of synthesis or accumulation must exceed the rate of degradation. The fractional rate of growth is high in early life.

The phenomenon of growth includes processes which change the size, shape and composition of farm animals over a period of time and is fundamental to all aspects of production and reproduction in farm animals. Growth is the process by which an animal becomes larger over time, and may be measured in different ways, such as physical height or length, but the most common measure is the body weight change. Growth occurs by processes of hyperplasia (increased cell numbers) and by hypertrophy (increased cell size). In all tissues of the body it is difficult to access the relative contribution of hyperplasia and hypertrophy to the overall increase in size. During the first stage of fetal growth hyperplasia generally precedes hypertrophy. Rapid rate of growth after a period of starvation is called compensatory growth.

Biochemical and Genetic Determinants of Growth

As animals were domesticated over the years, their growth and body composition patterns were altered to meet the needs of individuals who were responsible for their domestication. That is why there is so much genetic diversity among domestic animals. Livestock performance depends mainly on the genetic potential of the animal. On the other hand, optimum nutrition, good management and disease control etc, permit full expression of this genetic potential. Therefore, improvement in genetic capabilities as well as environment are both required for animal improvement. The maximum size of an animal is determined by its genetics, but nutrition and disease influence whether the animal reaches its genetic potential for size. Growth and development are continuous and dynamic processes requiring integration of numerous physiological functions, they are influenced by:

- Nutrition,
- Efficiency of metabolism and respiration,
- Hormonal regulation,
- Immune response,
- Physiological status of the animal,
- Diseases and parasites, and
- Maintenance of homeostasis.

The growth can be divided into two phases i.e. Prenatal Growth and Postnatal growth.

Prenatal Growth

Conception is the starting point of growth. The period of growth between the time of fertilization and the birth of the young one is called prenatal growth. In poultry 21 days are required for the fertilized egg to become a fully functional chick, but in farm animals it takes a long time. Prenatal growth and development are broken down into three stages:

- ovum development
- embryogenesis,
- organogenesis

A new individual arises from the union of a sperm and ovum, forming one cell with diploid number of chromosomes. The single fertilized cell divides as it passes down the oviduct but there is little increase in total size. In this cell division, the mother cell produces two daughter cells, which are capable of further division to form new cells.

The time of prenatal development has been divided into three stages: ovum, embryonic, and fetal stages. The ovum stage lasts from conception until hatching of the blastocyst from the zona pellucida. The embryonic stage involves the key process of differentiation from the three germ layers of the inner cell mass of the blastocyst (endoderm, mesoderm, and ectoderm) to formation of the tissues of the organs, muscles, skeleton, and skin. The fetal stage is the time of further growth of the fetus to parturition. The endoderm becomes the lungs, liver, pancreas, and esophagus and the lining of the stomach, intestines, and colon. The mesoderm becomes the muscles, bones, and other connective tissues; heart and circulatory system; and kidneys. The ectoderm becomes the brain and spinal cord, skin, and hair.

The size of the foetus is judged by the total foetal length, crown-rump length, curved crown-rump length or foetal weight.

In live conditions, the actual weight of the fetus is difficult to measure. The foetal body confirmation can easily be assessed by ultrasound or X-ray techniques. These foetal measurements can also be employed for estimating the growth rate or the age of the fetus.

The developing fertilized egg undergoes a process of differentiation in which the mother cell produces different kinds of daughter cells like brain cells and heart cells is called cytogenesis or histogenesis . This process is irreversible in which the brain cells cannot form the egg cells. As the development of embryo proceeds many organs are formed and then differentiation ceases. The organization of various dividing cells into different organs each with a particular structure and function is known as morphogenesis or organogenesis. During morphogenesis, the differentiated cells synthesize new proteins and enzymes, which are specific for each tissue formed.

PostNatal Growth

The period of postnatal growth extends from birth or hatching until death. The length of this period depends greatly on the species. Sheep and cattle tend to live to be around 15 and 30 years of age, respectively.

Somatic cells produced from cell division have a diminishing power to grow by hyperplasia. In highly differentiated cells, the power to produce is lost e.g., mature RBCs entering the circulation do not have nucleus and cannot divide and die after about 120 days but the bone marrow cells produce the RBCs continuously. But, the differentiated nerve or brain cells lose their ability to divide and there is no mechanism to create new cells.Muscle, bone, and fat are the three main types of tissues that develop as an animal grows.Growth of animal tissues results in formation of key food products such as meat which consists of muscle and connective tissues.

Muscle growth is the result of protein synthesis, and the rate of muscle growth slows as the animal reaches approximately half its mature size. Muscles contain a mixture of three types of muscle fibers: Type I (red), Type II β (white), and Type II α (intermediate). Red muscle fibers are used for sustained work, such as long-term locomotion, and are termed aerobic because they derive their energy from oxidative metabolism. White muscle fibers are larger in diameter than red fibers, are used for short-term, rapid bursts of activity such as quick movement, and are termed anaerobic because they derive their energy from the metabolism of glycogen. Intermediate muscle fibers utilize both oxygen and glycogen to generate ATP for muscle contraction. Selection for animals with larger muscles results in animals having a larger proportion of white and intermediate-type muscle fibers.

The two types of bone found in the body are cortical (dense) bone or spongy bone. Cortical bone is found in the shafts of long bones of the appendicular skeleton and is responsible for the strength of the long bones. Both compact and spongy bones are produced by endochondral ossification or conversion of cartilage to bone. The layered bones of the skull are produced by intramembranous ossification, a process of direct deposition of bone onto a connective tissue network. Bone is deposited by osteoblasts and mobilized by osteoclasts, whereas osteocytes are relatively inactive bone cells found isolated in the bone matrix. Longitudinal growth of long bones occurs at the epiphyseal plates, a region of chondrocyte production and cartilage synthesis at the junction of the epiphysis and diaphysis. The relative degree of ossification of cartilage of spinal vertebrae and epiphyseal plates is used as an indicator of maturity of beef and lamb carcasses, respectively. Bone growth is stimulated by growth hormone, thyroid hormones, and IGF-I, and bone growth is inhibited by estrogens and a deficiency of vitamin D.

Development of fat tissue occurs at each of the four growth stages, but the majority of fat tissue is deposited in the end of the third and fourth growth stages. The fat is deposited in a highly organized order through genetic control mechanisms. Subcutaneous fat, intermuscular fat, and intramuscular fat are examples of the building blocks for the fat depots. When adipocytes (fat cells) are developed and enlarged, they are filled by the synthesis of fatty acids. This process takes place in each growth stage.

The adipose tissue is a very active physiological tissue that produces substances that regulate fat deposition and fat reduction. Resistin and leptin are examples of hormonal control substances released from the fat tissue that control fat deposition. The rate of fat deposition is also influenced by genetics, the rate of animal growth, energy and nutrient intake, efficiency of growth, and animal age. The fat components of the carcass can influence meat flavor positively and negatively, meat processing, meat marketing, and to some degree, meat tenderness.

Several hormones are responsible for regulation of growth in the body which include the peptide growth factors, leptin, prostaglandins etc. Hormone regulation of growth involves multiple hormones acting in concert.

Isometric growth:When an organ grows at the same rate as that of the general body growth it is known as isometric growth.

Allometric growth: When an organ grows at the different rate than the general body growth it is known as allometric growth. Allometry is the study of relative growth, of changes in proportion with increase in size. Sir John Hammond, one of pioneers in the study of farm animal growth,used a method of growth analysis by making photographic prints of animals at magnifications giving a constant skull length. To estimate meat yield in live animals it is necessary to visualize the muscle mass beneath the animal's outward shape.

At birth, meat animals tend to have large heads and long slender limbs. Subsequent growth is marked by an increase in body length and depth until, finally, the hams fill out convexly. Hammond's technique showed the animal shape that would be most likely to yield the greatest mass of edible meat.

Regulation of Growth, Metabolic and Hormone Interactions

Cellular and molecular mechanisms that control farm animal growth, including development and body composition are important. A multitude of hormones, local growth factors and gene transcription factors regulate growth and differentiation of skeletal muscle, bone and adipose tissue of animals. Hormone regulation of growth involves multiple hormones acting in concert. The main hormones concerned with growth are pituitary growth hormone, thyroid hormone,insulin, the sex hormones testosterone and estrogen, and the pituitary gonadotropic (sex-gland-stimulating) hormones and two newly discovered hormones Leptin and Ghrelin.

Growth hormone (GH) is essential for postnatal somatic growth, maintenance of lean tissue at maturity in domestic animals and milk production in cows. Two hormones principally regulate the secretion of GH: growth hormone-releasing hormone (GHRH) stimulates, while somatostatin (SS) inhibits the secretion of GH. Pituitary growth hormone (GH) has considerable potential as an anabolic agent in animal production.

The other hormones essentially required for normal growth and development are thyroid hormones, and gonadal steroid hormones.

Myostatin also known as GDF-8 is a negative regulator of skeletal muscle growth, responsible for double muscling in animals including sheep. In double muscling, muscle mass is increased which results in the decreased weight of bones, fat and digestive tract. The decrease in weight of other body components results in heavier carcasses and a higher proportion of leaner and expensive cuts of meat.

Insulin

Insulin is a very important hormone involved in muscle growth and development. It stimulates the transport of certain amino acids into muscle tissue and is active in reducing the rate of protein degradation. Growth hormone (GH) and insulin-like growth factor-I (IGF-I) control growth in cattle and swine. Insulin has been shown to have an impact on both prenatal and postnatal growth. Specific mechanisms of insulin action on adipose cell function and lipid storage are well defined. Insulin probably acts in concert with other anabolic factors (i.e., growth hormone and somatomedins) to stimulate muscle protein anabolism and suppress protein catabolism. Insulin also plays a role in energy balance regulation by the hypothalamus.

Leptin and Ghrelin

Leptin and ghrelin seem to be the big players in regulating appetite, which consequently influences body weight/fat. Leptin decreases hunger and in contrast to leptin,ghrelin increases hunger. Leptin and Ghrelin play a central role in the neurohormonal regulation of food intake and energy homeostasis

Jeffrey Friedman cloned the ob gene in mice and its homolog in humans in 1994. In 1995, Friedman purified the gene product, a hormone he called leptin. Friedman's discovery of leptin showed that there is a robust physiologic system that regulates food intake and metabolism, that fat is an endocrine organ, and that obesity is a problem of biology. Leptin acts to maintain homeostatic control of fat mass .

Leptin is a hormone predominantly made by adipose cells and the small intestine that helps to regulate energy balance by inhibiting hunger. This hormone acts on receptors in the arcuate nucleus of the hypothalamus. In obesity, a decreased sensitivity to leptin occurs (similar to insulin resistance in type 2 diabetes), resulting in an inability to detect satiety despite high energy stores and high levels of leptin.

Leptin, is a 16 kD protein consisting of 146 amino acids which is synthesized primarily by adipose tissue and is secreted into the bloodstream after cleavage of the 21 amino acid signal peptide. The hypothalamus is the primary site of action, since leptin receptors are located within hypothalamic areas associated with control of appetite, reproduction and growth.

Ghrelin

Ghrelin hormone is known for potent growth hormone releasing and appetite stimulating activities which is maximally secreted by stomach and duodenum but there are many more sources of ghrelin secretion in the body. Ghrelin is a 28 amino acid peptide that is the natural ligand for the growth hormone secretagogue (GHS) receptor. Ghrelin receptors are expressed in a wide variety of tissues, including the pituitary,stomach, intestine, pancreas, thymus, gonads, thyroid, and heart. Ghrelin is a potent stimulator of growth hormone secretion from the anterior pituitary gland.

Factors Affecting Efficiency of Growth and Production in Ruminants and Single Stomach Animals

The growth and development of animals depend on several factors like environment, management practices, and genetics. The growth and development of domestic animals are largely affected by two important factors. The first one is genetic, which includes disease resistance, feed conversion efficiency, breed etc. The second most important factor is non-genetic in origin and it encompasses factors like nutrition, management, disease control, and environmental conditions.

Heredity : The efficiency of growth and production depends to a great extent on the genotype of the individual animal. There are variations in the species, individuals and breeds. The maternal contribution to variability in fetal size is greater than the paternal contribution.

Generally, non ruminants are more efficient utilizers of concentrates than ruminants, in which concentrate feeds are fermented by bacteria in the rumen before the main sequence of digestion, thus reducing efficiency. Similarly the high meat or milk producers are better at efficient conversion of feed to meat or milk, as it decreases the proportion of feed energy lost to maintenance.

Protein metabolism in the rumen is the result of metabolic activity of ruminal microorganisms. Ruminal protein degradation is affected by pH and the predominant species of microbial population. Dietary protein is divided into rumen-degradable and undegradable protein with RDP composed of nonprotein and true protein N. True protein is degraded to peptides and AA and eventually deaminated into ammonia N or incorporated into microbial protein. Nonprotein N is composed of N present in DNA, RNA, ammonia, AA, and small peptides with the N from peptides, AA, and ammonia being used for microbial growth. Microbial protein synthesis in the rumen provides the majority of protein supplied to the small intestine of ruminants, accounting for 50 to 80% of total absorbable protein.

The most important factors affecting microbial protein degradation include the type of protein, interactions with other nutrients (mainly CHO within the same feedstuff and within the rumen contents), and the predominant microbial population (dependent on the type of ration, ruminal passage rate, and ruminal pH). Solubility of proteins is a key factor determining their susceptibility to microbial proteases and, thus, their degradability. Some of the key factors affecting the efficiency of growth are

Nutrition: The influence of the plane of nutrition is very important because of its relation to economics of milk and meat production. Varying the nutritional status of the animals during various periods of growth can alter the carcass composition of meat animals.

The effect of a plane of nutrition depends on the stage of growth. If a low plane of nutrition is fed during the accelerating phase of growth it induces retardation of growth. Since feed costs constitute the most important parameter of efficiency of animal production, the nutrients hold the supermost position in the factors affecting growth.

All vitamins especially Vitamin B complex, A and C are needed for normal growth hence affect the efficiency of growth in domestic animals. The feed additives also are important factors.

Sex : Generally males grow faster and reach better rates man females of equivalent ages even if both the sexes are provided with same nutrition.

Hormones : Lot of studies have been conducted on the effect of castration on the growth rate of domestic animals but the results have been conflicting. IGF-1 has been reported to be key anabolic hormones in beef cattle due to altered sex steroid production.

Litter size has a strong effect on behavior, eating patterns and body weight in animals with large litter size.In heat stressed animals, there is a reduction in food consumption which reduces substrate availability for growth and development processes in the body.

Environmental effect on growth are very profound and important. The primary environmental factors that affect animal growth and development are temperature extremes, either heat or cold, arid or humid climates, altitude and photoperiod effects. Climate influences growth by influencing indirectly the availability of fodder and directly the animal itself. Summer in the tropics offers poor quality and quantity of fodder thereby reducing the growth rate. In the temperate zone fodder is scarce during winter therefore decreasing the growth rate. Heat tolerant animals perform better than non heat tolerant animals under heat stress. Zebu cattle are better heat tolerant as compared to exotic cattle.

The effect of cold temperatures, or cold stress, are pronounced in newborn animals as the low temperatures during the early neonatal period greatly increases the morbidity and mortality of neonates. Cold stress puts increased stress on body processes involving body heat conservation and heat production. Peripheral vasoconstriction is one such process which redirects the blood flow from the periphery to body core.

Diseases retards growth of animals by directly interfering with metabolism and absorption or indirectly by affecting the appetite of the animal. If the animals are immunized it will prevent occurrence of diseases and help in optimum growth of animals.

Tissue specific growth factors affect the growth of animals by affecting the proliferation and development of specific types of cells.

- **Insulin-like growth factor**- The main effector of growth hormone (GH) is insulin-like growth factor-1 (IGF-1), an endocrine mediator of growth and development under physiological conditions. Besides this important function, IGF-1 also plays a prominent role in the regulation of immunity.
- Epidermal growth factor (EGF)
- Nerve Growth Factor (NGF)
- Erythropoietin (EP)
- Promine and Retine
- Chalones

Growth in Meat Producing Animals & Birds

As the world's population increases, the need for reliable protein sources is growing. Meat is well-considered a good source of high biological value protein. Meat is an important source of nutrition for many people around the world. Global demand for meat is growing: over the past 50 years, meat production has more than quadrupled. The world now produces more than 320 million tonnes each year.As animals were domesticated over the years, their growth and body composition patterns were altered to meet the needs of individuals who were responsible for their domestication.

There is a difference in priority of different tissues for nutrient utilization. Nervous tissues gets the most priority and fat tissue gets the least. In between lies the skeletal muscle or what we call growth in meat producing animals.Similarly the body area which gets the most priority is Head followed by neck and shoulder. The rib and loin are the least priority. The perinephric fat gets the most priority and intramuscular the least with intermuscular and subcutaneous fat in between.

The proportion of muscle, bone and fat ratio changes with age, species, plane of nutrition and many other factors. Muscle growth is the result of protein synthesis, and the rate of muscle growth slows as the animal reaches approximately half its mature size. Muscles contain a mixture of three types of muscle fibers: Type I (red), Type II β (white), and Type II α (intermediate). Red muscle fibers are used for sustained work, such as long-term locomotion, and are termed aerobic because they derive their energy from oxidative metabolism. White muscle fibers are larger in diameter than red fibers, are used for short-term, rapid bursts of activity such as quick movement, and are termed anaerobic because they derive their energy from the metabolism of glycogen. Intermediate muscle fibers utilize both oxygen and glycogen to generate ATP for muscle contraction. Selection for animals with larger muscles results in animals having a larger proportion of white and intermediate-type muscle fibers.

Efficiency of Growth

The efficiency of growth of meat producing animals is sometimes measured by Feed conversion ratio (FCR)- Quantity of animal feed required to produce one kilogram of meat, egg or milk product. This is measured as dry matter feed in kilograms per kilogram of edible weight output. For broiler producers, an FCR of 1.6 means that their chickens gain 1 kilogram of weight for every 1.6 kilograms of feed consumed. The proportion of feed in a broiler's ration ranges from 40 to 70% of the cost of production. The lower the FCR, the more efficient animals are at converting feed into food. FCR is a function of the animal's genetics and age, the quality and ingredients of the feed,and the conditions in which the animal is kept. Comparisons of FCR among different species may be of little significance unless the feeds involved are of similar quality and suitability. The best way to improve FCR is to provide poultry with good nutrition, reliable systems of feed procurement and production, good care and husbandry, and disease control to ensure efficient poultry and egg production. The feed conversion ratio of broilers has been increased by various means e.g. feed modifications such as feeding of additives, prebiotics, probiotics or exogenous enzymes and genetic improvement. Improving feed efficiency is critical when attempting to reduce production costs in poultry.

Growth rate and FCE (feed conversion efficiency) are higher in intact males than in castrates.

Growth Curves

Growth is an increase in body height, length, girth and weight that occurs when a healthy young meat animal is given adequate food, water and shelter.

Anabolism versus catabolism:Anabolism is the building up of body components, while catabolism is their destruction.All live animals show both anabolism and catabolism.

- If anabolism exceeds catabolism, the animal is growing.
- If catabolism exceeds anabolism, the animal is wasting away.
- If anabolism equals catabolism, animal weight is constant.

There are various ways of measuring growth, as actual weight, percentage increment, or weight per day gained. Average daily weight gain is generally the most common method to measure growth rate, as it forms a basis for daily food requirements and, conversely, also enables the rate of growth to be controlled exactly by regulation of the food intake. The live-weight growth curve of the animal as a whole is made up of the sum of the different parts and tissues of the body, each of these growing at different rates. Growth curves of animals were widely used to evaluate and predict animal growth.

A common definition of growth is an increase in live weight gain per unit of time and these two concepts are plotted to develop the growth curve. If animal height or weight are measured from conception to senescence, the data usually follow a flattened "S" shape called the sigmoid curve.

The animal growth rate is closely related to the ability for nutrient absorption in the small intestine.

The patterns and stages of growth are associated with nutrition and environmental interactions, genetic regulations, and production traits. A common definition of growth is an increase in live weight gain per unit of time and these two concepts are plotted to develop the growth curve.

Growth curves are often divided into four stages.

- The first stage reflects the early development of the head and neck region as well as the internal organs.
- The second growth stage results in an increase in body length, major increases in bone and muscle, and organ growth is almost completed.
- The third growth stage results in a deepening and thickening of the body with a major increase in muscle and the start of significant fat deposition.
- The fourth growth stage involves greater development of the loin and hindquarter, an increase in depth of the body, an increase in intramuscular fat, the muscle growth greatly declines, and waste fat is the major tissue deposited.

Intramuscular fat (marbling), however, is deposited in both the early and later growth stages.

Growth curve can also be obtained by plotting the average daily weight gain against the age of the animal. This curve shows that the rapid growth rates are seen during the postnatal period, culminating in the high growth rate during the time of maturation , followed by a slow decline in growth rate until mature size is reached.

Recombinant Gene Transfer Technologies for Growth Manipulation- Advantages and Limitations

Genes contain the codes for the growth, development, and function of all living organisms.Gene is a segment of DNA that codes RNA for polypeptide molecules. Since the initial descriptions in the early 1970s of methods to successfully generate recombinant DNA molecules, recombinant DNA technology has advanced to the point that researchers now have the ability to routinely introduce DNA into the genome of animals to experimentally alter patterns of gene expression in vivo. This gene transfer capability provides a powerful tool with which to evaluate the function of genes within the intact animal and to study the interplay of genes in tissue and organ systems. Gene transfer is a relatively rapid way of altering the genome of domestic livestock. The basic objective of gene transfer is to modify phenotype through modification of gene expression. The use of these tools will have a great impact toward improving the efficiency of livestock production and animal agriculture in a timely and more cost-effective manner. Gene transfer is to transfer a gene and DNA segments from one organism to another. This area of genetic manipulation makes important contributions to domesticated animals in relation to immunology, vaccines, aging, and cancer.Gene transfer technology provides the ability to genetically manipulate the cells of higher animals.

Gene transfer technologies include electroporation, microinjection, macroinjection, biolistics or microprojectiles for DNA transfer, liposome mediated gene transfer, calcium phosphate mediated DNA transfer, DEAE-Dextran for gene transfer, gene transfer by polycation-DMSO, polyethylene glycol mediated transfection and gene transfer through peptide.

The extraordinary potential of altered DNA molecules is to give rise to new life-forms that may be better than the original in terms of productivity, disease resistance and adaptability and sustainability.Gene transfer methods have been used in gene therapy and gene manipulation attempts.

The advent of molecular biology has initiated the search for use of molecular genetic markers as selection criteria in farm animals. The single locus markers such as genes for the hormones leptin, growth hormone and insulin-like growth hormones are suitable candidates as these hormones are associated with body composition, growth rates and birth and weaning weights.

Farm animal proteomics has been implemented and successfully applied to optimize welfare and productivity in the farm and food industry. Meat and milk are major sources of proteins in the human diet. Both are raw materials of high value, but are economically fully exploited only through processing by the dairy and meat industries. The quality of the multiple end-products (e.g.cheese and cured meat) is highly dependent on the quality of the raw materials, hence directly associated with the structure and function of the constituent protein. Proteome-based markers for meat and milk quality are in great demand,because these markers allow scoring and ranking raw materials. Quality ranking allows optimal use of the entire product range by assessing the specific suitability of the individual products for further industrial processing. Moreover, proteome markers are useful for monitoring and optimizing the industrial processes in the dairy and slaughter industry. Such technological markers are thus important tools for maximizing the gains of the food industry.

Variations in meat quality characteristics, like tenderness,juiciness, flavour and odour, are closely related biological traits and genetic variations of the live animals. Hence a broad selection of studies including genetics,physiology, cell biology and biochemistry has been aiming at characterizing biological traits and molecular mechanisms behind observable variations in meat quality. In particular, the biology of muscle differentiation and growth, carcass composition, and fat deposition patterns have been characterized in detail at the proteome level.While intramuscular fat deposition increases the taste and juiciness of meat, the subcutaneous fat deposition is a waste in meat production. Hence, optimizing pigs through breeding towards deposition of intramuscular rather than subcutaneous fat is a major goal. Proteomics is an important tool for finding candidate genes that may influence this fat deposition.

As these traits are complex, and multigenic in nature, molecular characterization greatly benefits from correlated proteome and transcriptome analyses.

Proteome Markers for Animal Health

As in human pathology, proteome based bio-markers are important for early diagnostics in veterinary medicine. Diseases prevailing in farm animals, however, are very different from those that commonly challenge human health (like cancers and cardiovascular diseases). Thus, dedicated bio-marker studies on farm animals are needed to monitor animal health and welfare, and to investigate type and state of disease, for ensuring animal welfare as well as for monitoring quality and safety of animal products.

Protein Deposition in Animals and Poultry

The ultimate goal of animal production is to convert various feedstuffs into edible meat and milk for human consumption. Thus, enhancing the efficiency of the bio-transformation of feed mass into body mass, especially, the lean body mass, is the bottom line for improving the profitability, as well as the sustainability, of meat and production in animals. Protein deposition in animals and poultry affects the practical aspects of animal production and concern mainly the muscle synthesis and deposition in ruminants and egg proteins in poultry. Skeletal muscle is a major reserve of protein in large animals. There is a large turnover of skeletal muscle protein taking place in the body all the time because of substantial exchange between plasma and muscle free amino acids. Protein deposition in animals is because of net positive balance of nitrogen retention in the muscles. This positive nitrogen balance depends on nitrogen intake, protein quality and dietary energy. Protein accretion and growth of skeletal muscle may be constrained by inadequate intake of protein or energy.

The quality of the dietary protein is an important determinant of the efficiency of deposition of dietary nitrogen within the body. The substrates for protein accretion and secretion in the mammal are the amino acids which are absorbed from the small intestine. Digestible Crude Protein was initially used to predict the protein availability in ruminants. Besides the supply of amino acids through absorption from the small intestine, the protein deposition in muscle tissue is also governed by the factors which decide how these amino acids are utilized by the animals. Because of microbial digestion in the rumen, the quantity and quality of amino acids ingested from the intestine may be different from the consumed amino acids.

Another important mechanism in nitrogen handling by ruminants is that proteolytic enzymes in the rumen lead to ammonia production in the rumen and absorbed ammonia is converted to urea in the liver and either excreted by the kidneys into the urine or recycled back into the rumen via the saliva (Urea recycling.).

Amino acids are the building blocks of proteins and polypeptides that are the major component of animals' muscles and tissues. In addition to being building blocks of body proteins, amino acids play a significant role in various important biochemical and metabolic processes in the cells of animals. So, from growth to production and reproduction, amino acids play a large part in the productivity of farm animals and can contribute significantly to the profitability of a farm.

Essential amino acids: These are amino acids that the animal cannot make by itself and must be provided through dietary intake to ensure normal function of the animal. They include phenylalanine, valine, threonine, tryptophan, isoleucine, methionine, histidine, arginine (sometimes considered to be non-essential), leucine and lysine.

Non-essential amino acids: These are amino acids that can be synthesized within the animal's body, usually from other amino acids or other compounds. They include alanine, aspartic acid, cysteine, cystine, glutamic acid, glycine, hydroxyproline, proline, serine and tyrosine.

Animal need sufficient amounts of all amino acids to meet their metabolic needs, whether they need to produce milk, build muscle and tissues or reproduce. The protein-producing potential of an animal is limited by the quantities of amino acids in its body. Supplementing amino acids to ruminants (cows, goats and sheep) in the rumen is special in the sense that some limiting amino acids are fed as protected proteins to increase the protein synthesis capacity of ruminants.

Hormones and Growth Factors Responsible for Protein Deposition

There are several factors which are responsible for nitrogen retention by domestic animals. Several hormones and a variety of growth and differentiation factors which have hormone-like activity affect the extent and rate of protein metabolism in animals. The predominant factors responsible for protein deposition are hormonal. Insulin, growth hormone, the thyroid hormones, the glucocorticoids, and steroids with anabolic activity are some of the hormones responsible for affecting the protein deposition. Animals administered somatotropin (Growth Hormone) have experienced large increases in protein deposition in growing animals. Exogenous pST treatment consistently improves ADG, feed conversion efficiency and protein deposition, and reduces fat deposition in pigs. Dose-dependent increases in lean deposition and reductions in feed intake, fat deposition, and carcass fat have been observed. no growth responses are observed because the reduction in fat deposition may offset the increase in protein deposition.

Based on the study of the role of hormones on protein deposition, anabolic agents have been developed to manipulate protein deposition in domestic animals. Anabolic agents are substances with physiological functions similar to those of the sex steroids which increase nitrogen retention and protein deposition in farm animals.These analbolic agents are either steroids and non steroids.

Anabolic agents

Amino acids or metabolites

Glutamine

Arginine

Hydroxy methyl butyrate

Anabolic hormones

Insulin

Insulin-like growth factor-1 (IGF-1)

Testosterone

Anabolic steroids-eg synthetic anabolic steroid Oxandrolone

Human growth hormone

Genetic Regulation of Protein Deposition

A number of candidate genes have been identified as potentially relevant to meat quality traits. The Ryanodine receptor 1 (RYR1) gene has been reported as the main cause of PSE in various pig breeds. The PRKAG3 gene is primarily expressed in white skeletal muscle fibers. The functional mutation in PRKAG3 gene is correlated with increased glycogen content in skeletal muscle. Heart fatty acid-binding protein gene (H-FABP) is involved in fatty acids transport. Melanocortin-4 receptor gene (MC4R) plays an important role in energy homeostasis and is associated with growth rate and feed intake. MYF-5 has been associated with intramuscular fat (IMF).

Questions on Growth and Its Regulation

1. Factor influencing prenatal growth
2. Factor influencing postnatal growth
3. Direct growth regulators
4. Measurement of postnatal growth

Summary

- Growth is a correlated increase in the mass of the body in definite intervals of time, in a way characteristic of the species i.e. increase in size and weight.
- Growth process involves both an increase in the size of cells called as hypertrophy and an increase in the number of the body cells called as hyperplasia.
- A multitude of hormones, local growth factors and gene transcription factors regulate growth and differentiation of skeletal muscle, bone and adipose tissue of animals.
- The growth and development of domestic animals are largely affected by two important factors. The first one is genetic, which includes disease resistance, feed conversion efficiency, breed etc. The second most important factor is non-genetic in origin and it encompasses factors like nutrition, management, disease control, and environmental conditions.
- Anabolism is the building up of body components, while catabolism is their destruction. If anabolism exceeds catabolism, the animal is growing. If catabolism exceeds anabolism, the animal is wasting away.
- There is a difference in priority of different tissues for nutrient utilization.
- Farm animal proteomics has been implemented and successfully applied to optimize welfare and productivity in the farm and food industry.

18

Physiology of Temperature Regulation

Domestic animals –including chicken and mammals, belong to the category of *homeotherms*, as opposed to *poikilotherms*. Homeotherms or warm blooded animals are those which are able to maintain constant body temperature in the face of varying environmental temperature. The poikilotherms or the cold blooded animals change their body temperature according to the temperature of the surroundings. Most invertebrates and lower vertebrates belong to the category of poikilotherms.

Two Types of Animals

1. *Homeotherms* or endotherms or warm blooded animals
2. *Poikilotherms* or ectotherms or cold blooded animals

Homeotherms have a high metabolic rate and therefore their heat production is 7-10 times greater than that of the poikilotherms.

Why do animals have to maintain constant body temperature? As we are aware that enzymatic reactions in the body are temperature sensitive. In fact, a 10 degree centigrade increase in temperature can result in doubling of the reaction rates. In order to maintain optimum functioning of the enzymatic reactions in the body a constant temperature is required. This constant body temperature is not very constant in the sense that it varies somewhat during exercise and also when the animal is exposed to extremes of temperature of the surroundings. That means that the temperature regulation mechanisms in the body are not 100 percent perfect.

At this stage it is desirable to clarify the distinction between surface temperature and core temperature. The surface temperature, in contrast to the core temperature rises and falls with the temperature of the surroundings. It is the temperature of the deep tissues or internal organs which remains constant. The temperature of the rectum is usually taken as a useful indicator of core temperature because of the ease of measurement.

Abnormal core temperature deviations of even a couple of degrees will challenge the body's thermoregulatory mechanisms, and swings in temperature outside the normal range can prove fatal.

The relative lability of body temperature is also dependent on species. The camel is able to increase its body temperature by several degrees without any ill effect. Such an increase is an adaptation in response to counteract heat stress, as the body can store and dissipate more heat at higher body temperature. Kangaroo, desert donkey and goat also have a relatively labile body temperature, albeit of a lesser magnitude.

Heat Balance

The ability to maintain body temperature is a function of the body to maintain a balance between heat gain and heat loss from the body. Heat is continually being produced in the body as a by-product of metabolism. By the oxidation of the constituents of food (carbohydrates, fat, or proteins), energy is transformed into heat in the body.The rate of heat production is a function of basal metabolic rate and also the increase in the rate of metabolism by the body during exercise and as a result of actions of hormones. Heat is produced in all body cells from the conversion of metabolic energy into mechanical and thermal energy. This process is very inefficient and thus approximately 30–70% of the energy liberated during muscle contraction appears as thermal energy. Thyroxine, epinephrine and norepinephrine are some of the hormones which enhance the metabolic rate and in consequence heat production by the body.

Both the heat gain and heat loss are centrally regulated by the centres situated in the hypothalamus and also by peripheral receptors. There is a high degree of coordination between the central temperature receptors and peripheral receptors.

Zone of Thermal Comfort/Thermoneutrality: The body temperature of domestic animals is maintained constant within a certain thermal limit called zone of thermal comfort. The animals in this zone are put to least amount of thermal stress and the animal has to make minimum efforts to maintain the body temperature. The range of temperature within which the animal uses no additional energy to maintain its body temperature is called the zone of thermoneutrality.It is this zone within which the physiological costs to maintain body temperature are minimal and productivity is maximum.The most comfortable environmental temperature range for temperate dairy cattle is between 5 and 25°C. Above this temperature, dairy cows increase respiratory frequency and rectal temperature that causes a decline in milk yield and reproductive performance.A rise in the core temperature also increases heat loss by panting and sweating.

Newtonian Heat Loss

Non-evaporative heat loss also known as Newtonian heat exchange. The body is able to lose heat from the body through conduction, convection and radiation and also from surface evaporation. The loss of heat by conduction, convection and radiation are governed by Newton's law, hence called Newtonian heat loss. Loss of heat by radiation means loss in the form of infrared heat rays, a type of electromagnetic wave. All objects that are not at absolute zero radiate such rays. The animal radiates heat waves in all directions and in turn heat rays are being radiated by surrounding objects towards the body. If the temperature of the body is greater than the temperature of the surroundings, a greater quantity of heat is radiated from the body than is radiated to the body.

Evaporative Heat Loss- Surface Evaporation

In order to maintain body temperature, the loss of heat by means of surface evaporation is also an important means of heat loss in animals including domestic animals. This stems from the fact that water has a high heat of evaporation, that means, one gram water evaporated causes the body to lose 584 cal (2443 Joules). The water from the body is lost through two means. Sweating from the sweat glands of the body surface and through panting, from the respiratory passages. Heat dissipation is faster in young than adult animals due to higher body surface area per unit of body weight.

Most species of mammals possess sweat glands, but their activity varies greatly. There are species differences in the number of sweat glands per unit area and also sweat gland activity.Variations in sweat gland density and shape explain only a part in the efficiency of sweating.Cattle use cutaneous evaporation as the primary route of water loss in temperature regulation. The sweat glands density in cattle is on an average 2000 glands/cm^2.The main source of evaporation in the camel is via the skin. A characteristic of the camel is that there is no copious flow of sweat or obvious wetting of the fur. On an average there are about 200 glands/cm^2 in the camel.

The relative contribution of sweating and panting to total evaporation varies with species. Birds, dogs, cats, pigs and the water buffalo are essentially non sweating species. Sheep and goats use sweating as well as panting equally effectively. The cattle are much better sweaters. The camel and horse are very good at sweating and use it very effectively. The zebu cattle (*Bos indicus*) use sweating to a much greater extent as compared to the exotic cattle (*Bos taurus*).

Sweat glands are tubular in shape and comprise a body and a long straight duct. The sympathetic nervous system is involved in the control of sweating. As most species respond to adrenaline in terms of sweat output, this hormone acts as a transmitter.

- ***Apocrine***: Controlled by adrenergic nerve fibers
- ***Eccrine***: Controlled by cholinergic sympathetic fibers

The evaporation takes place at the surface of the skin and body cools because of latent heat of evaporation.

Van't Hoff effect: Metabolic rate and thus heat production approximately double with every 10°C increase in body temperature.

Warm and cold receptors located in the core of the body (core receptors) present in hypothalamus and in the spinal cord are 5-10 times more sensitive than those in the skin.

The sweating rate is a function of sweat gland number and activity. The activity of the different sweat glands also varies. The sweating rate is measured in domestic animals by a simple technique called sweat gland prints. This technique uses cobalt chloride impregnated filter paper in which the weight of the filter paper is taken before and after application of the paper to a measured area of shaved skin. The filter paper is covered by a cellophane tape to prevent absorption of moisture from the environment. The sweat gland density in different species of domestic animals is given in Table 18.2. There is evidence that zebu cattle originating from the Indian subcontinent have 50-100% more sweat glands per unit area than breeds originating in Europe. Thus secretion of sweat serves through evaporation to cool the body.

Heat loss via skin is more in cows and heat loss by respiration is higher in buffaloes. Buffaloes contain less number of sweat glands as compared to exotic cattle and much less as compared to zebu cattle. The sweat gland of buffaloes have surface of 0.247

cm^2 each which is about twice the size of those for cattle (0.124 cm^2); but buffaloes have fewer glands so the glandular surface area per cm^2 of skin surface is about 1.07 in buffaloes and 3.08 in cattle.

Wallowing in animals is a comfort behaviour during which an animal rolls its body about in mud, water.To compensate for less water evaporation, the buffaloes during summer use wallowing in a pond or river. Wallowing is defined as to roll about or lie in mud or water, especially to keep cool or avoid biting insects. The greater proportion of wallowing in buffaloes occur between sunrise and sunset, particularly when the intensity of solar radiation is high. Buffaloes are more sensitive than cattle to high ambient temperature and direct solar radiations.

The dark body color of buffaloes is conductive to heat absorption when the animals are exposed to direct rays of sun. The thick epidermal layer of buffalo skin also reduces heat loss by conduction and radiation.Pigs lack functional sweat glands and are almost incapable of panting. To thermoregulate, they rely on wallowing in water or mud to cool the body. In Haryana, India the buffalo owner often apply mustard oil massage to the buffaloes. The oil massage also helps to retain water on the body for longer period by forming a water oil colloid and helps in thermal comfort.

Modern housing management for buffaloes requires a wallowing pond to be constructed near the buffalo paddock. However, the wallow should be one with clean water and not far from the farm. Spending time walking in the sun to and from the wallowing costs more than it saves. Showering of the buffaloes with cool water for 3 minutes twice a day has proven to be an efficient way for them to get rid of excess heat.

Elephant's skin is without sweat glands, therefore they suck water with their trunks and spray it over their bodies. When water is not available, they aspirate their own saliva and sprinkle it over their bodies to facilitate evaporative cooling in the hot summer season. A marked decline in the sweating rate or sweat gland fatigue occurs in man, goat, sheep during prolonged exposure to severe heat stress. Sweating in some species is accompanied by loss of salts from the body. Miner's or stoker's cramps result from salt loss under hot and humid environments, and can be prevented by incorporating small amounts of salt in drinking water.

Panting in most animals takes the form of very rapid shallow breathing, chiefly, through the nose at rates which may exceed about 300 per minute in case of sheep, or about 15 times minimum resting levels. During panting the respiration rate is increased several times. The air exhaled from the respiratory tract is saturated with water. During panting there is an increase in the amount of air exhaled and consequently the amount of water evaporating from the respiratory passages. As this process requires heat, which is taken up from the body, resulting in a cooling effect.

Continued heat exposure in some animals, after respiration rates have reached a maximum, results in a change to a deeper slower type of open mouthed breathing (second phase breathing).

Exposure of the animal to high environmental temperature stimulates the peripheral and core core body receptors in the hypothalamus, to help in preventing the rise in body temperature.

Heat Tolerance

Heat tolerance can be defined as the ability to maintain thermal stability at warm temperatures. Heat tolerance of animals is related to their heat dissipation ability and metabolic heat production at warm temperatures. The zebu cattle (*Bos indicus*) breeds are better adapted to thrive in warm climates as compared to exotic cattle (*Bos Taurus*). The zebu breeds are morphologically differentiated by the presence of a thoracic or cervicothoracic hump in Bos indicus (Zebu or Humped) which is absent in Bos Taurus cattle. The Bos indicus and Bos Taurus have been recognized as separate subspecies that evolved from the wild oxen Bos primigenius.The Bos indicus is presumed to be better adapted to heat owing to its evolution in hot climates.

Relative heat tolerance of different animals and different breeds is assessed on the basis of changes in respiration rate, pulse rate and rectal temperature when subjected to similar heat stress. Several heat tolerance indexes have been developed to measure relative heat tolerance of cattle in hot climates. Most of these indexes now are based on THI (Temperature Humidity Index).

Heat dissipation is determined by relative surface area, sweating rates, external insulation and respiratory heat loss.Higher heat tolerance in zebu and crossbred cattle is because of their lower metabolic rate. It has been postulated that higher heat tolerance is inversely related to milk yield.

Hypothermia and Hyperthermia

When the animal is exposed to cold, the body temperature is maintained by two mechanisms.

Heat Production

When the animal is exposed to cold, the heat is produced by increased metabolic activities and also by shivering. The primary motor center for shivering is situated in the posterior hypothalamus near the wall of the third ventricle. During exposure to cold, the heat production center activates the motor center and shivering occurs. Enormous heat is produced during shivering due to severe muscular activities.

Prevention of heat loss

Prevention of heat loss is due to vasoconstriction of the skin. Due to reduced blood flow to the skin, sweat secretion is decreased and heat loss is prevented. The heat gain centre of the body is situated in posterior hypothalamus and gets stimulated by cold exposure.

For each species, strain and individuals within species, there is a range of environmental temperatures, defined as zone of thermal comfort or thermoneutral zone, within which the metabolic heat production is unaffected by temperature change and homeothermic animals can maintain a fairly constant body temperature (heat loss is equal to heat gain) and an efficient level of growth, reproduction and lactation by its lower and upper ends by the lower critical temperature and upper critical temperature.

The lethal body temperature of most organ systems is approximately 43-45°C, at which temperature enzyme systems begin to denature.

Temperature-humidity index (THI) is an index for assessment of the potential of an environment to induce heat stress in humans and farm animals.

Lower Critical temperature : The ambient temperature below which the rate of heat production of an animal under resting state increases to maintain body heat balance is the lower critical temperature.

Thermo-regulation in Farm Animals

Body temperature represents the balance between heat production and heat loss. All metabolising body cells manufacture heat in varying amounts. Therefore, body temperature is not evenly distributed across the body. In ruminant animals the temperature in the rumen is considerably higher than the rectal temperature due to fermentative action in the rumen. Phulia, Upadhyay, Jindal and Misra, recorded the surface body temperature of goats using infrared tele temp thermometer and found that skin surface temperature increased with increasing intensity of solar radiation at noon. Body sites directly exposed to solar radiation had significantly higher skin surface temperature than unexposed parts. Core body temperature is found in the blood supplying organs such as the brain and those in the abdominal and thoracic cavities. Peripheral temperature is recorded in tissues such as the skin, where environmental factors and a lack of insulating connective tissue influence temperature.

Body temperature is a vital sign and it is important to measure it accurately.A thermometer is used to measure the temperature of the body. Body temperature of animals is measured by placing a thermometer in the anus and is called as rectal temperature. In the case of human beings the temperature is measured by placing a mercury thermometer at sublingual level for one minute. Average oral temperature for healthy adults has been considered 37.0 °C (98.6 °F), while normal ranges are 36.1 °C (97.0 °F) to 37.8 °C (100.0 °F).

Body temperature is centrally controlled by the hypothalamus. The thermoregulatory centre is located in the hypothalamus in the brain. It consists of the heat-loss centre, the heat-promoting centre and the preoptic region, which analyse and coordinate responses to maintain body temperature within the homeostatic range. The anterior part of the hypothalamus is concerned with heat loss while the posterior part is concerned with heat production. Signals arrive at the thermoregulatory centre via afferent pathways from the sensory receptors in the skin and organs. The centre's response is propagated along efferent neural pathways to the target organ or blood vessel to elicit a response to gain or lose heat The hypothalamus is in concurrence and aided by peripheral (cutaneous) thermosensors and the thermoregulatory response by the animal is a consolidated response of the two. Any change in the set point of the hypothalamus or changes in the temperature of the external environment can elicit the thermoregulatory response.

Role of skin

The skin is a protective barrier, and an endocrine, sensory and thermoregulatory organ. Skin is the layer of usually soft, flexible outer tissue covering the body of a vertebrate animal.

The skin has four major functions.

1. ***Protection*** : Against invasion by foreign organisms, such as bacteria and viruses : against dehydration and against some wavelengths of electromagnetic radiation.
2. ***Perception***: The detectors of changes in the environment are located in the skin.
3. ***Thermoregulation***: The skin is having thermoregulatory function as the heat loss from the body is regulated via skin. Sweat secretion evaporating from the skin accelerates heat loss.
4. ***Excretion*** : Glands in the skin excrete salts, nitrogenous end products and other wastes, making the skin a site of exchange with the environment.

Skin however has its limitation as a protective organ. Most irritant and cellular poisons are unable to penetrate it, but there are a few notable exceptions, including mustard gas and the irritant of poison ivy. Several kinds of bacteria can cross the skin and several kinds of fungi can form colonies on the surface of it. Nevertheless the skin does offer a rather high degree of protection against invasion. The mean thickness of the skin of water buffalo is reported to be 5.45 mm. Skin thickness increases as age advances and dorsal regions show more thickness as compared to other regions.

The skin is a complex structure, consisting of an avascular epidermis, a vascular dermis and subcutaneous fat. The skin layers vary greatly in thickness in various regions of the body. Skin blood flow is reflexly controlled by two distinct branches of the sympathetic nervous system, including an adrenergic vasoconstrictor branch and a cholinergic active vasodilator branch. The dermis is usually divided into two parts or layers. (1) The superficial papillary layer and (2) Deep reticular layer. The superficial papillary layer is thinner and is composed of collagen, elastic and reticular fibres. The dermis is composed of dense irregular connective tissue. The general arrangement of two layers of skin namely epidermis and dermis is found throughout the body, including areas of modified epidermal structures such as hair, horns, and hooves. The epidermis is composed of a deep growing layer, the stratum germinativum and superficial layer of cornified dried cells called stratum corneum.

The population of hairs on skin surface varies with the site. The hairs are generally shed during the summer whereas large fur develop during the winter. However this tendency varies with the species in its intensity. The average number of hairs in buffaloes has been reported to be 85.9/ mm^2.

The skin is the largest sense organ and can detect several types of environmental changes through the basic sense of touch. The sense of touch allows us to detect cutaneous sensations, or skin sensations. These cutaneous sensations include pressure, pain, and temperature. The skin detects changes in temperature through the use of specialized receptors known as thermoreceptors.

Changes in environmental temperature are detected by thermoreceptors localized in cutaneous endings of primary somatosensory nerve fibers.Thermoreceptors are specialized nerve cells that are able to detect differences in temperature. Temperature is a relative measure of heat present in the environment. Thermoreceptors are able to detect heat and cold and are found throughout the skin in order to allow sensory reception throughout the body. The location and number of thermoreceptors will determine the sensitivity of the skin to temperature changes.

Heat receptors are closer to the skin's surface, while cold receptors are found deeper in the dermis. This means that sensitivity to hot temperatures will be higher than lower temperatures based on the location. Additionally, different sections of the skin will have more receptors than others. The hand, for example, has more thermoreceptors than the thigh or shin (the front part of the leg from the knee to the ankle. the lower part of the foreleg in cattle), which means it will be more sensitive to temperature changes.

Cold is detected by specific thermoreceptor neurons that innervate the surface of the body. Cold-sensitive neurons (CSNs) from trigeminal ganglia (TG) and dorsal root ganglia (DRG) detect environmental temperature decreases with exquisitely temperature-sensitive molecular machinery, concentrated in the free axonal endings that innervate superficial layers of the skin and mucosae. Cold thermoreceptors in the hypothalamus are 3.5 times more common than heat receptors.

Role of skin in thermoregulation: The skin is the major organ that controls heat and moisture flow to and from the surrounding environment. The body's heat exchange mechanisms include sensible heat transfer at the skin surface (via conduction, convection, and radiation (long-wave and short-wave)), latent heat transfer (via moisture evaporating and diffusing through the skin, and through sweat evaporation on the surface), and sensible plus latent exchange via respiration from the lungs. Two mechanisms contribute to this action: control of skin blood flow and thermal sweating. Only mammals have sweat glands. Sweat glands produce moisture that evaporates on the skin to cool the body when it is overheated. Sweating is controlled from a centre in the preoptic and anterior regions of the hypothalamus where thermosensitive neurons are located. The heat regulatory function of the hypothalamus is also affected by inputs from temperature receptors in the skin. High skin temperature reduces the hypothalamic set point for sweating and increases the gain of the hypothalamic feedback system in response to variations in core body temperature.

As sweat also contains ions in addition to water, sweating requires the intake of salts and water to maintain fluid homeostasis. Not all animals can sweat, however, and they must therefore use a different method of cooling when the environmental temperature is very high. Dogs, for example, pant to increase their heat loss. Heat loss via skin is more in cows and heat loss by respiration is higher in buffaloes. This is due to less number of sweat glands in buffaloes. Pigs do not have sweat glands.

When an animal sweats, electrolytes and salt are lost with the water, but they are not lost via the respiratory route.

Responses of Animals to Heat and Cold

Heat Stress

The primary factors that cause heat stress in dairy animals are high ambient temperatures and relative humidity. In addition, radiant heat from the sun contributes to stress, if animals are not properly shaded. Homeothermic animals respond to high temperatures by increasing heat loss and reducing heat production in their attempt to avoid increased body temperature (hyperthermia).

It is done by several mechanisms, these are as follows

- Decrease in insulation
- Increase in evaporation from skin (sweating and diffusion)-
- Increase in evaporation form respiratory tract-As ambient temperatures rise, the respiratory rate increases with panting progressing to open-mouth breathing.
- Relationship between cutaneous and respiratory evaporation
- Decrease in heat production
- Reflectance of hair coat to solar radiation
- Integration of all heat defensive mechanism
- Immunesuppression due to Heat Stress : The immune system has evolved as a complex of mechanisms to protect the host from invasion by pathogenic organisms. A number of factors may affect the proper functioning of the immune system. Heat stress may impair the function of the immune system in food-producing animals. Effects of heat stress on immune function are not always straightforward and may depend on the species, breed, genotype, age, social status, acclimation level, and intensity and duration of the exposure to the unfavorable conditions.

Severe heat stress reduces colostral immunoglobulins (IgG and IgA) in dairy cows with negative consequences on immunization and survival of newborn calves. High temperatures impair the functionality of neutrophils, which have a central role in the protection of the mammary gland against infections. There is an increased occurrence of mastitis during the summer months.

High ambient temperature is the major constraint to buffalo productivity due to poor heat tolerance capacity because of low sweat gland density and black coat colour. Under excess thermal loads of heat and work, buffaloes employ moderate levels of sweating and resort to open mouth panting. High temperatures may cause heat stroke, heat exhaustion, heat syncope, heat cramps, and ultimately organ dysfunction.

Defense Against Cold

By

- Conservation of heat (insulation) i.e. by increased insulation
    - Tissue insulation (by vasoconstriction and subcutaneous fat)
    - Hair coat insulation

   - Air insulation
- Production of more heat
- Combination of both

Adaptation in Cold Region

Phylogenetic adaptation (more economic)– High body insulation chiefly by hair coat and normal heat production

Ontogenetic adaptation – Increased heat production

Adaptation to Water Scarcity

Breeds of ruminants native to arid lands are able to with-stand prolonged periods of water deprivation and graze faraway from watering sites at times 50 km or more far apart. Desert goats have been reported to be the most efficient among ruminants in terms of ability to withstand dehydration.Such goats in addition minimize water loss through urine and feces.

Temperature Regulation

Regulators of Body Temperature

There are 3 Components of Temperature Regulating System

1. Sensors
2. Thermostatic control unit (in hypothalamus)
3. Thermoregulatory effectors
   - Can be subdivided into heat exchange by conduction, convection or radiation.
   - The system is approximately 50% efficient for glucose oxidation, the remainder of the energy (335 Kcal) appearing as heat.

Heat Exchange

There are several ways that an animal can absorb or lose heat from or to the environment: conduction, convection, radiation, and evaporation.

(a) ***By conduction***: Heat is transferred by conduction form higher temperature to lower temperature through either solids or fluids without movement of molecules.

(b) ***By convection***: Heat loss by convection is achieved by the movement of fluid or gas in contact with the skin, whether this be air or water.

Convection is of 2 Types

1. **Free convection** e.g. changes in density of water or air associated with the transfer of heat causes it to move under the influence of gravity.
2. ***Forced convection*** : Caused by wind or motion of water

Heat transfer within the body is both by conduction and convection . Convective heat transfer by the circulation is the main mode of heat distribution within the body.

(c) By Radiation : Is the transfer of heat through electromagnetic radiation without objects coming into contact. An example of radiation is the warming that can occur to animals in sunlight.

(d) Evaporative Heat Loss

There are four strategies used in animals and birds to increase evaporative heat loss.

1. Panting
2. Sweating

3. Wallowing

4. Saliva spreading

Panting

Panting is defined as rapid shallow breathing.

- Increased respiratory frequency and decrease in tidal volume
- Increased dead space ventilation and no change in alveolar ventilation

Fever

Fever is a physiological condition characterized by an elevated core body temperature. Warm blooded animals produce fever by increasing heat production (through shivering) or reducing heat loss (by peripheral vasoconstriction). Fever is an adaptive mechanism for controlling infection. Fever is commonly caused by the presence in the blood of certain chemicals called pyrogens. One type of pyrogen is derived from microorganism and is produced by the body tissues and has been isolated from Leukocytes. Fever is produced by certain exogenous (largely microbial) stimuli that activate bone-marrow-derived phagocytes to release a fever-inducing hormone (endogenous pyrogen). Endogenous pyrogen, in turn, circulates to the thermoregulatory center of the brain (preoptic area of the anterior hypothalamus) where it causes an elevation in the "set-point" for normal body temperature. Pyrogenic substances increase the set point at which the body temperature is regulated.

At the onset of fever, the body responds as if to cold stress. Heat loss is reduced by vasoconstriction in the peripheral tissues, and the heat production is increased. The sensation of chills occurs and the body responds by shivering. The core body temperature rises to some new level where it will be regulated as long as fever- producing pyrogen is present. After the pyrogen is removed, the set point in the hypothalamus is lowered and the body responds as if to heat stress. Cutaneous vasodilation and sweating are common during this phase and the body gradually returns to normal levels.

Fever is an important feature for the diagnosis of disease in domestic animals. The body temperature of animals, which is taken rectally, is different from one species to another. For example, a horse is said to have a fever above 101 °F (38.3 °C). Medications that lower fevers are called antipyretics. Ibuprofen and paracetamol are two most commonly used antipyretics.

Body temperature and hibernation

Hibernation is a state of inactivity and metabolic depression in endotherms. Hibernation is a way animals conserve energy to survive adverse weather conditions or lack of food.It involves physiological changes such as a drop in body temperature and slowed metabolism. When hibernating, an animal's metabolism slows significantly: its heartbeat slows, it breathes more slowly and its body temperature drops—in some extreme cases to below the freezing point of water (zero degrees Celsius). And here we get to the reason why animals hibernate: reducing their metabolism allows them to conserve energy. It most commonly occurs during winter months.

Hibernation functions to conserve energy when sufficient food is unavailable. To achieve this energy saving, an endothermic animal decreases its metabolic rate and thereby its body temperature. Before entering hibernation, animals need to store enough energy to last through the duration of their dormant period, possibly as long as an entire winter.

Waking up from hibernation is related to a *Tau protein* (Tau or tubulin binding proteins was one of the first microtubule-associated proteins (MAPs) to be characterized) which also builds up in the brain of people with Alzheimer disease. The fact that hibernating animals don't experience muscle deterioration after long periods of not moving, can help us prevent muscle deterioration during ageing or to treat muscle disorders. The lack of bone deterioration in hibernating animals can lead to new ways of treating degenerative bone problems or diseases.

Hibernation is a way of evolution by most animals to survive harsh winters. Hibernation is like sound sleep. Most warm and cold blooded animals have the capacity to hibernate during winter months. The animal chooses a safe and well hidden place in order to avoid predators. The process of hibernation differs from one species to another species. Some start migrating towards warmer regions, others produce thick fat layer and fur coat over their body and some just sleep. Domestic animals hibernate as a result of natural instinct, but with more active periods in between

Temperature Regulation in Birds

Birds have a higher internal body temperature (> 40^0C) under thermoneutral conditions which provides them with an advantage as the thermal gradient between the animal and environment is increased, facilitating heat loss from the bird and maintenance of homeothermy.

Peripheral Regulation

The hypothalamus, which provides the highest level of endocrine control, integrates the activities of the nervous and endocrine systems. The hypothalamus plays an important role in regulating the body temperature. This function is carried out by the anterior hypothalamus and the posterior hypothalamus.

Adaptation in Response to Cold

When surroundings get too cold, skin plays a role in preserving body heat so that body temperature doesn't drop below a certain level. It is important that the body maintains an optimum temperature for the enzymes in our body (around 37 degrees celsius). The insulation of the tissue and hair coat prevents heat loss from the body under cold stress. The air present in the hair coat also acts as a good insulator. Thus fleece of unshorn adult wool sheep forms a very effective barrier to the transfer of heat into and out of the body. Animals also react by increasing the heat production by the body. Reflex cutaneous vasoconstriction is an early and sustained response to whole body cold exposure, limiting convective heat loss to the environment.

The other adjustments include the increase in food intake. If all these mechanisms fail the body increases its body metabolism by shivering thermogenesis.

Adaptation in Response to Heat Stress

Different animals are able to withstand high degrees of heat stress because of various adaptation mechanisms. Camel, sheep, goat and zebu cattle, are especially adapted to withstand heat stress for long periods. Some of the mechanisms include decrease in heat production, reduction in feed intake. Most desert adapted animals like camel, donkey, sheep and goat, conserve water by excreting drier faeces under heat stress. Although the mechanism of water withdrawal from the digestive tract has aroused much interest, little is known about the control of this process.

When water is lost to the environment during exposure to high temperatures and dry air, the volume of blood is affected before the fluids in the other body compartments. Only the camel has an ability to maintain a relatively high, almost unchanged blood volume in the face of severe dehydration. Mechanisms controlling the plasma proteins and thereby the osmotic pressure of the blood as well as the permeability of blood capillaries contribute to this ability.

Although most livestock possess well-developed mechanisms of thermoregulation, they may not be able to adequately maintain homeothermy under heat stress, esspecially the high producing animals. Among the genetic adaptations that have developed in Zebu cattle during its evolution has been the acquisition of genes for thermotolerance. Zebu breeds are better able to regulate body temperature in response to heat stress than are cattle from Bos Taurus breeds of European origin.

Heat Shock Proteins/ Stress Proteins

Recently several proteins have been identified to help in adaptation in response to thermal stress. These proteins are known as heat shock proteins. Heat shock proteins (HSP) are a class of functionally related proteins whose expression is increased when cells are exposed to elevated temperatures or other stress. Heat-shock proteins are named according to their molecular weight. HSPs play important physiological roles in normal conditions and situations involving both systemic and cellular stress. The principal HSPs that have chaperone activity (supervisory activity) belong to five conserved classes: HSP60, HSP70, HSP90, HSP100 and the small HSPs. HSPs are molecular chaperones that oppose stress induced denaturation of other proteins.

HSP60 is mostly found in the mitochondria. It helps in refolding of proteins and prevents aggregation of denatured proteins. HSP70 is mostly found in the cytosol and nucleus. Its functions are nascent protein folding, cytoprotection and as molecular chaperones. HSP90 is mostly found in the cytosol, ER and nucleus. Its main functions are protein translocation and regulation of steroid hormone receptors.

Heat shock protein β1 (HSPB1) is one of the major genes of the HSP family that helps in cell survival during stress, regulates apoptosis, cellular development and differentiation.

Questions on Physiology of Temperature Regulation

1. Thermoregulation in mammals
2. Thermoregulation in birds

Summary

- Most domestic animals are homeotherms, i.e. they keep their body temperature constant.
- Animal body loses heat through sensible losses by radiation, conduction and convection from their body surfaces and evaporative losses of water from the body surface and lungs.
- The ability to maintain body temperature is a function of the body to maintain a balance between heat gain and heat loss from the body.
- In order to maintain body temperature, the loss of heat by means of surface evaporation is an important means of heat loss in animals.
- The water from the body is lost through two means. Sweating from the sweat glands of the body surface and through panting, from the respiratory passages.
- Homeothermic animals respond to high temperatures by increasing heat loss and reducing heat production in their attempt to avoid increased body temperature (hyperthermia)
- Fever is a physiological condition characterized by an elevated core body temperature. Fever is an adaptive mechanism for controlling infection.
- Hibernation is a way animals conserve energy to survive adverse weather conditions or lack of food.It involves physiological changes such as a drop in body temperature and slowed metabolism.

19

Ecophysiology

Ecophysiology is the branch of physiology which aims to define the adaptive features of an organism which fits it to its environment. Most of the time the environment in which the animal lives is a difficult one, hence the requirement of adaptation to environment. Environment is defined as the surroundings in which the organism lives. The environment may be the physical environment, the chemical environment or the biological environment. Environment has two components - abiotic and biotic. The abiotic environment includes the air (atmosphere), water (hydrosphere) and land (lithosphere). Biosphere— Narrow zone where land water and air interact. The biotic environment includes the plants, animals and the microbes. The branch of biology, which deals with the relationship of organisms with their environment is known as 'ecology'. The aberrant climatic conditions, including vagaries of rainfall, hailstorms, cyclones, flood, extremes of weather etc., are adversely affecting productivity of livestock particularly poor farmers. Abiotic stresses like drought, temperature extremes, flood, salinity, acidity, mineral toxicity and nutrient deficiency are threatening agricultural, livestock, fisheries and other production systems globally posing challenges in sustaining even the current productivity levels. In recent years, abiotic stresses have become aggravated by climate change.

Climatology-various Parameters and Their Importance

Climate is a long term pattern of weather in a particular area. Different parts of the world have different climates. Atmospheric climate is the one which is most variable and also the one which affects livestock productivity The most common elements of atmospheric climate include average temperature and rainfall(precipitation). Climate is further divided into Micro climate and Macro climate.

Macro-climate is the Climate of a Larger Area

Micro-climate the variations in localized climate around or inside a building. Most animal or poultry housing attempts to change the microclimate inside the housing area by various means eg sprinkling or installation of coolers or fan or air conditioning.

The animal's environment is complex. Scientists attempt to define and measure it in terms of a single parameter or a small group of parameters considered of primary importance.

Various environmental weather elements are:

Temperature:Temperature affects most of the critical factors for livestock production, such as water availability, animal production, reproduction and health.High ambient temperature is a major constraint on animal productivity in tropical climates since it evokes series of drastic changes in the animal's physiological functions that include depression in feed intake, efficiency and utilisation; disturbances in metabolism of water, protein, energy and mineral balances, enzymatic reactions, hormonal secretions and blood metabolites. Homeothermic animals respond to high temperatures by increasing heat loss and reducing heat production in their attempt to avoid increased body temperature (hyperthermia). Such responses include an increase in respiratory and sweating rates and a decrease in feed intake. Environmental temperature also affects the reproduction of the farm animal in both sexes. In the case of male animals different semen parameters are decreased like motility, live and dead percentage concentration, abnormal sperm count, etc.

Wind Velocity

Wind Speed (or Wind Velocity) is an air moving from high to low pressure. Wind velocity is typically measured with an anemometer, which is a common weather station instrument. The normal unit of wind speed is the knot (nautical mile/hour) or miles per hour. The speed at which air flows over the surface of water affects the rate at which the water evaporates.

Humidity

Relative humidity refers to the amount of water in the air, as a fraction of the total amount the air can hold, when it is saturated. Once the air reaches 100 percent relative humidity, it is no longer able to hold water, which then condenses out of the atmosphere. The amount of humidity in the air directly affects the speed at which water will evaporate.

Wet and dry bulb thermometer, an instrument used to measure the relative humidity of the atmosphere. It consists of a thermometer with a bulb that is wet or moist and one that is kept dry. The relative humidity is calculated from the difference in readings of the thermometers when water evaporates from the wet bulb, decreasing its temperature.

A sling psychrometer is an instrument that measures the relative humidity and dew point in an area. A sling psychrometer has two thermometers: a wet bulb and a dry bulb. The wet bulb has a cotton wick over the bulb of the thermometer, which is moistened with room temperature water. The dry bulb is simply a thermometer. When the sling psychrometer is spun rapidly in the air, the evaporation of the water from the wick causes the wet bulb thermometer to read lower than the dry bulb thermometer. After the psychrometer has been spun long enough for the thermometers to reach equilibrium temperatures, the unit is stopped and the two thermometers are quickly read. A psychrometric chart (or table) is then used to convert the dry bulb temperature and the wet bulb temperature into humidity information.

Precipitation

Precipitation is any form of liquid or solid water particles that fall from the atmosphere and reach the surface of the Earth. Precipitation occurs when water vapour cools. When the air reaches saturation point (also known as condensation point and dew point) the water vapour condenses and forms tiny droplets of water. Precipitation forms in the clouds when water vapor condenses into bigger and bigger droplets of water. When the drops are heavy enough, they fall to the Earth.

Sunshine

Sunshine duration is the length of time that the ground surface is irradiated by direct solar radiation. A sunshine recorder is a device that records the amount of sunshine at a given location or region at any time. The crystal ball is typically 10 cm (4 inches) in diameter, and is designed to focus the rays from the sun onto a card mounted at the back and is set on a stand. The card is held in place by grooves of which there are three overlapping sets, to allow for the altitude of the sun during different seasons of the year. The unit is designed to record the hours of bright sunshine which will burn a hole through the card.

Cloud cover

Of various measures of the biological environment, dry bulb temperature is generally considered to be the principal thermal measure. High humidity or solar radiation worsens the effect of high temperature.

Temperature–Humidity Index is one of the most popular index of meteorological variables affecting livestock production. Temperature–humidity index (THI) is an index for assessment of the potential of an environment to induce heat stress in humans and farm animals. It is a simple index, which indicates the degree of heat stress on dairy animals which incorporates the effect of climate parameters like, temperature and relative humidity. It has been extensively used for estimation of degree of heat stress in dairy cattle. There are a number of models for formulating THI the index. A few are as below.

- Bianca 1962 $((0.15 \times T_{db} + 0.85 \times T^{wb}) \times 1.8 + 32)$
- NRC 1971
- Yousef, 1985
- Mader et al., 2006
- Berman et al., 2016

Climatic environment affects animal productivity both directly and indirectly. Directly through affecting the body metabolism and indirectly by affecting the changes in the supply of nutrients, occurrence of diseases and parasites etc.

The evaluation of the adaptability and tolerance to heat are determined mainly by the physiological parameters measurement such as body temperature and respiratory rate. Recently infrared thermography technique has been introduced to study the adaptability and tolerance to heat. Infrared thermography technology is a noninvasive method that has been used to indicate thermal bio-metric changes in animal metabolism resulting from increased body temperature and changes in blood flow in response to environmental or physiological conditions.

Effect of Different Environmental Variables Like Temperature, Humidity, Light, Radiation, Altitude on Animal Performance

To account for the combined effects of relative humidity and temperature, the temperature humidity index (THI) is widely used to provide an accurate assessment of the effects of the thermal environment on poultry and livestock. THI has also been used to establish thresholds for heat stress in domestic animals.

For most mammalian species the acceptable range of relative humidity is 30–70% (NRC 2011), and the optimum range of relative humidity for chicken during and after brooding is 60–80 and 50–70%, respectively. High relative humidity affects animal bedding, which results in increased litter moisture and ammonia concentrations.

The occurrence and prevalence of infectious diseases is sensitive to relative humidity, not only because the impaired trachea and bronchi in the respiratory system provides an environment favorable for pathogen infection, but also because the abnormal levels of humidity increase the infectivity of pathogens.

The net effect of a stressful environment on both the hot and cold extreme is to decrease productivity be it in terms of meat, milk, fibre or eggs production or in terms of decreased growth and reproductive potential.

Cold Stress

Goats exposed to cold reduce their milk secretion which is due to a reduced blood flow to the mammary gland.

Heat stress

Heat stress negatively impacts livestock performance in most areas of the world, as it reduces milk production in animals with high genetic merit. Buffaloes and high-producing cows suffer most at high ambient temperatures, and severe heat stress often leads to loss in their reproductive and productive performance.

Cattle kept at high environmental temperatures have shorter lactation periods and lower milk and butter fat production as compared to their twins kept on the same ration at low environmental temperature.

Indirectly, in most animals, semen is poorer and lesser in volume during heat stress. The ability of semen to survive cold storage freezing also varies with the environmental temperature. The season of birth is known to affect the age at puberty in female domestic animals. Some of the domestic animals have well defined sexual seasons, which correspond well with the compatibility of the environmental temperature to the body of the animal.

During the wet or rainy season, there is a good growth of grasses which is adequate for milk production and live weight gain in meat animals. But after the cessation of the rainy season, the poor quality of the forages become a limiting factor in the productivity of these animals. One of the first noticeable responses of most livestock to heat stress is a decrease in feed intake. However, there occurs important differences among breeds of cattle in their changes in feed consumption with rising environmental temperature. In one experiment it was shown that the feed intake of lactating Jersey, Brown Swiss and Holstein cows was depressed at 27°C while that of Brahman cows did not decline until 38°C.

Although it is clear that reduced intake of feed results in lower performance of animals in warm climate regions. However, the mechanism of reduced feed intake is not very clear. Several explanations include.

(1) Direct regulation by heat regulation centres.

(2) Interference with feeding by high respiration rates.

(3) Changes in behaviour directed towards decreased heat production or removal of the animal from the proximity of feeding areas, such as seeking shade.

The direct influence of high temperature brings about a reduction in efficiency in the utilization of feed energy for productive purposes. Not only do animals eat less, but they retain less per unit of intake. Although the best temperature for lactating cows is 10°-18°C, no significant decline in milk yield is usually evident under cold conditions until the temperature drops to about -12°C. On the other hand, the level of milk yield is very sensitive to elevated temperatures, with measurable decline occurring in high producing cows at 24°C. The level of temperature at which significant depressions will occur is, of course dependent upon the level of production and the animals size, stage of lactation and genetic potential for milk yield.

Buffaloes are more prone to heat stress because of their dark coloured skin, sparse hair coat and scanty sweat glands which compromises their heat dissipation capacity. Although the buffalo can adapt to harsh environments and live on poor quality forage, reproductive efficiency is often compromised by such conditions, resulting in late sexual maturity, long postpartum anoestrus, poor expression of oestrus, poor conception rates and long calving intervals. Severe thermal stress causes a cessation of oestrus and ovulation in cattle and sheep. Summer anoestrus in buffaloes is quite common. Level of body temperature of the cow and buffaloes at the time of insemination is considered important in conception. That is why, it is generally recommended that buffaloes be bred in cooler hours of the morning.

Global Climate and Animal Productivity

Climate change has far reaching effects on animal productivity. We will particularly concern ourselves with two aspects important for animal health and production. First is the effect of global climate change or warming on productivity of our livestock and second the environmental aspects of pollution from livestock waste and ways and means to ameliorate the situation using modern biotechnological tools. India is a low latitude tropical country highly vulnerable to the consequences of temperature increase. Weather variability, a major constraint on growth and welfare of India, will increase with global warming. Temperature increases in the Tibetan plateau, the Hind Kush and the Himalayas will affect the volume and timing of river flows in north India. Projected precipitation changes will also increase the variability of water availability in peninsular India. Rise in sea level will affect all coastal settlements. A Intergovernmental Panel on Climate Change has been constituted to look into the various issues related to global climate change.

Governments are seeking a global commitment to limit the risk of temperature increase by imposing a limit on harmful emissions (Greenhouse Gases). It has been estimated that a 2°C goal implies a limit of 450ppm on GHG concentration in the atmosphere which will require at least a halving of global emissions by 2050.Climate change is one of the biggest and urgent issues of the present world and overwhelming scientific consensus is concerned with climate change. The earth's climate is rapidly changing mainly as a result of increase in greenhouse gases caused by human activities. Over the last 100 years (1906-2005), global temperature has increased by 0.74°C and it is expected to increase by about 0.2°C per decade over the next two decades.

Climatic environment affects animal productivity both directly and indirectly. Directly through affecting the body metabolism and indirectly by affecting the changes in the supply of nutrients, occurrence of diseases and parasites etc.

The net effect of a stressful environment on both the hot and cold extreme is to decrease productivity be it in terms of meat, milk, fibre or eggs production or in terms of decreased growth and reproductive potential. Goats exposed to cold reduce their milk secretion which is due to a reduced blood flow to the mammary gland.

The threat of climate change and global warming is now recognized worldwide and some alarming manifestations of change have occurred. We all know, the earth is surrounded by a cover of gasses as atmosphere. This atmosphere allows most of the light to pass through, which reaches the surface of earth. This light from the sun is absorbed by the earth surface and converts into heat energy. This heat energy is re-emitted by the surface of the earth during night. Due to excessive presence of some gasses in the atmosphere, this escape of heat from earth's surface is prevented, resulting in heating of earth called 'global warming'. The gasses which are responsible for causing global warming are called 'greenhouse gasses'. Carbon dioxide is one of the most important greenhouse gases. This carbon dioxide mostly comes to the atmosphere as air pollution from vehicles, coal-fired power plants and other industries burning fossil fuels. Human population increase and large scale deforestation are also responsible for carbon dioxide generation. Thus, Global Warming adds energy to the Earth's biosphere. The climate change which we are experiencing is due to global warming. Heat is the fuel of weather systems. More heat, more extreme weather. Thus, it shouldn't be surprising that the result is more extreme weather. More rain, more drought and more storms.

Animal health may be affected by climate change in four ways: heat-related diseases and stress, extreme weather events, adaptation of animal production systems to new environments, and emergence or re-emergence of infectious diseases, especially vector-borne diseases critically dependent on environmental and climatic conditions.

Acclimation and adaptation

Acclimation and adaptation are different processes.

Animals are considered acclimated to a given ambient temperature when body temperature returns to pre-stress levels. Systemic, tissue and cellular responses associated with acclimation are coordinated, require several days or weeks to occur, and are therefore not homeostatic in nature.

Adaptation, on the other hand, requires modifications of the genetic structure and is a process involving populations, not individuals. Genetic improvement is an evolutionary action; evolution should be defined as a continuous process of adaptation of the populations of organisms to the ever-changing geological, biological and climatic conditions.

Acclimatization to a stressor is a two-stage process. The first stage is driven by homeostatic responses to environmental change and the second stage is a homeorhetic process driven by the endocrine system which enables animals to respond to stress. The resulting cellular, metabolic, and systemic changes associated with acclimatization is to reduce the impact of the stress on the animal and allow it to function more effectively in the stressful environment. These changes are lost if the stress is removed so the process is not based on changes in the genome. However, if the stressful environment is not removed over successive generations these changes will become "genetically fixed" and are referred to as adaptations. A better understanding of genetic differences between adapted animals will contribute useful information on the genes associated with acclimation.

Little attention has been paid to the genetic aspects of the adaptation of livestock to their environment, however. It has generally been considered faster and easier to improve production through alterations of the environment and most of the research efforts have been focused on environment modification. Study of gene expression changes during acclimatization will assist in identifying genes associated with improved thermotolerance.

Acclimatization -general Adaptive Syndrome

Animals have developed coping mechanisms to minimize the impact of these environmental stressors on their biological systems. These responses are termed acclimation, acclimatization, and adaptation. Acclimatization or acclimatisation (also called acclimation) is the process in which an individual organism adjusts to a change in its environment (such as a change in altitude, temperature, humidity, photoperiod, or pH), allowing it to maintain performance across a range of environmental conditions.

Animals acclimatize in many ways. Sheep grow very thick wool in cold, damp climates. The salt content of sweat and urine decreases as people acclimatize to hot conditions.

Clinical effect on endocrine -reproductive function

Climate change exerts an overwhelming negative effect on livestock health and welfare. The negative effects of climate change on animal health and welfare will be the consequence of combined changes of air temperature, precipitation, frequency, and magnitude of extreme weather events and may be both direct and indirect.

The direct effects of climate change may be due primarily to increased temperatures and frequency and intensity of heat waves. Depending on its intensity and duration, heat stress may affect livestock health by causing metabolic disruptions, oxidative stress, and immune suppression causing infections and death. Rumen volatile fatty acid (VFA) production decreases under conditions of extreme heat.

The indirect effects of climate change are primarily those linked to quantity and quality of feedstuffs and drinking water and survival and distribution of pathogens and/or their vectors.

Heat Cramps and heat stroke

Increased sweating as a result of heat exposure results in loss of water as well as salts. Large quantities of loss of water and salt from the body can result in severe painful cramps in human beings. Heat stroke (sunstroke, heat hyperexia, insolation) is the most common heat disorder in the dog. Heat stroke is a severe and often fatal illness which occurs when the body is exposed to extreme heat and the body temperature rises above 41^{0}c (106 ^{0}F). Under such circumstances, hypothalamus loses the power of regulating body temperature. Heat exhaustion should be treated by placing the animal in a cool environment and administering IV fluids and electrolytes.

The threat of climate change and global warming is now recognized worldwide and some alarming manifestations of change have occurred. We all know, the earth is surrounded by a cover of gasses as atmosphere. This atmosphere allows most of the light to pass through, which reaches the surface of earth. This light from the sun is absorbed by the earth surface and converts into heat energy. This heat energy is re-emitted by the surface of the earth during night. Due to excessive presence of some gasses in the atmosphere, this escape of heat from earth's surface is prevented, resulting in heating of earth called 'global warming'. The gasses which are responsible for causing global warming are called 'greenhouse gasses'. Carbon dioxide is one of the most important greenhouse gases. This carbon dioxide mostly comes to the atmosphere as air pollution from vehicles, coal-fired power plants and other industries burning fossil fuels. Human population increase and large scale deforestation are also responsible for carbon dioxide generation. Thus, Global Warming adds energy to the Earth's biosphere. The climate change which we are experiencing is due to global warming. Heat is the fuel of weather systems. More heat, more extreme weather. Thus, it shouldn't be surprising that the result is more extreme weather. More rain, more drought and more storms.

Global warming is likely to impact productivity of buffaloes due to their sensitivity to temperature changes (Upadhyay et al., 2007). Both milk production and reproductive functions of Murrah buffaloes are likely to be affected due to warming effects. Severe thermal stress causes a cessation of estrus and ovulation in cattle and sheep. Summer anoestrus in buffaloes is quite common. Level of body temperature of the cow and buffaloes at the time of insemination is also considered important in conception. It is generally recommended that buffaloes be bred in cooler hours of the day.

One of the ways to deal with the effects of global warming is to introduce species that are not only more productive but also can cope with the higher temperatures. Researchers have been looking to tap into the genetic diversity of livestock in tropical countries to create heat-tolerant breeds that can also produce more milk. However, improvements in the housing systems such as better hygiene and more space would reduce stress on stock and the incidence of disease. According to a study published in the June issue of the Journal of Animal Science, today's dairy producers use only 10 percent of the land, 23 percent of the feedstock and 35 percent of the water that was used to produce the same amount of milk in 1944. However, to further optimize the animal production due to new challenges of global warming is to be worked out. Recent research at CIRG has shown that a thatch or asbestos housing is more helpful in maintaining the physiology of goats during comfortable weather as compared to goats kept in the open. Similarly, breeds like Sirohi have been shown to be more heat tolerant as compared to Barbari and therefore more suitable to be selected for combating the adverse effect of heat stress. Therefore, proper housing is going to play an important role in mitigating the adverse effect of climate change on animal productivity. More efforts need to be carried out to quantitate the heat tolerance ability of different breeds of livestock vis-a-vis productivity, so that optimum breed selection can be made to optimize production.

The harmful effects of the presence of greenhouse gasses in the atmosphere are global warming, climate change, ozone depletion, sea level rise, adverse effects on biodiversity etc. Abnormal rise in greenhouse gas, methane, in the earth atmosphere has been causing arctic ice to vanish in time to come.

The domestic animal population has increased by 0.5 to 2.0 percent per year during the last century. One result of this population increase is that emissions from livestock have become a significant source of atmospheric methane. In fact, domestic animals currently account for about 15 percent of the annual methane emissions. Much of the world's livestock are ruminants--such as sheep, goats, camel, cattle, and buffalo--who have a unique, four-chambered stomach. In the chamber called the rumen, bacteria break down food and generate methane as a by-product. The production rate is affected by factors such as quantity and quality of feed, body weight, age, and exercise, and varies among animal species as well as among individuals of the same species. It is estimated that ruminants on low quality feeds produce more than 75 percent of the total livestock methane emissions. Fortunately, there are ways to reduce greenhouse gas emissions from livestock production through management strategies that improve production efficiency and result in lower emissions per unit of milk or meat produced. Globally, ruminant livestock produce about 80 million metric tons of methane annually, accounting for about 28% of global methane emissions from human-related activities. An adult cow may be a very small source by itself, emitting only 80-110 kgs of methane, but with about 100 million cattle in the U.S. and 1.2 billion large ruminants in the world, ruminants are one of the largest methane sources. In the U.S., cattle emit about 5.5 million metric tons of methane per year into the atmosphere, accounting for 20% of U.S. methane emissions.

Cattle emit methane through a digestive process that is unique to ruminant animals called enteric fermentation. Since methane represents a loss of carbon from the rumen and therefore an unproductive use of dietary energy, scientists have been looking for ways to suppress its production. The most promising approach for reducing methane emissions from livestock is by improving the productivity and efficiency of livestock production. Greater efficiency of livestock production can increase profitability and be good for the environment at the same time. This general approach has been demonstrated by the dairy industry over the past several decades as milk production increased and methane emissions decreased. Nutritional and genetic improvements are mainly responsible for making modern dairy cows more productive.

Animal health may be affected by climate change in four ways: heat-related diseases and stress, extreme weather events, adaptation of animal production systems to new environments, and emergence or re-emergence of infectious diseases, especially vector-borne diseases critically dependent on environmental and climatic conditions. To face these new menaces, the need for strong and efficient Veterinary Services is irrefutable, combined with good coordination of public health services, as many emerging human diseases are zoonoses. Climate driven and other changes in landscape structure and texture, plus more general factors, may create favourable ecological niches for emerging diseases. Changes in climatic patterns and in seasonal conditions may affect disease behaviour in terms of spread pattern, diffusion range, amplification and persistence in novel habitats. Pathogen invasion may result in the emergence of novel disease complexes, presenting major challenges for the sustainability of future animal agriculture at the global level. To face these new menaces, the need for strong and efficient Veterinary Services is irrefutable, combined with good coordination of public health services, as many emerging human diseases are zoonoses eg corona virus epidemic in human beings in 2020 which brought the whole world to a stand still lockdown state.

Livestock waste contributes to some extent to the environmental pollution in the form of sewage etc. Landfilling and incineration are popular ways to deal with biowaste but both cause negative environmental effects such as the use of valuable land and production of dangerous gases. The use of natural and genetically engineered microorganisms for domestic animal waste treatment is an emerging field to provide benefit to mankind and the environment. The structural components of cells, cellulose and hemicellulose, make biowaste very susceptible for bioproduct development and biowaste offers biotechnology an opportunity to assist in maintaining environmental quality.

Circadian Rhythm

A biological rhythm is a cyclical change in the biological or chemical function of the body. The biological rhythms are endogenously controlled by self-contained circadian clocks. Circadian rhythm-A circadian rhythm is a roughly 24 hour cycle in the physiological processes of living beings.Circadian rhythm are cyclic patterns of behaviour or of tissue activity (e.g. hormone secretion) that repeat with a period of approximately 24 hours, even when organisms are isolated from the normal daily environmental changes.The recurrence of any event within a biological system at more-or-less regular intervals can be considered a biological rhythm. Circadian rhythms are physical, mental, and behavioral changes that follow a daily cycle. They respond primarily to light and darkness in an organism's environment. A circadian rhythm is a natural, internal process that regulates the sleep-wake cycle and repeats roughly every 24 hours.

Sleeping at night and being awake during the day is an example of a light-related circadian rhythm. Circadian rhythms can influence sleep-wake cycles, hormone release, eating habits and digestion, body temperature, and other important bodily functions. The precise temporal relationships between day-night cycles and the activity rhythms of domestic animals are unknown. Biological clocks adapt an organism to environmental changes that vary depending on the time of day. Horses that travel across time zones for competitions also experience disruptions to this internal clock, which may affect athletic performance. Internal clock influences metabolism in nearly every cell in the body. The detoxifying functions of the liver and kidney fluctuate with the time of day, as does body temperature.

The circadian rhythm is set by the suprachiasmatic nucleus of the hypothalamus, which regulates the sleep-wake cycle. The suprachiasmatic nucleus projects to the pineal gland to release melatonin, which promotes sleep. The suprachiasmatic nuclei (SCN) in the hypothalamus are regarded as the anatomical loci of the circadian pacemaker. Suprachiasmatic nucleus (SCN)-a tiny region located in the hypothalamus, situated directly above the optic chiasm, is responsible for controlling circadian rhythms. The SCN is a very small structure consisting of a pair of pinhead-size regions, each containing only about 10,000 neurons out of the estimated 100 billion neurons in the brain.The most important synchronising trigger of circadian rhythm is environmental light/dark (LD) cycle.The daily alternation of light and dark is the main regulatory factor of the pineal hormone melatonin.

The stress hormone cortisol fluctuates depending on the time of day, which in turn has significant effects on the immune system. Lactation in cattle is influenced by the photoperiod (the length of day and nights). Under natural daylight, chickens start to lay eggs when day length increases in the summer/spring. Based on this tendency, chicken producers increase the light period for young laying hens to stimulate egg production.In 2017, Nobel prize has been awarded for discovery of molecular mechanisms controlling this circadian rhythm.

Daily fluctuations in plasma cortisol levels are dependent on the circadian clock within the adrenal cortex.

The circadian pacemaker in the mammalian SCN consists of a double complex of circadian genes (Per1/Cry1 and Per2/Cry2), which is able to maintain the endogenous rhythm.

Understanding what makes biological clocks tick may lead to treatments for sleep disorders, obesity, mental health disorders, jet lag, and other health problems.

Summary

- Environment is defined as the surroundings in which the organism lives.
- Environment has two components - abiotic and biotic. The abiotic environment includes the air (atmosphere), water (hydrosphere) and land (lithosphere). The biotic environment includes the plants, animals and the microbes.
- Acclimatization or acclimatisation (also called acclimation) is the process in which an individual organism adjusts to a change in its environment (such as a change in altitude, temperature, humidity, photoperiod, or pH), allowing it to maintain performance across a range of environmental conditions.
- Climate change exerts an overwhelming negative effect on livestock health and welfare. The negative effects of climate change on animal health and welfare will be the consequence of combined changes of air temperature, precipitation, frequency, and magnitude of extreme weather events and may be both direct and indirect.
- Heat stress may affect livestock health by causing metabolic disruptions, oxidative stress, and immune suppression causing infections and death.
- Circadian rhythms are cyclic patterns of behaviour or of tissue activity (e.g. hormone secretion) that repeat with a period of approximately 24 hours.

20

Neurophysiology of Behavior

Behavior can be defined as an expressed course of action produced in organisms in response to stimulus from a given situation. Alternatively, behaviour may be defined as the response by the animals to internal and external stimuli. Behaviour is a significant indicator of the health of animals. The goal of all behavioral responses is common i.e. to survive and reproduce. The value and performance of animals can be increased when managers can apply their knowledge of animal behavior. Knowledge of animal behavior is important to understanding the whole animal and its ability to adapt to various environments and management systems.

Behaviour varies with sex, breed, nutrition and climate and between individuals. Understanding the behavior is essential for good farm management. Monitoring behavioural activities of livestock can be helpful to livestock producers by identifying the problems and further implementation of potential solutions for better livestock management and welfare.

The brain and genes are major factors that control animal behavior. Scientific interest in animal behaviour has rapidly grown in recent years due to concerns related to animal welfare.

Neurophysiology of Behavior

Neurophysiology can provide insight into this area because of the similarities between human and non-human brains and therefore into the kind of emotions and perceptions that animals are likely to have. The group of structures responsible for the expression and sensation of emotions are often referred to as the limbic system. Animals unlike human beings cannot argue, talk or reason but like human beings can suffer pain. Pain fibres identical to those found in humans exist in domestic animals. Central nervous system structures that are responsible for the affective component of pain-such as the thalamus are well developed in all mammals. Many animal welfare problems in farm and companion animals arise from a mismatch between the animals' adaptive capacity and the housing and handling conditions they are exposed to.

Survival and well-being of humankind is inextricably bound to our domestic animals. Domestication process of animals has made important changes with respect to their behavior. Domestication has brought about adaptability to a captive environment which is usually accompanied by some genetic changes occurring over generations as well as environment induced changes. Certain behaviors may have been changed because of man's role between the animal and its environment. One of the most important behavioral changes due to domestication is the reduction in responsiveness to changes in the animal's environment. Man has also exerted more control on the breeding of domestic animals. Increases in productive capability of domestic animals can compromise thermal acclimation and plasticity, requiring greater investments in housing systems. Behavioural activities are often used as indicators of welfare.

Physiological causes of animal behaviour can be explained by two types of mechanisms ie neural and hormonal.

Farm animals rely on information about the external environment, which they receive from the sense organs and subsequently reflected in their behaviour. Behavior is a significant indicator of health in animals. Behavior is among the most labile of traits, and there are many different ways that behaviour can vary within individuals as a function of variation in external or internal stimuli. For example in colic and painful conditions in animals, loss of appetite is the first behavioural symptom.Behavioural signs and history of behavioural symptoms are a great help to the clinician in appraisal of animal's condition. Domestic animals live in a profoundly different habitat to their wild ancestors and in many cases their appearance and behaviour have changed substantially.Study of behaviour may be important in situations in which a domestic animal may be under stress or its welfare compromised. Abnormal behaviour in domestic animals is of great relevance for veterinary diagnosis as well as for animal production aspects. Abnormal Behaviour in some animals like dogs may include aggression, biting, growling, food aggression, destructive behaviours, house soiling, coprophagia.In case of cow aggression, kicking, biting are some of the symptoms of abnormal behaviour.

Ethology is the study of animal behavior in natural environments and the primary concern of the ethologists is instinctive or innate behavior. Chemical communication plays an important role in various social interactions which determine behavior. Neural mechanisms are important in understanding their natural behaviors in domestic animals.

Cerebral cortex of animals is less developed than in humans but domestic animals suffer less psychologically from the long-term consequences of pain (fear, depression). There exists a species difference in fear reactions. Amygdala acts as the fear center in the brain. Destroying the amygdala can make a wild rat tame and reduce its emotionality. Rats lose all of their fear of cats when the amygdala is lesioned. Heart rate, blood pressure, and respiration also change in animals when the flight or fight response is activated. All these autonomic functions have neural circuits to the amygdala.

Similarly an example of reproductive behaviour modification is ram's presence affects ovarian activity in the ewe. The involvement of the hypothalamus in feeding behaviour was first tested in the fowl by Lepkovsky and his co-workers. Behavioural studies of farm animals can provide insight into the adaptation of the animals to their housing and management. Poultry under non-traditional lighting regimes are claimed to improve production efficiency but may affect the poultry behaviour.

Feeding behaviour is also important. Herbivores masticate for a longer time before swallowing compared to carnivores. Herbivores rely heavily on their lips and tongue, carnivores rely more on their teeth. Olfaction is not highly developed in cattle and does not seem to play a major role in selection of feed although they possess the vomeronasal organ. Olfactory substances reach it during Flehmen response.

Types of Behavior

The animal behavior can be classified as normal as well as abnormal behavior.

Normal Behavior

Social Behavior

Domestic animals are social animals and exhibit social behavior.Social behaviour is an animal's ability to communicate with each other. Social hierarchy is formed in a well established group. Introduction of new animals into a group or the mixing of groups will normally lead to fighting until a new social order is established . Aggression at mixing a new animal in the group is common in domestic animals. Aggression is partly because of limited supply of food and space and also competition among animals for breeding.

Mating Behavior

Domesticated ruminants exhibit promiscuous mating systems, in which no individuals have exclusive breeding rights, and in which little or no interaction between the sexes occurs other than during mating. Promiscuity may have resulted from generations of breeding in captivity, though a more plausible explanation is that this behavioral trait was a pre-adaptation that facilitated successful domestication.

Pain Behavior

Pain is an unpleasant sensory and emotional experience associated with actual or potential tissue damage or described in terms of such damage. In response to painful stimuli animals have sensory experiences which change their biochemistry, physiological parameters and behaviour and they try to avoid such stimuli in future. Farm animals may show no major apparent symptoms when in pain because such individuals (sick or injured) are more prone to predation; thus, hiding signs of painful events has become a strategy of survival in many species.Currently it is advocated that the domestic animals should enjoy freedom from Pain, Injury or Disease by prevention or rapid diagnosis and treatment.

Although in companion animals successful pain management is becoming widespread, it has been reported that farm animals are frequently given no analgesic drugs for treatment of a whole range of unambiguously painful procedures such as tail docking in pigs, sheep and cattle , castration in male calves, sheep, pigs or dehorning in cattle.

Painful states are caused particularly by tissue or nerve damage, inflammatory processes, viral infections and are characterized by pain hypersensitivity.

Pain is often classified in two parts.

- **Somatic Pain**- Somatic pain originates in the skin and is called superficial pain. Somatic pain refers to pain originating from the periphery and can in most cases be well localized.
- **Deep pain**-If it originates in the muscles, bones, joints or connective tissues it is called deep pain.

The main glucocorticoid hormone that is released in response to stresses including pain is cortisol.Plasma cortisol concentrations depend on circadian rhythms. Changes in plasma immunoreactive beta-endorphin can also be used as an indicator of pain.

Some types of behaviour in dogs has been associated with pain eg changes in posture (anxious glances, tail between legs), vocalising (howls, distinctive bark), changes in temperament (aggression or cringing and extreme submissiveness) and other changes (penile protrusion and frequent urination and defecation). Pain has been associated with increased locomotor activity and consequently increased restlessness, kicking, stamping, rolling, jumping, easing quarters, licking or biting at the damaged site and tail wagging being observed in few animals.

Sexual Behavior

Various patterns of courtship, display, motor activities and postures are shown by various species to ensure that male and female of a species come together so that fertilization, pregnancy and propagation of the species can occur.

Animals in the wild or field show a territorial behavior. Acoustical signals are important in organization of social behavior. The sense of smell is also important and well developed in domestic animals. The carpal glands of pig produce characteristic body odor involved in sexual behavior of pig.Endocrine mechanisms are important in exhibition of sexual behavior.Biogenic amines are involved in behavioral activities as neurotransmitters. Environmental factors like season, climate are known to influence sexual behavior of domestic animals. The intensity of sexual behavior is reduced in hot climates. Several abnormal sexual behavior have been reported in domestic animals such as homosexuality, hypersexuality and hyposexuality etc.The most common abnormal sexual behavior in female cattle is nymphomania.

Flehmen's Response

Flehman response is a mammalian behavior (Bull, Buffalo bull, camel, horses or cats) in which the animal inhales with the mouth open and upper lip curled to facilitate exposure of the vomeronasal organ to a scent or pheromone. The flehmen response draws air into the Jacobson's organ, an auxiliary olfactory sense organ that is found in many animals. This organ plays a role in the perception of certain scents and pheromones. This behavior helps them identify what they smell, especially the scent of animals they don't know and sexy scents, like females in heat. Male individuals commonly use the flehmen response as an olfactory mechanism for identifying the reproductive state of females of the same species based on pheromones in the female's urine or genitals.

Maternal and Neonatal Behavior

The behavioral events at birth and shortly afterward have an important influence on the survival of the newborn. Milk is let down in response to suckling behavior of the young one. Suckling excites a nervous reflex that augments secretion of hormones from the posterior pituitary. The incidence of licking and other maternal behaviour depends upon the characteristics of the calf and upon the state of the mother. The eating of the afterbirth is considered to be anti-predator behaviour. Calves of primiparous dams spent more time suckling and suckled from more quarters than did calves of older cows. Failure of the maternal and neonatal behavior patterns results in death of the offspring, loss of a reproductive season to the dam and a reduction of profit to the producer.

Foraging Behavior

One of the most important animal behaviors is foraging or the search for food within an animal's environment because without this ability, the animal's not likely to be able to survive and reproduce. Herbivores are able to select a balanced diet, when given choices, even though their nutritional requirements vary with age, physiological state, and environmental conditions. Knowing grazing and feeding behaviours of farm animals is of importance for efficient use of ranges and pastures and also for preventing feed waste.

Altruistic Behavior

Form of social behaviour whereby one organism puts itself either at risk or personal disadvantage for the good of other members of the species.

Aggressive Behavior

Aggression is a serious behavioral illness with numerous unlying causes and is dangerous both to humans and to other animals. Species-specific behaviours associated with attacks with the objective of causing physical injury. Besides farm machinery, animals are considered to be the second leading cause of injury in some livestock farms. Understanding of behaviour patterns of cattle, sheep, pigs, etc., can help in development of a production programme to minimize aggression, livestock injury and maximize safety to stock men.Camels have little aggressive behavior except among males during breeding season.

Management of Aggression in Domestic Livestock should Include

1. Animals should be raised in groups for better control.
2. Provision of adequate housing/holding area as well as wallowing area for pigs.
3. Provision of adequate feed/water & pasture: Location of feed in the environment is very important.
4. The stockman should maintain a dominant role with farm animals because animals form social relationships with caretakers who provide shelter and care for animals.

5. Stock men should be alert when handling animals during the most active time at dawn or dusk.
6. Some short-term treatments sometimes used to minimize aggression between newly mixed pigs include the use of tranquillizers (azaperone).

Eliminative Behavior

The neonate cannot voluntarily urinate and defecate. Instead, eliminative behaviors are controlled for several weeks by the urogenital reflex. Cattle, sheep, and goats eliminate their feces and urine indiscriminately. Cattle defecate 12 to 18 times per day and horses 5 to 12 times per day. Both urinate 7 to 11 times per day. The leg-raised (elevate) posture is typically associated with adult male dog urination.

Behavioral Adaptations in Temperature Regulation

Many animals have special mechanisms that enable them to control their body temperatures, such as sweating, panting and shivering. These activities involve the use of materials that may be in short supply, such as water in a desert climate. Modifications of behavior patterns, however, may be sufficient to enable an animal to survive a potential environmental stress without involving these other mechanisms. For example, cattle shift their grazing time from day to night hours under heat stress, solar radiation etc.

Animals exhibit remarkable patterns of thermoregulatory behaviour. They tend to seek the micro environment in which they find themselves most comfortable.

Cattle exposed to solar radiation, reduce their heat load by seeking shade. The tendency is more in case of exotic cattle as compared to zebu cattle. Shade seeking behaviour is prevalent even in birds and other domestic animals. Piglets are known to huddle together in cold stress to escape the rigours of cold. Under heat stress, they spread their limbs while they hold them close to the body during cold. Sheep look for shade particularly for the head, but if none is available, they face away from the sun and cease walking or grazing.

Water buffaloes and pigs have an additional behavioral wetting of skin under heat stress. Mud wallows by pig are more effective, as the cooling effect is prolonged by the water held in the mud. For water buffaloes, which have very less number of sweat glands, a wallow in clean water is essential for survival. Buffaloes who have no access to wallows, must be sprinkled with water several times from taps or showers, in order to maintain them in good health.

Abnormal Behaviour

Abnormal behaviour in domestic animals is of great relevance for veterinary diagnosis as well as for animal production aspects. Behaviors that lie outside the normal range and are considered pathologic. Some behaviors are definitely abnormal. Abnormal behavior may be expressed because of monotonous environment, overcrowding, suppression of natural instincts, inadequate exercise or movement, malnutrition etc and some of them can be injurious or destructive. In the cow, abnormal behavior may include kicking, biting and aggression.

Abnormal behavior is also known as anomalous behavior. In abnormal behavior the behavioral aberrations get repeated.The examples of abnormal behavior include tail-biting in pigs, tongue rolling and inter-suckling in calves,crib-biting and sucking by horse and feather pecking in hen. The neurophysiological changes responsible for abnormal behavior in domestic animals has not been studied to a great extent. Abnormal behavior serves not only as an indicator of poor welfare, but often also as an indicator of stress.

Anxiety, fear and phobic disorders are some of the most common unwanted and undesirable behaviors in dogs and cats. More than one anxiety disorder may be present at the same time and dogs and cats need to be examined in totality.In order to develop a suitable treatment plan , compulsive and repetitive behaviors may also be considered. Many behavioral illnesses occur in conjunction with other concomitant medical disorders and can have a negative impact on the animal's welfare and quality of life. Other abnormal behavior in pets can be attention-seeking behavior eg excessive licking behavior, compulsive behavior,separation anxiety, frustration, stress, fly-snapping, and partial seizures. Coprophagy is another abnormal behavior seen in dogs or cats.

Sometimes such disorders benefit from serotonin-enhancing medications (fluoxetine, sertraline) alongwith monoamine oxidase inhibitors.

Communication

Communication is when one animal transmits information to another animal causing some kind of change in the animal that gets the information.Communication is usually between animals of a single species, but it can also happen between two animals of different species. Animals communicate using signals, which can include visual; auditory, or sound-based; chemical, involving pheromones; or tactile, touch-based, cues. Domestic animals have less developed communication ability through language as compared to human beings.This is because of the fact that coordinated behavior of coordinated activities of central and peripheral speech apparatus are not as developed as in case of humans to have a developed speech and sound mechanism. However, some systems do exist to varying degrees of perfection in different domestic animals.

Communication behaviors can help animals find mates, establish dominance, defend territory, coordinate group behavior, and care for young.

Different animals communicate using a wide range of stimuli, known collectively as signals. Animals generally communicate using four methods: visual, auditory, tactile (touch) and chemical(Pheromones). Some species rely more on one form of communication over another.

But man himself cannot express love and humility by external signs, so plain as does a dog, when with drooping ears, hanging lips, flexuous body, and wagging tail, he meets his beloved master. Nor can these movements in the dog be explained by acts of volition or necessary instincts, any more than the beaming eyes and smiling cheeks of a man when he meets an old friend.' (Darwin, 1872: 10–1)

Here are some of the most common functions of communication:

Obtaining mates: Many animals have elaborate communication behaviors surrounding mating, which may involve attracting a mate or competing with other potential suitors for access to mates. Domestic animals often initiate mating by grooming, stroking or rubbing against each other. This provides the opportunity to apply chemical signals and to assess those excreted by the potential mate.

Establishing dominance or defending territory: In many species, communication behaviors are important in establishing dominance in a social hierarchy or defending territory.

Coordinating group behaviors. In social species, communication is key in coordinating the activities of the group, such as food acquisition and defense, and in maintaining group cohesion.

Caring for young. Among species that provide parental care to offspring, communication coordinates parent and offspring behaviors to help ensure that the offspring will survive.

Learning and Memory

Learning and memory are closely related concepts. Learning is the acquisition of skill or knowledge, while memory is the expression of what has been acquired by the animal. Learning refers to a neural mechanism by which the individual changes his or her behavior on the basis of the past experience. Memory refers to the acquisition, storage and retrieval of sensory information; while learning is the change in behaviour based on the sensory information stored in the brain. Brain has different sites and mechanisms for handling different types of information.

Learning is one of the ways in which animals are affected by their environment. Learning is an important way for animals to cope with and adapt to changing environments. Learning is defined as the neural mechanism by which an individual changes behavior on the basis of past experience. Learned behavior is one that an organism develops as a result of experience. Learned behaviors contrast with innate behaviors, which are genetically ingrained and can be performed without any prior experience or training. Of course, some behaviors have both learned and innate elements. Learning is a change in the brain as a consequence of information from outside the brain which results in modification in behavior.

Learning in domestic animals involves discriminating individuals, learn about food, feeding places, danger, risks associated with places or environmental variables. learning and memory are modulated by hormones released by aversive experiences. In the absence of verbal communication, those involved in the assessment of pain in animals have to rely on other strategies to establish the nature and intensity of the painful or nociceptive experience. From anatomical and physiological perspectives, all animals have the necessary receptors, nerves, neurotransmitters, and comparative central nervous system anatomy to be able to experience what humans describe as pain.

Instinct

An instinct is a behavior that animals exhibit independent of the wide range of learning and experiences of different individuals.Instinctual behaviors have evolved over evolutionary time to ensure the survival and reproduction of that species.

Habituation is a simple form of learning in which an animal stops responding to a stimulus, or cue, after a period of repeated exposure. Prairie dogs typically sound an alarm call when threatened by a predator. At first, they will give this alarm call in response to hearing human steps.However, the prairie dogs gradually become habituated to the sound of human footsteps, as they repeatedly experience the sound without anything bad happening. Eventually, they stop giving the alarm call in response to footsteps.

Conditioned behaviors are the result of associative learning, which takes two forms: classical conditioning and operant conditioning. The most famous example of classical conditioning comes from Ivan Pavlov's experiments in which dogs were conditioned to drool—a response previously associated with food—upon hearing the sound of a bell.As Pavlov observed, dogs salivate, or drool, in response to the sight or smell of food.

Operant conditioning is a bit different from classical conditioning in that it does not rely on an existing stimulus-response pair. Instead, whenever an organism performs a behavior—or an intermediate step on the way to the complete behavior—it is given a reward or a punishment. At first, the organism may perform the behavior—e.g., pressing a lever—purely by chance. Through reinforcement, the organism is induced to perform the behavior more or less frequently.

Memory is one of the most fundamental mental processes. The brain is the organ that is responsible for all learning and memory. It is the basis for thinking, feeling, wanting, perceiving, learning and memory, curiosity, and behavior.

Memory is defined as a behavioral change caused by an experience. Memory involves acquisition,storage and retrieval of sensory information. Learning is defined as a process for acquiring memory. There are different kinds of memory. Short term memory, intermediate term memory and long term memory. Prefrontal cortex refers to the portion of frontal lobes in front of the motor cortex is the site of working memory and thought processes. This area, like other association areas, is better developed in man than in any other species.

The nature and mechanisms of short-term memory are important to know because of the clear training and welfare implications in domestic animals such as horses. Training involves the development of desirable responses and deletion of unwanted responses. Animal training is the act of teaching animals specific responses to specific conditions or stimuli. Training may be for purposes such as companionship, detection, protection, and entertainment.

Training animals involves the improvement of timings of cues. An animal trainer should consider the natural behaviors of the animal and aim to modify behaviors through a basic system of reward and punishment. Top trainers know when and how to reward their subjects. Frequent rewards prevent development of improved responses. Reinforcement schedules are very important in animal training. Motivation encompasses a variety of factors that modify the extent and nature of any behavioural response.

- Companion bird training
- Hunting bird training
- Companion dog training
- Show dog training
- Race horse training-There are limitations in recall abilities in horses, in that they may not possess a prospective type of memory
- Mahout elephant training
- Circus elephant training
- Zoo elephant training
- Zoo exotic animal training

Behavioral Plasticity

Behavior can change in response to changes in internal or external stimuli. Behavioral plasticity refers to a change in an animal's behavior that results from exposure to stimuli, such as changing environmental conditions. When animals are confronted by new conditions, behavioral changes often occur in advance of physiological or morphological changes. Behavioral plasticity includes adaptation, learning, memory and changes in adult behavior as a result of experience during development.

One of the most intriguing features of the brain is its ability to be malleable, allowing it to adapt continually to changes in the environment. Specific neuronal activity patterns drive long-lasting increases or decreases in the strength of synaptic connections, referred to as long-term potentiation and long-term depression, respectively. Signaling cascades causes the synthesis of new plasticity-related proteins, which ultimately enable sustained changes in synaptic strength. By using the global gene expression methods as well as the candidate gene approach, it is now possible to link the function of genes to social behaviors. It is becoming increasingly clear that some candidate genes and gene networks are involved in complex social behaviors across even divergent species.

Study of neural plasticity and synaptic plasticity can pave way for the treatment of various behavioral disorders and to devise better ways of animal training. Human-induced environmental change currently represents the single greatest threat to global biodiversity. Species are typically adapted to the local environmental conditions in which they have evolved. Changes in environmental conditions initially influence behaviour, which in turn affects species interactions, population dynamics, evolutionary processes and, ultimately, biodiversity.

Plasticities can be divided into two broad categories, 'exogenous plasticity' and 'endogenous plasticity', where exogenous plasticity describes how behaviour varies within agents (individuals or genotypes) in response to variation in external factors, and endogenous plasticity describes how behaviour varies within agents in response to spontaneous changes in their internal state. Range of behavioural responses increase with increase in environmental variability. Knowledge concerning the ability of animals to adjust to environmental fluctuations is important for making predictions about population viability.

Domestication involves adaption of domestic animals to a captive environment imposed by the humans. Behavioural changes have occurred during the domestication process of domestic animals and involves some genetic changes occurred over generations. The transition from free-living to captive status is often accompanied by changes in availability and or accessibility of shelter, space, food and water, and by changes in predation and the social environment. Behavioral development in animals undergoing domestication is characterized by changes in the quantitative rather than qualitative nature of responses. Domestic phenotypes vary widely according to selection pressures favoring specific characteristics of use to humans. However, there are also shared features typical of domestic animals that include diminished "fight or flight" responses and high social tolerance. Accompanying changes may include increased attentiveness to human cues, greater promiscuity, reduced maternal care, and retention of playfulness into adulthood. Such changes reflect behavioral plasticity in response to human contributions to survival and reproductive success, including provisioning with food, protection from predators, and care of offspring.

The genetic phenomena with the greatest potential impact on the domestication process are inbreeding, genetic drift, and selection. Effects of cultivation by humans appear rapidly (within a few generations) suggesting that, in addition to changes in gene frequency, transgenerational epigenetic changes and gene–environment interactions during early development play an important role in generating domestic phenotypes.

Summary

- Behaviour is defined as the response by the animals to internal and external stimuli.
- The brain and genes are major factors that control animal behavior.
- The animal behavior can be classified as normal as well as abnormal behavior.
- Abnormal behavior serves not only as an indicator of poor welfare, but often also as an indicator of stress.
- Behavioral plasticity is defined as change in an animal's behavior that results from exposure to stimuli, such as changing environmental conditions.
- Learning is the acquisition of skill or knowledge, while memory is the expression of what you've acquired. Learning is an important way for animals to cope with and adapt to changing environments.
- Knowledge of animal behavior is important to understanding the whole animal and its ability to adapt to various environments and management systems.

27

Appendices

Appendix 1 : Syllabus

(For the Degree of Bachelor Of Veterinary Science And Animal Husbandry (B.V.Sc. & A.H.)

Unit- 1 (Blood, Cardiovascular, Nervous and Muscular Systems)

Introduction to Blood; Properties of blood as a body fluid, metabolism and fate of R.B.C; Hemoglobin-chemical structure, synthesis, physiological functions, derivatives of hemoglobin;

Heart- morphological characteristic, systemic excitability conduction and transmission processes. Cardiac Cycle: Regulation of cardiac output; coronary circulation; properties of pulse; metabolism and energetic of working myocardial cell, extrinsic and intrinsic regulation; Electro Cardio Graph and its significance in Veterinary Sciences -Echocardiography. Haemorrhage haemostasis. Haemodynamics of circulation, circulatory mechanics, resistance to flow,vasoconstriction, nervous and circulating fluid volume controls of blood pressure, neurohormonal control of vascular smooth muscle. Circulatory controls- shock stresses, regional and fetal circulation. Capillary exchange, control of blood pressure. Adjustment of circulation during exercise.

Muscle Physiology-basic muscle unit characteristic-electrical phenomenon in muscle cell - muscle action potential,excitation and propagation of impulse characteristics- latent period refractive ness, threshold level-all and none characteristics - contractile mechanism - excitation - contraction coupling-neuro-muscular transmission, types of muscle contraction, phenomenon of fatigue, rigor mortis.

Organization of nervous system- Mechanism of information processing, hierarchical control. Major function system- sensory, consciousness, emotion, motor and visceral control and basic functional unit - neuron structure, type- functional characteristics of sub-units of neurons. Membrane potential -ionic basis of resting membrane potential (RMP) nerve action potential, excitation and propagation of impulse characteristics- latent period- refractive-ness, threshold level-all and none characteristics. Degeneration and regeneration of nerve fibre. Synaptic and junctional transmission. Functions of nervous system-reflexes-control of posture and movements, autonomic nervous system and visceral control. Neurotransmitter wakefulness, sleep cycle. Higher function of neurons system - learning, memory, electroencephalography.

Sense organs and receptors physiology of special senses- Eye: functional morphology, nourishment and protection neural pathway, receptors- optics, ocular muscles and movements, photochemistry, Vision defects Ear: Physiology of hearing and common hearing impairment. Vestibule apparatus. Physiology of olfaction and taste

Unit-2 (Digestive and Respiratory Systems)

Morphological characteristics of mono gastric and polygastric digestive system. Prehension, rumination; defecation; vomition; regulation of secretory function of saliva, stomach, intestine, pancreas; bile secretion; hunger, appetite control,developmental aspects of digestion; luminous, membranous and microbial digestion in rumen and intestine; permeability characteristics of intestine, forces governing absorption, control intestinal transport of electrolyte and water, enzymatic digestion in monogastric and fermentative digestion in rumen, modification of toxic substances in rumen. Digestion in birds.

Functional morphology of respiratory apparatus. Mechanics of breathing. Transport of blood gases, foetal and neonatal oxygen transport, dissociation curves, pressures, recoil tendency, elasticity, surfactants, pleural liquid, compliance,exchanges of gases in lungs and tissues, neural and chemical regulation of breathing, diffusion, perfusion, hypoxia.Frictional resistance to air flow, airways smooth muscle contraction, respiratory muscle work, panting, adaptation of respiration during muscle exercise, high altitude hypoxia, Non-respiratory lung functions. Respiration in birds.

Unit-3 (Excretory and Endocrine Systems)

Kidney- Functional morphology of nephrons, factors determining filtration pressure, determination of glomerular filtration rate (GFR) and renal plasma flow – Re-absorption mechanisms for glucose, protein, amino acids, electrolytes; ammonium mechanism, glomerulo-tubular balance, methods of studying renal functions; urine concentration;micturition, uremia.

Fluid, water balance, fluid therapy, dehydration, water concentration mechanisms. Acid base balance and H^+ regulation, correction and evolution of imbalances, total osmotic pressure. Formation and excretion of urine of Birds.

Cerebrospinal fluid, synovial fluids - composition, formation and flow; Joints. Regulation of bone metabolism and homeostasis.

Hormone cell interaction, subcellular mechanisms-metabolism of hormones-methods of study of endocrine system; Receptors- mechanism of regulation; Chemistry of hypothalamo- hypophyseal hormones, target organ, pineal, thyroid,thymus, pancreas, adrenal, prostaglandins, hormones of calcium metabolism, disorders, renin-angiotensin system, atrial natriuretic factors, erythropoietin, GI hormones, pheromones.

Unit-4 (Reproduction, Lactation, Growth and Environmental Physiology)

Genetic and endocrine control of gonadal development, modification of gonadotropin release, ovarian functions,follicular development, dynamics, endocrine and receptor profiles, sexual receptivity, ovarian cycle, postpartum ovarian activity, ovum transport, capacitation, fertilization, reproductive cycles in farm animals- hormones present in the biological fluids during pregnancy and their uses for the diagnosis of pregnancy-maternal foetal placental participation in pregnancy and parturition, immunology of gestation, periparturient endocrine status.

Spermatogenic cycle and wave- function of sertoli cell-leydig cell-semen - composition- evaluation; Testosterone -function and regulation - cryptorchidism. Puberty - photoperiod - uses of androgens, progestogens, estrogens.

Functional and metabolic organization of mammary glands - structure and development; effect of estrogens and progesterone; hormonal control of mammary growth; lactogenesis and galactogenesis; biosynthesis of milk constituents, secretion of milk, and metabolism, prolactin and lactation cycle.

Biochemical and genetic determinants of growth, regulation of growth, metabolic and hormone interactions, factors affecting efficiency of growth and production in ruminants and single stomach animals. Growth in meat producing animals and birds, growth curves. Recombinant gene transfer technologies for growth manipulation-advantages and limitations. Protein deposition in animals and poultry.

Heat balance, heat tolerance, hypothermia, hyperthermia, thermo-regulation in farm animals, role of skin, responses of animals to heat and cold, fever, body temperature and hibernation. Temperature regulation in birds.

Climatology- various parameters and their importance. Effect of different environmental variables like temperature,humidity, light, radiation, altitude on animal performance. Acclimation, acclimatization - general adaptive syndrome.Clinical aspects of endocrine - reproductive functions, circadian rhythm.

Neurophysiology of behaviours, types of behaviour, communication, Learning and memory, behavioural plasticity.

Appendix 2: Selected Textbooks in Physiology

Anand, B.K . and Manchanda ,S. K .(1976) Textbook of Physiology. Tata McGrawHill, New Delhi.

Anthony, C.P. and Thibodeau, G.A. (1979) Textbook of Anatomy and Physiology, 10th Edition, CV Mosby Co. St. Louis.

B. Bhattacharya (2015) Textbook of Veterinary Physiology, 3rd Edition, Kalyani Publishers.

Bolis, L., K. Schmidt Nielson and S.H.P. Maddrell (1973) Comparative Physiology. American Elsevier, New York.

Bone, J.F. (1999) Animal Anatomy and Physiology. 3rd Edition Reston Pub. Co. Reston, Virginia, U.S.A.

Breazile, J.E. (1972) A Textbook of Veterinary Physiology. Harcourt, Philadelphia.

Brobeck, J.R. (1979) (Ed.) Best and Taylors Physiological Basis of Medical Practice, 10th Ed. William and Wilkins.

Chatterjee, C.C. (2018) Human Physiology,Vol. 1, 2. 12th Edition CBS Publishers & Distributors

Crouch, J.E. and McClintic, J.R. (1971) Human Anatomy and Physiology, John Wiley, New York.

Dowben, R.M. (1969) General Physiology: A Molecular Approach. Harper and Row, New York.

D'amour, F.E. (1961) Basic Physiology. University of Chicago Press, Chicago.

Davson, H. (1959) A textbook of General Physiology, 2nd Edition Little Brown and Co, Boston.

DeCoursey, R.M. (1961) The Human Organism, 2nd Edition, McGrawhill Book Co. New York.

Eric P. Widmaier, Hershel Raff, Kevin T. Strang (2010) Vander's Human Physiology. McGrawhill, N.Y.

Evans, C.L. (Ed.) (1956) Starlings Principles of Human Physiology 12th Ed. Lea and Febiger, Philadelphia.

Evans, W.F. (1976) Anatomy and Physiology, Prentice Hall, N.J.

Florey, E. (1966) An introduction to general and comparative Physiology. W.B. Saunders Company, Philadelphia.

Gottam, G.S., Mittal, P.K., Barkha Gupta, S.K. Jindal and Bilochi, D.R. (2020) Practical Veterinary Physiology, I.B.S. , New Delhi

Hall, John, E. (2015) Guyton and Hall Textbook of Medical Physiology, 13th Edition, W.B. Saunders, Philadelphia.

Hoar, W.S. (1983) General and Comparative Physiology, 3rd Edition, Prentice Hall Inc., Englewood Cliff, N.J.

Houssay, B.A. (1955) Human Physiology, 2nd Ed. McGrawhill Co. New York.

Indu Khurana (2015) Textbook of Medical Physiology, 2nd Edition, Elsevier.

Jain, A.K. (2017)Text Book of Physiology 7th Edition. Avichal Publishing Company

Kelle, C.A. and Neil, E. (1971) Samson Wrigh'ts Applied Physiology, 12th Edition, Oxford University Press.

Kim E. Barrett Susan M. Barman Scott Boitano Heddwen L. Brooks Ganong, W.F (2009) Ganong's Review of Medical Physiology, 23rd Edition (Lange Basic Science), California.

Klein, B.G. (2019) Cunningham Textbook of Veterinary Physiology, 6th Edition, Elsevier.

Lamn, J.F., C.G. Ingram, I.A. Johnston and R.M. Pitman (1980) Essentials of Physiology. Blackwell Scientific Publication Oxford.

Langley, L.L. and E. Cheraskin (1958) The physiology of man. 2nd Ed. McGrawhill, New York.

Lauralee Sherwood (2009) Human Physiology: From Cells to Systems, Brooks/Cole Pub Co.

Mountcastle, V.B. (1974) Medical Physiology. Ed. 13, C.V. Mosby Co. St. Louis.

Nagabhushnam,R., M.S.Kodarkar and S.Sarojini(1983) Textbook of Animal Physiology.2nd Edition,Oxford and IBH.NewDelhi.

Pantelouris, E.M. (1967) Introduction to Animal Physiology and Physiological Genetics, Pergamon Press, Oxford.

Phillis, J.W. (1976) (Ed.) Veterinary Physiology, John Wright, Bristol. pp 892.

Prosser, C.L. (1973) (Ed.) Comparative Animal Physiology, 3rd Edition. W.B. Saunders Company, Philadelphia.

Ralph, C.L. (1978) Introductory Animal Physiology, McGrawhill Book Company, N.Y.

Rastogi, S.C. (2007) Essentials of Animal Physiology. New Age Publishers.

Reece, William O. (2004) (Ed.) Duke's Physiology of Domestic Animals, 12th Edition, Comstock Publishing Assoc. Ithaca, New York.

Rogers, T.A. (1961) Elementary Human Physiology. John Wiley and Sons, New York.

Rowen D. Frandson, W. Lee Wilke, Anna Dee Fails (2009) Anatomy and Physiology of Farm Animals. 7th Edition. Wiley, John & Sons.

Ruch, T.C. and Patton, H.B. (1973) (Ed.) Physiology and Biophysics, 20 th Ed. 3 Vols . W . B. Saunders Company, Philadelphia.

Scheer, B.T. (1963) Animal Physiology, John Wiley, N.Y.

Schmidt-Nielson, K. (1994) Animal Physiology, 3rd Ed. Cambridge University Press, New York.

Schotellius, B.A. and Schotellius, D.B. (1978) Textbook of Physiology. 18th Edition, C.V. Mosby Co, St. Louis.

Sembulingam K., Sembulingam Prema (2016) Essentials of Medical Physiology, 7th Edition Jaypee Brothers Medical Publishers (P) Ltd.

Sharma, I.J. (2008) Physiological Basis of Veterinary Practice, Kalyani Publishers.

Sturkie, P.D. (Ed.) (1981) Basic Physiology. Springer Verlag New York.

Svendson, Par. (1984) An Introduction to Animal Physiology. 2nd Editions, MTP Press (Lancaster Lancashire and Boston)

Tartora, G.J. and Anagnostakos, N.P. (1981) Principles of Anatomy and Physiology, 3rd Ed., Harper and Row, New York.

Whittow, G. (1999) Sturkie's Avian Physiology 5th Edition, Academic Press.

Wilson, J.A. (1972) Principles of Animal Physiology. McMillan Co., New York.

Youmans, W.B. (1954) Human Physiology, McMillan Co, N.Y.

Other classic and Related Books on Physiology

Aggarwal, Anjali, and Ramesh Upadhyay.(2012) Heat stress and animal productivity. Springer Science & Business Media,.

Brody, S. (1945). Bioenergetics and growth; with special reference to the efficiency complex in domestic animals.Reinhold Publishing Co,

Cole, H. H., & Cupps, P. T. (Eds.). (2013). Reproduction in domestic animals. Elsevier.

Cowie, A. T., Forsyth, I. A., & Hart, I. C. (2012). Hormonal control of lactation (Vol. 15). Springer Science & Business Media.

Folley, S. J. (1956). The physiology and biochemistry of lactation. The physiology and biochemistry of lactation.

Hafez, E. S. E. (1976). Human semen and fertility regulation in men. Mosby.

Hafez, E.S.E (Ed) The Behaviour of Domestic Animals,3rd Ed. Bailliere-Tindale

Hafez, E.S.E. (Ed)(1968) Adaptation of domestic animals, Lea & Febiger

Hafez, E. (1969). Animal Growth and Nutrition, Lea & Febiger.

Hafez, E.S.E. and Hafez, B. (Ed.) (2000). Reproduction in Farm Animals, 7th Edition, Wiley, John & Sons.

Hammond, J. (1932). Growth and the development of mutton qualities in the sheep. A survey of the problems involved in meat production. Growth and the development of mutton qualities in the sheep. A survey of the problems involved in meat production.

Hammond, J. (1952). Farm animals: their breeding, growth, and inheritance. Farm animals: their breeding, growth, and inheritance., (2nd Edit).

Hammond, J. (1960). Farm animals. Their breeding, growth, and inheritance. Farm animals. Their breeding, growth, and inheritance.

Ian R. Gordon (2004) Reproductive Technologies in Farm Animals, CABI.

Kleiber, M. (1961). The fire of life. An introduction to animal energetics. The fire of life. An introduction to animal energetics.

Kleiber, M. (1975). The fire of life. An introduction to animal energetics. Krieger Pub Co

Lawrence TLJ. (1997). Growth of Farm Animals, CABI.

Mann, T. (1964). The biochemistry of semen and of the male reproductive tract. The biochemistry of semen and of the male reproductive tract.

Mann, T. and Lutwak Mann, C. (1981). Male Reproductive Function and Semen: Themes and Trends in Physiology, Biochemistry and Investigative Andrology. Springer Verlag, Berlin.

Marshall, F. H. A. (1952). Marshall's physiology of reproduction (Vol. 1). Longmans, Green.

Mauricio Pineda and Michael P. Dooley (Ed.) (2008). McDonald's Veterinary Endocrinology and Reproduction, 5th Edition, Wiley-Blackwell.

McDowell, L. R. 2000. Vitamins in animal and human nutrition. Iowa State University Press, Ames, IA. 793 pp.

McDowell, R. E. (1972). Improvement of livestock production in warm climates. Improvement of livestock production in warm climates.

Nalbandov, A.V. (1975) Reproductive Physiology 3rd Edition, W.H. Freeman, San Francisco.

Pineda, M. H., & Dooley, M. P. (2003). McDonald's veterinary endocrinology and reproduction (Ed. 5). Iowa state press.

Preston, T. R., & Leng, R. A. (1987). Matching ruminant production systems with available resources in the tropics and sub-tropics. Penambul Books.

Puniya A., Singh R., Kamra D. (2015)(eds) Rumen Microbiology: From Evolution to Revolution. Springer, New Delhi

Roberts, S.J. (1986). Veterinary Obstetrics and Genital Diseases. 3rd Ed. Published by the author. Ann Arbor, Michigan, Edwards Brothers.

Salisbury, G. W., VanDemark, N. L., & Lodge, J. R. (1978). Physiology of reproduction and artificial insemination of cattle(No. Ed. 2). WH Freeman and Company.

Tizard, I.R. (2009) Veterinary Immunology: an introduction. 8th ed., St. Louis, Saunders

Wagner, A. F. and Folkers, K. 1962. Vitamins and Coenzymes, Wiley (Interscience), New York, NY

Watson, J. D. (2004). Molecular biology of the gene (Vol. 1). Pearson Education India.

Appendix 3 : List of Nobel Prize Winners in Physiology or Medicine

The Nobel Prize in Physiology or Medicine is awarded annually by the Swedish Karolinska Institut to scientists and doctors in the various fields of physiology or medicine. It is one of the five Nobel Prizes established by the 1895 will of Alfred Nobel (who died in 1896), awarded for outstanding contributions in chemistry, physics, literature, peace, and physiology or medicine.

110 Nobel Prizes in Physiology or Medicine have been awarded since 1901. It was not awarded on nine occasions: in 1915, 1916, 1917, 1918, 1921, 1925, 1940, 1941 and 1942.

1901	E.A. Von Behring (Germany)- Emil von Behring, was a German physiologist who received the 1901 Nobel Prize in Physiology or Medicine, the first one awarded in that field, for his discovery of a diphtheria antitoxin.
1902	Sir Ronald Ross (England)- Sir Ronald Ross was a British medical doctor who received the Nobel Prize for Physiology or Medicine in 1902 for his work on the transmission of malaria.
1903	N.R. Finsen (Denmark)- Niels Ryberg Finsen was awarded the Nobel Prize for his invention of light therapy for skin tuberculosis (lupus vulgaris).
1904	Ivan P. Pavlov (Russia)- Ivan Petrovich Pavlov was a Russian physiologist known primarily for his work in classical conditioning.
1905	Robert Kock (Germany) for his investigations and discoveries in relation to tuberculosis
1906	S. Romon Cajal (Spain) & Camillo Golgi (Italy) in recognition of their work on the structure of the nervous system
1907	C.L.A. Laveran (France)
1908	Paul Ehrlich (Germany) & E. Metchnikoff (France) in recognition of their work on immunity"
1909	T-Kocher (Sweden) for his work on the physiology, pathology and surgery of the thyroid gland
1910	A. Kossel (Germany) in recognition of the contributions to our knowledge of cell chemistry made through his work on proteins, including the nucleic substances"
1911	A. Gullstrand (Sweden) for his work on the dioptrics of the eye
1912	Alexis Carrel (USA) in recognition of his work on vascular suture and the transplantation of blood vessels and organs
1913	Charles Richet (France) in recognition of his work on anaphylaxis
1914	R. Barany (Austria) for his work on the physiology and pathology of the vestibular apparatus"
1915-18	No Award
1919	J. Bordet (Belgium) Factors in blood serum work with antibodies to destroy bacteria, and Bordet's discovery of these complement proteins allowed the creation of tests that could diagnose many dangerous infectious diseases.

1920	August Krogh (Denmark) for his discovery of the capillary motor regulating mechanism
1921	No Award
1922	A.V. Hill (England) for his discovery relating to the production of heat in the muscle and Mtto Meyerhoff (Germany) for his discovery of the fixed relationship between the consumption of oxygen and the metabolism of lactic acid in the muscle
1923	Frederic G. Banting and J.J.R. MacLeod (Canada) for the discovery of insulin
1924	W. Einthoven (Holland)- Willem Einthoven was a Dutch physician and physiologist. He invented the first practical electrocardiogram in 1895.
1925	No award
1926	Johannes Fibiger (Denmark)- Danish pathologist for achieving the first controlled induction of cancer in laboratory animals
1927	J. Wagner-Jauregg (Austria)- His Nobel award was "for his discovery of the therapeutic value of malaria inoculation in the treatment of dementia paralytica"
1928	Charles Nocolle (France) for his work on typhus
1929	Sir F.G. Hopkins (England) and C. Eijkman (Holland)- for the discovery of vitamin B1
1930	Karl Landsteiner (USA) - Landsteiner's discovery of human blood groups, and his system for typing blood, allowed blood transfusions to be carried out without the risk of adverse reactions.
1931	Otto H. Warburg (Germany)- his discovery of the nature and mode of action of the cellular respiratory enzyme in normal and cancer cells.
1932	Sir C.S. Sherrington and E.D. Adrian (England) or their discoveries regarding the functions of neurons
1933	T.H. Morgan (USA) for his discoveries concerning the role played by the chromosome in heredity
1934	G.R.Minto, W.P. Murphy and G.H. Whipple (USA) -Vitamin B12
1935	Hans Spemann (Germany) for his discovery of the organizer effect in embryonic development
1936	Sir Henry H. Dale (England) and Otto Loewi (Austria) - Chemical Control of heart rate-discovered that nerve cells communicate with each other, and with their target organs, using chemicals.
1937	A. Szent Gyorgyi (Hungary) for his discoveries in connection with the biological combustion processes, with special reference to vitamin C and the catalysis of fumaric acid
1938	C. Heymans (Belgium) for the discovery of the role played by the sinus and aortic mechanisms in the regulation of respiration"
1939	G. Domagk (Germany) for the discovery of the antibacterial effects of prontosil
1940-42	No Award
1943	C.P. Henrik Dam (Denmark) and Edward A. Doisy (USA) for his discovery of vitamin K

1944	Joseph Erlanger and Herbert Gasser (USA)- constructed a recording device which revealed that different nerve fibres transmit different kinds of impulses
1945	Sir Alexander Fleming, Sir Howard W. Florey (England) and E.B. Chain (Germany) for the discovery of penicillin and its curative effect in various infectious diseases.
1946	H.J. Muller (USA) for the discovery of the production of mutations by means of X-ray irradiation
1947	Carl F. and Getty T. Cori (USA) for their discovery of the course of the catalytic conversion of glycogen and Bernardo A. Houssay (Argentina) for his discovery of the part played by the hormone of the anterior pituitary lobe in the metabolism of sugar
1948	Paul Mueller (USA) for his discovery of the high efficiency of DDT as a contact poison against several arthropods
1949	Walter R. Hess (Switzerland) for his discovery of the functional organization of the interbrain as a coordinator of the activities of the internal organs and Antonia, C.A.F. Moniz (Portugal)
1950	Edward C. Kendall, Philip S. Hench (USA) and T. Reichstein (Switzerland) for their discoveries relating to the hormones of the adrenal cortex, their structure and biological effects
1951	Max Theiler (USA - b, Africa) for his discoveries concerning yellow fever and how to combat it"
1952	S.A. Waksman (USA) for his discovery of streptomycin, the first antibiotic effective against tuberculosis
1953	Hans A. Krebs (England) for his discovery of the citric acid cycle and F.A. Lipmann (USA) for his discovery of coenzyme A and its importance for intermediary metabolism
1954	J.F. Enders, F.C. Robbins and T.H. Weller (USA)
1955	A.H.T. Theorell (Sweden) for his discoveries concerning the nature and mode of action of oxidation enzymes
1956	Andre F. Courn and D.W.Richards (USA) and W. Frossmann (Germany) for their discoveries concerning heart catheterization and pathological changes in the circulatory system
1957	Daniel Bovet (Italy) for his discoveries relating to synthetic compounds that inhibit the action of certain body substances, and especially their action on the vascular system and the skeletal muscles
1958	G.W. Beadle, Joshua Lederberg and E.L. Tatum (USA) or their discovery that genes act by regulating definite chemical events
1959	Severo Ochoa and Arthur Kornberg (USA) for their discovery of the mechanisms in the biological synthesis of ribonucleic acid and deoxyribonucleic acid
1960	Sir M. Burnet (Australia) and Peter B. Medawar (England) The concept of immunological tolerance showed how the body learns to recognize its own cells and tissues, which prevents the immune system from mounting a response against itself.

1961	George von Bekesy (USA) for his discoveries of the physical mechanism of stimulation within the cochlea
1962	Francis, H.C. Crick, Maurice, H.F. Wilkins (England) and James D. Watson (USA) for their discoveries concerning the molecular structure of nucleic acids and its significance for information transfer in living material
1963	Sir John C. Eccles (Australia), Andrew F. Huxley, A.L. Hodgkin (England)- Waves of charged atoms flowing in and out of cells provide the spark that fires electrical impulses through nerves.
1964	Konrad E. Bloch (USA) and Feodor Lyhen (West Germany) for their discoveries concerning the mechanism and regulation of the cholesterol and fatty acid metabolism
1965	Francis Jacob, Andre Lwoff and Jacques Monod (France) for their discoveries concerning genetic control of enzyme and virus synthesis
1966	Francis P. Rous and Charles B. Huggins (USA) for his discoveries concerning hormonal treatment of prostatic cancer
1967	Ranger Granit (Sweden), Haldon Keffer Hartline and George Wald (USA) for their discoveries concerning the primary physiological and chemical visual processes in the eye
1968	Har Govind Khorana (USA), Robert W. Holley and Marshall W. Nirenberg (USA)- for their interpretation of the genetic code and its function in protein synthesis.
1969	Max Delbruck (USA), Alfred, D. Hershey (USA) andSalvador Luria (USA) for their discoveries concerning the replication mechanism and the genetic structure of viruses
1970	Bernard Katz (England) Ulf von Euler (Sweden) Julis Axelrod (USA)- how chemical neurotransmitters can send information from one nerve cell to another within the blink of an eye.
1971	Earl Wilbur Sutherland (USA) for his discoveries concerning the mechanisms of the action of hormones
1972	Gerald Edelman (USA), Rodney Porter (Britain)-The two scientists independently deciphered the structure of antibodies, which revealed how seemingly identical-looking molecules can target specifically any one of a countless number of invaders for destruction.
1973	Karl von Frisch (West German), Zacharian Lorenz (Austria), Nicholas Tinbergen (Netherlands) for their discoveries concerning organization and elicitation of individual and social behaviour patterns
1974	Albert Claude (Luxembourg), George E. Palade (Hungary), Christian de Duve (Belgium) for their discoveries concerning the structural and functional organization of the cell
1975	David Baltimore (USA), Renato Dulecco (Britain), Howard M. Temin (USA) for their discoveries concerning the interaction between tumour viruses and the genetic material of the cell
1976	Baruch S. Blumberg (USA), D. Carleton Gajdusek (USA)

1977	Rosalyn S. Yalow (USA) for the development of radioimmunoassays of peptide hormones, Roger C. Guillemin (USA) Andre V. Schally (USA) for their discoveries concerning the peptide hormone production of the brain"
1978	Werner Arber (Switzerland), Daniel Nathans (USA), Hamilton O. Smith (USA) for the discovery of restriction enzymes and their application to problems of molecular genetics
1979	Godfrey Hounsfield (Britain) Allan McCormack (USA) for the development of computer assisted tomography
1980	Buruf Benacerraf (USA) George Shell (USA) Jean Dausset (France)- Breakthroughs from the three researchers helped to build a picture for how a specific set of proteins found on the surface of cells can regulate the immune response.
1981	Roger Sperry (USA) for his discoveries concerning the functional specialization of the cerebral hemispheres David Hubel (USA) Torsten Wiesel(USA) for their discoveries concerning information processing in the visual system
1982	S. Bergstroem (Sweden), B. Samuelson (Sweden) John Vane (Britain) for their discoveries concerning prostaglandins and related biologically active substances
1983	Barbara McClintock (U.S.A) for her discovery of mobile genetic elements..
1984	Nils Jerne, Georges Kohler and César Milstein Jerne's theories provided a clearer image of how the immune system engages antibodies to fight invaders, Köhler and Milstein's techniques for producing specific antibodies on demand helped to create better diagnostic tests and new treatments against diseases.
1985	Michael S. Brown & Joseph Goldstein (USA) for their discoveries concerning the regulation of cholesterol metabolism
1986	Stanley Cohen and Rita Levi-Mondalcini (USA)- nerve cells release growth factors that stimulate and regulate the development of the fantastically complex nervous system.
1987	Susumu Tonegawa (Japan) By uncovering the genetic mechanism for the construction of antibodies, Tonegawa revealed how the body can generate millions and millions of antibody proteins from a much smaller number of genes.
1988	James Black (UK), Gertrude Elion & George Hitchings (USA)- for their discoveries of important principles for drug treatment.
1989	J.Michael Bishop, Harold E Varmus (USA)
1990	Joseph E Murrey, E.Donnall Thomas (USA) for their discoveries concerning organ and cell transplantation in the treatment of human disease
1991	Erwin Neher and Bert Saksmann (Germany)- nerve cell membranes have individual ion channels through which tiny currents pass.
1992	Edmond Fischer & Edwin Krebs (USA) for their discoveries concerning reversible protein phosphorylation as a biological regulatory mechanism"
1993	Richard J Roberts (UK) Philip A. Sharp (USA) for their discoveries of split genes

1994	Alfred Gilman (USA) and Martin Rodbell (USA) for their discovery of G-proteins and the role of these proteins in signal transduction in cells
1995	Edward Lewis (USA), Christiane Nusslein Volhard (Germany) and Eric F. Wieschaus (USA) for their discoveries concerning the genetic control of early embryonic development
1996	Peter Doherty and Rolf Zinkernagel Doherty and Zinkernagel's discovery of how the immune system recognizes virus-infected cells uncovered the general mechanisms used by the cellular component of the immune system to distinguish foreign agents from its own cells and tissues.
1997	Stanley Prusiner (USA) for his discovery of Prions – a new biological principle of infection
1998	Robert F Furchgott, Louis J Ignarro and Ferid Murad (USA) for their discoveries concerning nitric oxide as a signalling molecule in the cardiovascular system
1999	Günter Blobel, for the discovery that proteins have intrinsic signals that govern their transport and localization in the cell
2000	Arvid Carlsson, Paul Greengard and Eric Kandel -deciphered the chemical messages passed across nerve cells that regulate some of the brain's most important functions.
2001	Leland H. Hartwell, R. Timothy Hunt and Paul M. Nurse for their discoveries of key regulators of the cell cycle
2002	Sydney Brenner, H. Robert Horvitz and John E. Sulston for their discoveries concerning genetic regulation of organ development and programmed cell death
2003	Paul C. Lauterbur, and Sir Peter Mansfield for their discoveries concerning magnetic resonance imaging
2004	Richard Axel, and Linda B Buck for their discoveries of odorant receptors and the organization of the olfactory system
2005	Barry J. Marshall, and J. Robin Warren for their discovery of the bacterium Helicobacter pylori and its role in gastritis and peptic ulcer disease
2006	Andrew Z. Fire, and Craig C. Mello for their discovery of RNA interference – gene silencing by double-stranded RNA
2007	Mario R. Capecchi, Sir Martin J. Evans, and Oliver Smithies for their discoveries of principles for introducing specific gene modifications in mice by the use of embryonic stem cells
2008	Harald Zur Hausen for his discovery of human papilloma viruses causing cervical can-cer , Francoise Barre Sinoussi, and Luc Montagnier for their discovery of human im- munodeficiency virus
2009	Elizabeth H. Blackburn, Carol W. Greider, Jack W. Szostak- "how chromosomes are protected by telomeres and the enzyme telomerase"
2010	Robert G. Edwards- "for the development of *in vitro* fertilization"
2011	Bruce A. Beutler United States "for their discoveries concerning the activation of innate immunity" Jules A. Hoffmann France Ralph M. Steinman Canada "for his discovery of the dendritic cell and its role in adaptive immunity" (awarded posthumously)

2012	John Gurdon United Kingdom "for the discovery that mature cells can be reprogrammed to become pluripotent" Shinya Yamanaka Japan
2013	James E. Rothman United States "for their discoveries of machinery regulating vesicle traffic, a major transport system in our cells" Randy Schekman United States Thomas c südhof United States
2014	John O'Keefe (neuroscientist) United States United Kingdom "for their discoveries of cells that constitute a positioning system in the brain" May-Britt Moser 2014. Norway Edvard Moser. Norway
2015	William C. Campbell Ireland United States "for their discoveries concerning a novel therapy against infections caused by roundworm parasites"Satoshi Ōmura Japan Tu Youyou China "for her discoveries concerning a novel therapy against malaria"
2016	Yoshinori Ohsumi Japan "for his discoveries of mechanisms for autophagy"
2017	Jeffrey C. Hall United States "for their discoveries of molecular mechanisms controlling the circadian rhythm" Michael Rosbash United States,Michael W. Young United States
2018	James P. Allison United States ,Tasuku Honjo Japan "for their discovery of cancer therapy by inhibition of negative immune regulation"
2019	Gregg L. Semenza- United States "for their discoveries of how cells sense and adapt to oxygen availability."

Appendix 4 : Physiological Literature

The physiological literature is vast in size. We cite here some of the more familiar sources of information.

Review Publications

- Physiological Reviews (https://journals.physiology.org/journal/physrev)
- Annual Review of Physiology(https://www.annualreviews.org/journal/physiol)

Research Journals

- Journal of Physiology (London)(https://physoc.onlinelibrary.wiley.com/journal/14697793)
- Journal da Physiologie (Paris)(https://www.journals.elsevier.com/journal-of-physiology-paris)
- American Journal of Physiology-Cell Physiology
- American Journal of Physiology-Endocrinology and Metabolism
- American Journal of Physiology-Gastrointestinal and Liver Physiology
- American Journal of Physiology-Heart and Circulatory Physiology
- American Journal of Physiology-Lung Cellular and Molecular Physiology

- American Journal of Physiology-Regulatory, Integrative and Comparative Physiology
- American Journal of Physiology-Renal Physiology
- Physiology (https://journals.physiology.org/journal/physiologyonline)
- Canadian Journal of Physiology and Pharmacology
- Acta Physiologica Scandinavica
- Pflugers Archives (European Journal of Physiology) (https://www.springer.com/journal/424)
- Japanese Journal of Physiology
- Acta Physiological Latinomerica
- Physiologics Bohemoslav
- Indian Journal of Physiology and Pharmacology
- Quarterly Journal of Experimental Physiology and Cognate
- Medical Sciences (Now ceased Publication, 1981)
- IRCS Journal of Medical Science (Physiology)
- International Journal of Animal Sciences (discontinued)
- Indian Journal of Animal Science.
- Journal of Dairy Science
- Journal of Animal Science
- Canadian Journal of Animal Sciences
- Asian Australasian Journal of Animal Sciences

In addition there are a lot of journals specialised in the respective fields of Physiology.

Reproduction

- Reproduction (Formerly Journal of Reproduction and Fertility)
- Reproduction, Fertility and Development
- Biology of Reproduction
- Andrologia
- Journal of Andrology
- International Journal of Andrology
- Fertility and Sterility International Journal of Fertility
- Indian Journal of Animal Reproduction
- Animal Reproduction Science Elsevier
- Theriogenology

Endocrinology

- Endocrinology (https://academic. oup.com/endo) Journal of Endocrinology (https://joe. bioscientifica. com/) General and Comparative Endocrinology (https://www.journals. elsevier. com general-and -comparative endocrinology
- Endocrinologica Experimentalis Hormone and Metabolic Research Hormone Research
- Acta Endocrinologica
- Endocrinologica Japonica
- Molecular endocrinology (https://academic.oup.com/mend)

Animal Physiology/ Animal/Dairy Science

- Journal of Animal Science
- Journal of Dairy Science
- Australian Journal of Science
- Physiological Zoology
- Comparative Biochemistry and Physiology
- Respiration
- Respiration Physiology
- Digestion
- British Journal of Nutrition
- Animal feed Science & Technology
- Journal of Nutrition
- Archiv fur Tiernahrung

In addition many articles of physiologists interest appear in

- Nature
- Science
- Federation Proceedings
- Physiologist
- Comp Rendes des Acad Sci.

Multivolume Publications in Physiology

- Handbook of Physiology
- Recent Progress in Hormone Research
- Vitamins and Hormones
- The Testis

- The Ovary
- Marshall's Physiology of Reproduction
- Sex and Internal Secretion
- Lactation : A comprehensive treatise.

Internet Resources.

- https://www.wikipedia.org/
- https://www.ncbi.nlm.nih.gov/pubmed/
- https://www.sciencedirect.com/
- http://cera.iari.res.in/index.php/en/
- https://krishikosh.egranth.ac.in/

Physiological Societies

- American Physiological Society
- International Union of Physiological Sciences
- The Physiological Society
- Society of Animal Physiologists of India
- Association of Physiologists and Pharmacologists of India

Appendix 5 : Model Questions

Model Questions for Examinations

- Climatic elements and their impact on growth, production and reproduction
- Describe the digestion of protein in ruminants?
- Describe the events in the estrous cycle with interplay of hormones
- Describe the mechanism of blood coagulation
- Describe the neuromuscular junction. Enlist at least five neurotransmitters and their actions.
- Describe the process of oogenesis and the hormones controlling it
- Describe the various events of cardiac cycle
- Describe the various stages of estrous cycle
- Different types of animal behaviour
- Differentiate between ruminant and non-ruminant saliva?
- Differentiate between serum and plasma?
- Direct growth regulators
- Draw a labelled figure of mammalian heart showing the different heart valves.
- Enumerate various functions of saliva in ruminants?
- Explain fate of erythrocytes.

- Explain spermatogenesis and the factors affecting it
- Explain the functions of testosterone and estrogen
- Explain the process of implantation and maternal recognition of pregnancy
- Explain the statement that Pancreas is exocrine as well as endocrine gland.
- Factor influencing postnatal growth
- Factor influencing prenatal growth
- Hormonal changes during estrous cycle
- Hormonal interactions during folliculogenesis
- How urine is concentrated in mammalian kidney
- Measurement of postnatal growth
- Mechanism of vision
- Physiological role of ovarian hormones
- Thermoregulation in birds
- Thermoregulation in mammals
- What are the characteristics of cardiac muscle ?
- What are the different lung volumes and capacities?
- What do you mean by isotonic and isometric contractions of skeletal muscle. Describe the changes occurring at the molecular level during muscle contraction.
- What is blood pressure? Explain factors affecting blood pressure
- What is cardiac output? Describe the various factors that affect cardiac output.
- What is ECG? Explain the PQRS complex.
- What is rigor mortis and how it occurs?
- Write a short note on Anaemia.
- Write in details the functions of the hypothalamus.
- Write the functions of blood
- Write the hormonal control of mammary gland development and lactogenesis.
- What are the three types of muscle and what are some of the general characteristics of each type?

Multiple Choice Questions

This vitamin is needed to make red blood cells

a. B_1 b. B_2
c. B_6 **d. B_{12}**

Which of these are fat soluble?

a. Vitamin K b. Vitamin E
c. Vitamin D d. Vitamin A
e. All of the above

While reading a blood test I notice a high level of creatinine, I could assume from this that

a. There is a possibility of a UTI

b. There is a possibility of diabetes

c. There is a possibility of kidney failure

d. There is nothing wrong, this is normal

If an animal is dehydrated than the body will increase

a. ATP

b. ADH

c. Diluted Urine

d. ADP

Nephrons

a. Eliminate wastes from the body

b. Regulate blood volume and pressure

c. Control levels of electrolytes and metabolites

d Regulate blood pH

e. All of the above

How are wastes carried to the kidney for removal?

a. in cells

c. in the urine

b. in blood

d. in interstitial fluid

The term used to describe, "cell eating" is?

a. Exocytosis

b. Phagocytosis

c. Pinocytosis

d. Diffusion

Which of the following requires energy?

a. Diffusion

b. Osmosis

c. Active transport

d. Facilitated diffusion

What is a melanoma?

a. The outermost layer of skin

b. A type of nail disease

c. A malignant tumor that originates

d. The lowermost layer of in melanocytes skin

Where is the body's "thermostat" found?

a. Within the nervous system, in the Hypothalamus

b. Within the integumentary system, in the skin

c. Within the brain, in the corpus callosum

d. Within the Urinary system, in the kidneys

The passage of food from the mouth to the stomach is called

a. Deglutition

b. Mastication

c. Vomiting

d. Prehension

S.A. node is located in the --------

a. Left atrium b. Right atrium
c. Left ventricle d. Right ventricle

The natural anticoagulant present in the body is -------

a. EDTA b. Citrate
c. Oxalate **d. Heparin**

Dialysis is performed to replace physiological function of

a. Kidney b. Heart
c. Lung d. Liver

Bile salts help in digestion of absorption of -----

a. Carbohydrates b. Proteins
c. Lipids d. VFAs

Every cell of the mammalian body has a nucleus with the exception of ?

a. Epithelial cell b. Nerve cells
c. Muscle cells **d. Erythrocytes**

The proteins that act as catalysts for biochemical reactions in the body are known as?

a. Hormones b. Enzymes
c. Acids d. Nucleic acids

The movement of a chemical substance from an area of high concentration and occurs mainly in gases,liquids and solutions?

a. Active transport **b. Diffusion**
c. Osmosis d. Dialysis

Fill in the Blanks

VFAs are end products of fermentation of --------

a. Carbohydrates b. Protein
c. Fat

Nature of rumen fermentation is --------------------

a. Aerobic b. Anaerobic

Rigor mortis occurs due to lack of --------------------

a. ATP b. Calcium ions

Respiratory centre is located in ---------------------

a. Hypothalamus b. Brain stem

Plasma proteins are synthesized in -------------------

a. Bone marrow b. Liver

The ADH is secreted from-----------------------------

a. Hypothalamus
b. Posterior pituitary
c. Anterior pituitary

Cerebrospinal fluid (CSF) is the fluid -------------------

a. In joints
b. In eyes
c. Secreted by choroid plexuses

The basic structural and functional unit of nervous system is --------

a. Neutron
b. Nephron
c. Neuron

Define or explain the following

- Acclimation
- Acclimatization
- Acrosome reaction
- Adaptation
- Allometric growth
- Anaemia
- Anoxia
- Autecology/Species ecology/Self ecology
- Axon
- Blastocyst
- Bioclimatology
- Bloat
- Brady cardi
- Capacitation
- Cardiogenic shock
  - Chemotaxis
- Climate
  - Compensatory growth
- Critical temperature
- Cryptorchidism
- Cyanosis
- Differentiation/Cytogenesis/Histogenesis
- Diuresis
- Diurnal variation
- Ecology
- Ectotherms

- EEG
- Electrocardiograph
- Emesis
- Emulsification
- Endotherms
- Epididymis
- Erythropoiesis
- Ethology
- False growth
- Functions of scrotum
- Ghrelin
- Gluconeogenesis
- Growth
- Hematocrit
- Hemolysis
- Hering-Breuer Reflex
- Heterotherms
- Homeorrhesis
- Homeotherms
- Hyperventilation
- Implantation
- Induced ovulation
- inner cell mass
- Isometric growth
- Labial cells/Renewing cells
- Leptin
- Lethal temperature
- Leydig cells
- LH surge
- Lymph
- Macro climate
- MCHC
- Metabolic acidosis
- Microclimate
- Micro climate
- Micturition

- Milk protein
- Morphogenesis/Organogenesis
- NK cells
- Pacemaker
- Period of estrus
- Peristalsis
- Permanent cells/Static cells
- Photoperiod influence on reproduction
- Placentome
- Poikilotherms
- Polycythemia
- Postnatal growth
- Prehension
- Prenatal growth
- Primordial follicle
- Rigor mortis
- Rumination
- Sarcomere
- Seminal vesicle
- Sertoli cells
- Shock
- Spermatogenic cycle
- Split estrus
- Stable cells/Expanding cells
- Synapse
- Synecology/Population ecology/Biocenology/Biosociology
- Syngamy
- Systolic pressure
- Thermoneutral zone/Comfort zone
- Trophoblast
- True growth
- Vagal escape
- Vital capacity of lungs
- Vitelline block
- Weather
- Zygote

True False (All the below statements are true)

- Nephron is the structural and functional unit of kidney

  True/False

- Albumin, globulins and fibrinogen are the major protein fractions of blood serum.

  True/False

- The average erythrocyte count in a cow is 5-6 millions / cu mm True/False
- In domestic animals blood volume is generally 5-8 percent of body weight.

  True/False

- Fibrinogen is the biggest blood serum protein having the highest molecular weight.

  True/False

- Herbivores have longer and capacious digestive tracts.

  True/False

- AV node is the pacemaker of the heart

  True/False

- Second heart sound is produced due to closing of the semilunar valve.

  True/False

- Serum is the liquid part of coagulated blood.

  True/False

Short Notes

- Calcium homeostasis
- Corpus luteum
- Descent of testes
- Differentiate between serum and plasma
- Endocrine control of lactogenesis
- Endocrine regulation of parturition
- Factors affecting onset of puberty
- Fertilization
- Folliculogenesis
- Follicular wave
- Galactopoiesis
- Hormones involved in mammogenesis
- Lactose synthesis in mammary tissue

- Maternal recognition of pregnancy
- Mechanism of ovulation
- Ovarian hormones
- Photoperiod on reproduction
- Placenta
- Pseudopregnancy.
- Puberty in females
- Role of FSH on ovarian follicular development
- Role of gonadotropins in spermatogenesis
- Role of hCG and PMSG in reproduction
- Role of hormones during gestation
- Sperm transport in female reproductive tract
- Spermiogenesis
- Synthesis of milk fat
- Thermoregulation in testes

Index

D

E

F

G

Glucagon 170, 171, 172, 276, 277, 278

H

I

J

K

L

M

N

O

P

R

S

T

U

V

W

Z